HIKE LIST

60 HIKES
WITHIN 60 MILES

MADISON
INCLUDES
DANE AND SURROUNDING COUNTIES

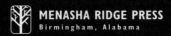

MENASHA RIDGE PRESS
Birmingham, Alabama

60HIKES
WITHIN60MILES

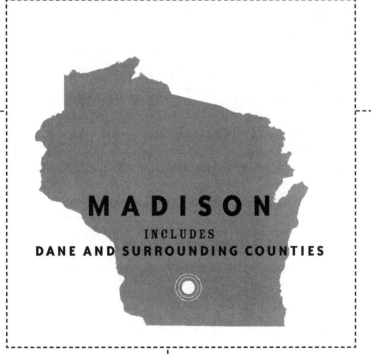

MADISON
INCLUDES
DANE AND SURROUNDING COUNTIES

KEVIN REVOLINSKI

DISCLAIMER

This book is meant only as a guide to select trails in the Madison area and does not guarantee hiker safety in any way—you hike at your own risk. Neither Menasha Ridge Press nor Kevin Revolinski is liable for property loss or damage, personal injury, or death that result in any way from accessing or hiking the trails described in the following pages. Please be aware that hikers have been injured in the Madison area. Be especially cautious when walking on or near boulders, steep inclines, and drop-offs, and do not attempt to explore terrain that may be beyond your abilities. To help ensure an uneventful hike, please read carefully the introduction to this book, and perhaps get further safety information and guidance from other sources. Familiarize yourself thoroughly with the areas you intend to visit before venturing out. Ask questions, and prepare for the unforeseen. Familiarize yourself with current weather reports, maps of the area you intend to visit, and any relevant park regulations.

Copyright © 2008 by Kevin Revolinski
All rights reserved
Printed in the United States of America
Published by Menasha Ridge Press
Distributed by Publishers Group West
First edition, fourth printing 2013

Library of Congress Cataloging-in-Publication Data

Revolinski, Kevin.
  60 hikes within 60 miles, Madison : including Dane and surrounding counties
/ Kevin Revolinski.
    p. cm.
  Includes index.
  ISBN-13: 978-0-89732-794-7
  ISBN-10: 0-89732-794-2
    1. Hiking—Wisconsin—Madison Metropolitan Area—Guidebooks. 2. Trails—
Wisconsin—Madison Metropolitan Area—Guidebooks. 3. Madison Metropolitan
Area (Wis.)—Guidebooks. I. Title. II. Title: Sixty hikes within sixty miles,
Madison.
  GV199.42.W62M34 2008
  796.5109775—dc22

                                                                    2008004604

Text and cover design by Scott McGrew and Steveco International
Cover photograph by Kevin Revolinski
Author photograph by Preamtip Satasuk
Cartography and elevation profiles by Tim Lohnes, Scott McGrew, and
  Kevin Revolinski

Menasha Ridge Press
P.O. Box 43673
Birmingham, Alabama 35243
www.menasharidge.com

TO MY FATHER, FOR RAISING ME TO LOVE THE OUTDOORS
— KEVIN REVOLINSKI

TABLE OF CONTENTS

ACKNOWLEDGMENTS

I couldn't have done this book without all the kind and generous contributions of so many people along the trail. Of course there are hundreds of park managers, trail volunteers, land owners and donors, and fellow hikers, some of whom I've met and others who have done or continue to do great things to preserve the natural beauty of Wisconsin. But in particular, I'd like to thank Sharon Kizer for a great starting list of recommendations. Thanks to Jen, Scott, and Evie Lynch for great suggestions for hikes for kids and a natural remedy for mosquito bites. The Ice Age Trail segments benefited from the information from Theresa Werner and Lorraine Lange, and Eric Sherman and Kevin Thusius of the Ice Age Park and Trail Foundation. Specifically for that great trail project, we all need to thank the private land owners who have been so kind as to allow us to tread upon portions of their property, as well as the many volunteers working hard to create the route.

I'm grateful to Danica for helping me sort out the labyrinth of an outdated map of a park full of uncharted trails. Cheers to Joel Green from the Department of Natural Resources and Sara Kehrli with Columbia County Parks for helping me find my way along some trails less traveled. More thanks go to Steve Johnston at New Glarus Woods State Park (and Badger State Trail), as well as David Borsecnik at the Department of Natural Resources (formerly at Lake Kegonsa State Park), and Chris James, Park Planner for Dane County. My gratitude to Molly and Russell and all the folks at Menasha Ridge Press, and a big thanks to Johnny Molloy, mentor and all-around outdoor sensei, for continued advice and mental and tech support.

I owe the continued health of my feet to Steve Schmitt of The Shoe Box in Black Earth, who was kind enough to donate a great pair of hiking boots to the cause. Still the best shoe store in Madison, though it isn't actually *in* Madison.

Thanks to Brian Babler for providing a backup when my GPS device seemed a little wonky, and my cousin Renee Lajcak for some wildflower identification support; Nicki Richmond, Kristin Abraham, and Mark Geske for some trail companionship. Thanks to Preamtip Satasuk for the author photo and for being a good sport when I found the road less traveled wasn't worth traveling and in fact was more akin to a bramble patch and not a good place to hike in shorts. My bad. Dave and Kate Sebastian for a couple great assists on pick-ups and drop-offs.

And to my parents for finally giving up on trying to tell me I should be teaching. Their continued support means a ton to me.

—KEVIN REVOLINSKI

ABOUT THE AUTHOR

Kevin Revolinski's love for the outdoors came from frequent childhood fishing trips and hikes in the woods of northern Wisconsin. He is also the author of *The Yogurt Man Cometh: Tales of an American Teacher in Turkey* and *The Wisconsin Beer Guide: A Travel Companion,* and coauthor of *The Best in Tent Camping: Wisconsin.* He has written for Rough Guides guidebooks, and his articles and photography have appeared in a variety of publications including *Chicago Tribune, Caribbean Travel and Life,* and *Miami Herald.* He has lived abroad in several places including Turkey, Italy, Guatemala, and Panama, but currently makes camp back in the homeland in Madison, Wisconsin.

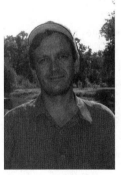

FOREWORD

Welcome to Menasha Ridge Press's *60 Hikes within 60 Miles,* a series designed to provide hikers with the information they need to find and hike the very best trails surrounding metropolitan areas.

Our strategy is simple: First, find a hiker who knows the area and loves to hike. Second, ask that person to spend a year researching the most popular and very best trails around. And third, have that person describe each trail in terms of difficulty, scenery, condition, elevation change, and other categories of information that are important to hikers. "Pretend you've just completed a hike and met up with other hikers at the trailhead," we told each author. "Imagine their questions, be clear in your answers."

An experienced hiker and writer, Kevin Revolinski has selected 60 of the best hikes in and around the Madison metropolitan area. From the towering bluffs of Devil's Lake to an urban stroll around the capital, Revolinski provides hikers (and walkers) with a great variety of outings—and all within roughly 60 miles of Madison.

You'll get more out of this book if you take a moment to read the Introduction explaining how to read the trail listings. The "Topographic Maps" section will help you understand how useful topos are on a hike, and will also tell you where to get them. And though this is a "where-to," not a "how-to" guide, readers who have not hiked extensively will find the Introduction of particular value.

As much for the opportunity to free the spirit as well as to free the body, let these hikes elevate you above the urban hurry.

All the best,
The Editors at Menasha Ridge Press

PREFACE

"I only went out for a walk and finally concluded to stay out till sundown, for going out, I found, was really going in."

—*John Muir*

Madison, the saying goes, is 76 square miles (an ever-changing number) surrounded by reality. The statement was meant as an attack on progressive-minded politics and perhaps the endless bickering that goes on here over what might be best for the community and Wisconsin at large. It's an impassioned population, to be sure. The reality that indeed surrounds us Madisonians, however, is some impressive land preservation, a great state park system, and ongoing restorations of forests, wetlands, prairie, savanna, and long-lost trout streams. Forward thinking has accomplished much in preserving the natural beauty of the area that might have otherwise been lost to reckless development.

So much of the region was once clear cut for farming; wetlands were drained for the same, trout streams dammed for mill ponds. But a long line of environmentalists including onetime resident and University of Wisconsin professor Aldo Leopold, land donors such as the Frautschi family, Edna Taylor, and Edward T. Owen, and a small army of concerned citizens and activist groups, have all worked hard to keep Madison's relationship with the land and the environment harmonious. The city's Arboretum is considered a mainstay of our green space, a symbol of our love of natural beauty, and yet less than a century ago, hardly any of what we see today existed. Traces of the failed urban development known as the Lost City can still be found in the preserve's soggy soil. From one park to the next, efforts are being made to restore prairies to the way they were before European settlers arrived. Oak savanna and forests have also made their comebacks.

The State of Wisconsin and the City of Madison, and all the neighboring communities from the Dells to Janesville and from Dodgeville to Delafield have put public resources into various trail and park projects, but more important than anything has been the contribution of the thousands of volunteers who maintain trails, compile maps, run Web sites, and organize events. The money of private donors and the easements granted by private land owners are what make something as magnificent and massive as the Ice Age National Scenic Trail possible. Much of what I've hiked on the IAT is someone's backyard or overgrown farmland.

In terms of hiking trails, there is something for everyone here. Treks range from easy strolls not far from home such as Picnic Point along Lake Mendota or the challenging 18-mile hike of the Ice Age Trail segment that climbs both 500-foot bluffs at Devil's Lake State Park. Within a 60-mile radius, you can find migrating birds and wetlands in Horicon Marsh, deer and prairie flowers in New Glarus Woods, trout flitting in the shadows of Rowan Creek, and the marks of the last advance of the glaciers in Kettle Moraine State Forest.

History hiked these trails as well, and you can visit the tragic battlegrounds of Sauk warrior Black Hawk, where he made a stand that allowed his people to escape, albeit temporarily, across the Wisconsin River in 1832. Find enchantment in the mysterious archaeological remains at Aztalan or the many Native American effigy mounds in several of the parks, or discover the remains of Civilian Conservation Corps projects or pioneer settlements.

Those fascinated by geology should be adequately impressed by the sandstone rock outcrops of Green, Rock, Dane, Columbia, and Sauk counties, which date back to between 460 million and 550 million years ago. All of that looks a bit recent, however, when compared to the quartzite of the Baraboo Hills and Devil's Lake bluffs in Sauk County, which is said to be 1.6 billion years old.

Southern Wisconsin is not the remote woods of Appalachia or the secluded mountains of the West, to be sure. But the reestablishment of the ecosystems of yesteryear and the outstanding state and county park systems provide places that seem a hundred miles away from the last human outpost and yet all lie within an hour of the front door.

CITY OF MADISON

In 1908, John Olin and the members of the Madison Park and Pleasure Drive Association brought in landscape architect John Nolen, who in turn set out much of the urban plan for parks in the City of Madison and even provided the foundations for the state park system. Nolen believed that "simple recreation in the open air amid beautiful surroundings contributes to physical and moral health, to a saner and happier life." Thanks to him and some like-minded Madisonians, we have a variety of excellent parks, including the Arboretum, which offers several escapes from the city in the very *heart* of the city along the shores of Lake Wingra.

The Ho Chunk tribe referred to the Madison area as Dejope, meaning "four lakes." The lakes define Madison, and the hike to Picnic Point is a classic, simply synonymous with the Madison Experience and one of the best ways to see Lake Mendota and the Capitol. Olin Park and Turville Point see the dome from the Lake Monona side. The Yahara River and its watershed feed the lakes and create wetlands such as Cherokee Marsh and Token Creek, which provide good wildlife viewing and easy strolls along grassy paths and boardwalks.

University Professor Edward T. Owen feared that reckless urban development would spoil the natural beauty of Madison. He did much to develop pleasure drives in the late 19th century, and he and his colleagues John Olin and Edward Hammersley donated land for that purpose. Now Owen's former summer retreat is a west-side conservation park, prime for birders and offering trails that make the surrounding cityscape seem nonexistent. Edna Taylor Conservation Park and the Aldo Leopold Nature Center do the same for the east side of town.

THE MECCAS

KETTLE MORAINE STATE FOREST

The most recent period of the Ice Age is known as the Wisconsin Glaciation. It came to its dwindling end in a jagged line across the state about 10,000 years ago. Thanks to the land-altering efforts of an ice sheet that was as much as a mile thick in some places, there is no better place to see the dramatic effects of continental glaciers than in Wisconsin. Two massive lobes of glacial ice left behind two ridges approximately 120 miles long in the southeastern part of the state. Melting ice buried within glacial deposits left kettle-like depressions that have since been overgrown with hardwood forests and in some cases filled in with bogs. The very ground beneath your feet is strewn with sand and broken rock, some of which may have originated all the way back in Canada.

THE ICE AGE TRAIL

This is a project in development. The ultimate goal is a 1,000-mile national scenic trail that roughly follows the terminal edge of the last glaciation. The trails are often rugged and secluded and tend to be some of the more challenging hikes. It is possible to camp along parts of the trail, and many hikers set out to hike it all either in increments or at a go. Roadways and a network of urban streets connect the wilderness segments, but the segments in this book are good out-and-back or one-way treks that can be done in as little as an hour or as much as an entire day.

DEVIL'S LAKE STATE PARK

Arguably this is the most popular of the area state parks. Nothing rivals the views from atop the two 500-foot rocky bluffs other than perhaps Gibraltar Rock State Natural Area. Though steep at times, the trails along the cliffs are nicely laid out with stone steps and asphalt. Between the two bluffs lies the lake. A whole network of trails explores the woods and prairies beyond the East Bluff, and great facilities make the park ideal for camping or having a swim at one of two beaches.

The tumbled quartzite talus along the slopes and the rock formations and glacial moraines will impress as well.

THE "DRIFTLESS" AREA

The stopping line of the last glaciers passes right through this book's territory, and crossing from Ice Age country, you enter the Driftless Area characterized by river valleys, rolling hills, caves, springs, and sinkholes. No natural lakes occur here as no glacial debris or "drift" was left to block springs and streams. At Blue Mound State Park, you can find an abundance of springwater bubbling its way down the rocky terrain in the forest. The view from the untouched bluff reaches to a far horizon and the mound itself is visible all the way back in Madison. Governor Dodge State Park has a hike through a sandstone canyon and around two lakes formed from the damming of a spring creek that should not be missed.

HIKING RECOMMENDATIONS

HIKES LESS THAN 3 MILES

1 Arboretum: Greene Prairie (page 16)
2 Arboretum: Wingra Marsh (page 20)
3 Arboretum: Wingra Woods (page 24)
5 Cherokee Marsh North (page 33)
11 Olin-Turville Park/Turville Point (page 62)
12 Owen Conservation Park (page 66)
16 Tom George Greenway (page 85)
17 Gibraltar Rock State Natural Area (page 92)
18 Ice Age Trail: Groves-Pertzborn Segment (page 96)
24 CamRock County Park: Area 2 (page 125)
44 Aztalan State Park (page 230)
50 Devil's Lake State Park: West Bluff (page 262)
53 Natural Bridge State Park (page 276)
54 Pewit's Nest (page 281)
55 Rocky Arbor State Park (page 285)

HIKES 3–6 MILES

6 Cherokee Marsh South (page 37)
7 Edna Taylor Conservation Park (page 43)
8 Elver Park (page 48)
9 Madison Capitol and Downtown (page 52)
10 Nine Springs E-Way Trail (page 57)
15 Tenney Park to Schenk's Corners (page 80)
21 Rowan Creek Trail (page 108)
22 Swan Lake State Wildlife Area (page 112)
25 Donald County Park (page 130)
26 Governor Nelson State Park (page 134)
27 Ice Age Trail: Table Bluff Segment (page 139)
29 Indian Lake County Park (page 149)
30 Lake Kegonsa State Park (page 154)
32 Pope Farm Park (page 164)
33 Stewart County Park (page 169)

HIKES 3–6 MILES *(continued)*

HIKES 6–9 MILES

HIKES GREATER THAN 9 MILES

HISTORIC SITES

WETLAND HIKES *(continued)*

GOOD FOR CHILDREN

GOOD FOR SOLITUDE

GOOD FOR BIRD-WATCHING

GOOD FOR BIRD-WATCHING (continued)

BEST MAINTAINED TRAILS

BUSY HIKES

EASIEST HIKES

FLAT HIKES

HIKES GOOD FOR RUNNERS

HIKES WITH DOGS

HIKES WITH DOGS *(continued)*

MOST DIFFICULT HIKES

MOST SCENIC HIKES

MOST SCENIC HIKES *(continued)*

STEEP HIKES

URBAN HIKES

WATERFALL HIKES

WHEELCHAIR-ACCESSIBLE HIKES

WILDFLOWER HIKES

WILDFLOWER HIKES *(continued)*

WILDLIFE HIKES

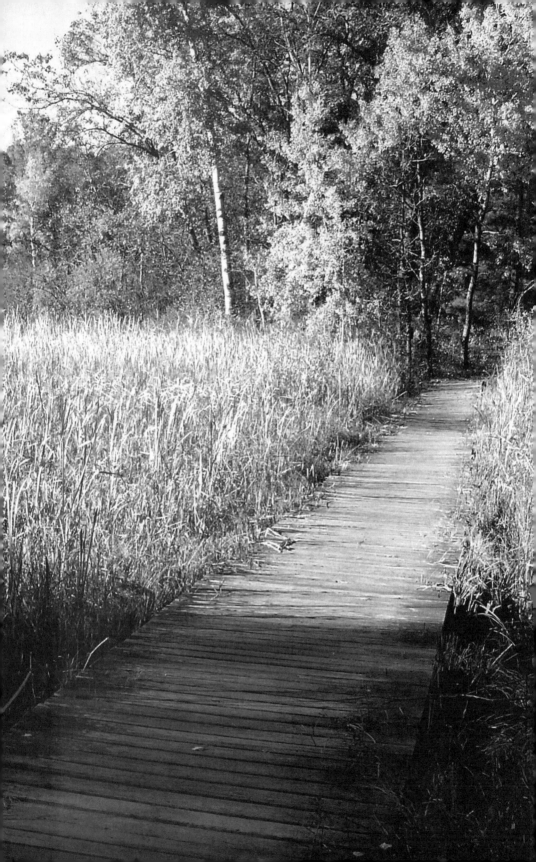

INTRODUCTION

Welcome to *60 Hikes within 60 Miles: Madison.* If you're new to hiking or even if you're a seasoned trailsmith, take a few minutes to read the following introduction. We explain how this book is organized and how to use it.

HOW TO USE THIS GUIDEBOOK

THE OVERVIEW MAP AND OVERVIEW MAP KEY

Use the overview map on the inside front cover to assess the exact locations of each hike's primary trailhead. Each hike's number appears on the overview map, on the map key facing the overview map, and in the table of contents. Flipping through the book, a hike's full profile is easy to locate by watching for the hike number at the top of each page. The book is organized by region as indicated in the table of contents. A map legend that details the symbols found on trail maps appears on the inside back cover.

REGIONAL MAPS

The book is divided into regions, and prefacing each regional section is an overview map of that region. The regional provides more detail than the overview map, bringing you closer to the hike.

TRAIL MAPS

Each hike contains a detailed map that shows the trailhead, the route, significant features, facilities, and topographic landmarks such as creeks, overlooks, and peaks. The author gathered map data by carrying a GPS unit, the Garmin eTrex while hiking. This data was downloaded into digital mapping program Delorme Topo USA 6.0 and processed by expert cartographers to produce the highly accurate maps found in this book. Each trailhead's GPS coordinates are included with each profile.

ELEVATION PROFILES

Corresponding directly to the trail map, each hike contains a detailed elevation profile. The elevation profile provides a quick look at the trail from the side, enabling you to visualize how the trail rises and falls. Key points along the way are labeled. Note the number of feet between each tick mark on the vertical axis (the height scale). To avoid making flat hikes look steep and steep hikes appear flat, height scales are used throughout the book to provide an accurate image of the hike's climbing difficulty.

GPS TRAILHEAD COORDINATES

To collect accurate map data, each trail was hiked with a handheld GPS unit (Garmin eTrex series). Data collected was then downloaded and plotted onto a digital USGS topo map. In addition to rendering a highly specific trail outline, this book also includes the GPS coordinates for each trailhead in two formats: latitude/longitude and UTM. Latitude/longitude coordinates tell you where you are by locating a point west (latitude) of the 0° meridian line that passes through Greenwich, England, and north or south of the 0° (longitude) line that belts the Earth, aka the equator.

Topographic maps show latitude/longitude as well as UTM grid lines. Known as UTM coordinates, the numbers index a specific point using a grid method. The survey datum used to arrive at the coordinates in this book is WGS 84 (versus NAD27 or WGS 83). For readers who own a GPS unit, whether handheld or onboard a vehicle, the latitude/longitude or UTM coordinates provided on the first page of each hike may be entered into the GPS unit. Just make sure your GPS unit is set to navigate using WGS 84 datum. Now you can navigate directly to the trailhead.

Most trailheads, which begin in parking areas, can be reached by car, but some hikes still require a short walk to reach the trailhead from a parking area. In those cases a handheld unit is necessary to continue the GPS navigation process. That said, however, readers can easily access all trailheads in this book by using the directions given, the overview map, and the trail map, which shows at least one major road leading into the area. But for those who enjoy using the latest GPS technology to navigate, the necessary data has been provided. A brief explanation of the UTM coordinates from Rowan Creek Trail (page 108) follows.

UTM Zone	16T
Easting	0304396
Northing	4805951

The UTM zone number 16 refers to one of the 60 vertical zones of the Universal Transverse Mercator (UTM) projection. Each zone is 6 degrees wide. The UTM zone letter T refers to one of the 20 horizontal zones that span from 80 degrees South to 84 degrees North. The easting number 0304396 indicates in meters how far east or west a point is from the central meridian of the zone. Increasing easting coordinates on a topo map or on your GPS screen indicate that you are moving east; decreasing easting coordinates indicate you are moving west.

The northing number 4805951 references in meters how far you are from the equator. Above and below the equator, increasing northing coordinates indicate you are traveling north; decreasing northing coordinates indicate you are traveling south. To learn more about how to enhance your outdoor experiences with GPS technology, refer to *GPS Outdoors: A Practical Guide for Outdoor Enthusiasts* (Menasha Ridge Press).

HIKE DESCRIPTIONS

Each hike contains seven key items: an "In Brief" description of the trail, a key at-a-glance box, directions to the trail, trailhead coordinates, a trail map, an elevation profile, and a trail description. Many also include a note on nearby activities. Combined, the maps and information provide a clear method to assess each trail from the comfort of your favorite reading chair.

IN BRIEF

A "taste of the trail." Think of this section as a snapshot focused on the historical landmarks, beautiful vistas, and other sights you may encounter on the hike.

KEY AT-A-GLANCE INFORMATION

The information in the key at-a-glance boxes gives you a quick idea of the statistics and specifics of each hike.

LENGTH The length of the trail from start to finish (total distance traveled). There may be options to shorten or extend the hikes, but the mileage corresponds to the described hike. Consult the hike description to help decide how to customize the hike for your ability or time constraints.

CONFIGURATION A description of what the trail might look like from overhead. Trails can be loops, out-and-backs (trails on which one enters and leaves along the same path), figure eights, or a combination of shapes.

DIFFICULTY The degree of effort an "average" hiker should expect on a given hike. For simplicity, the trails are rated as "easy," "moderate," or "difficult."

SCENERY A short summary of the attractions offered by the hike and what to expect in terms of plant life, wildlife, natural wonders, and historic features.

EXPOSURE A quick check of how much sun you can expect on your shoulders during the hike.

TRAIL TRAFFIC Indicates how busy the trail might be on an average day. Trail traffic, of course, varies from day to day and season to season. Weekend days typically see the most visitors. Other trail users that may be encountered on the trail are also noted here.

TRAIL SURFACE Indicates whether the trail surface is paved, rocky, gravel, dirt, boardwalk, or a mixture of elements.

HIKING TIME The length of time it takes to hike the trail. A slow but steady hiker will average 2 to 3 miles per hour, depending on the terrain.

DRIVING DISTANCE Indicates expected distance from an easily identified point.

ACCESS A notation of any fees or permits that may be needed to access the trail or park at the trailhead.

Trails in the state parks often require a permit for parking: a day pass is $7, and the annual sticker is $25. If you plan to hike or visit the parks frequently each year, it is worth buying the annual sticker. Stickers can be purchased at state park offices or Department of Natural Resources service centers; they also are available online through the Wisconsin Department of Natural Resources Web site (**www.dnr.state .wi.us/org/land/parks/fees**).

City and county parks typically do not require any permits or parking fees.

WHEELCHAIR ACCESSIBILITY What to expect in terms of access to trail and facilities.

MAPS Here you'll find a list of maps that show the topography of the trail, including Green Trails Maps and USGS topo maps.

FACILITIES What to expect in terms of restrooms and water at the trailhead or nearby.

DIRECTIONS

Used in conjunction with the overview map, the driving directions will help you locate each trailhead. Once at the trailhead, park only in designated areas.

GPS TRAILHEAD COORDINATES

The trailhead coordinates can be used in addition to the driving directions if you enter the coordinates into your GPS unit before you set out. See page 2 for more information on GPS coordinates.

DESCRIPTION

The trail description is the heart of each hike. Here, the authors provide a summary of the trail's essence and highlight any special traits the hike has to offer. The route is clearly outlined, including landmarks, side trips, and possible alternate routes along the way. Ultimately, the hike description will help you choose which hikes are best for you.

NEARBY ACTIVITIES

Look here for information on nearby activities or points of interest. This includes nearby parks, museums, restaurants, or even a brewpub where you can get a well-deserved beer after a long hike. Note that not every hike has a listing.

WEATHER

Madison enjoys all four seasons. Flowers and trees start to bloom by late April on into June. Colors change from late September through October, and snow might start to stick by the end of November. While each season brings exciting changes in the flora and fauna, the temperatures don't always abide by the start dates. Be prepared for a wide range of temperatures and conditions regardless of the season. Winters typically offer temperatures well below freezing and moderate snowfall with the occasional blizzard; summers go to the other extreme with high humidity and temperatures often reaching the upper 80s to 90s. The average annual precipitation is 37 inches, and it comes in a rather even distribution throughout the year. Typically June is the wettest month.

Average Temperature by Month

	Jan	Feb	Mar	Apr	May	Jun
High	26	31	43	57	70	78
Low	10	14	25	35	46	56

	Jul	Aug	Sep	Oct	Nov	Dec
High	82	79	71	60	43	30
Low	61	59	50	39	28	16

WATER

How much is enough? Well, one simple physiological fact should convince you to err on the side of excess when deciding how much water to pack: A hiker working hard in 90-degree heat needs approximately 10 quarts of fluid per day. That's 2.5 gallons—12 large water bottles or 16 small ones. In other words, pack along one or two bottles even for short hikes.

Some hikers and backpackers hit the trail prepared to purify water found along the route. This method, while less dangerous than drinking it untreated, comes with risks. Purifiers with ceramic filters are the safest. Many hikers pack along the slightly distasteful tetraglycine-hydroperiodide tablets to debug water (sold under the names Potable Aqua, Coughlan's, and others).

Probably the most common waterborne "bug" that hikers face is *Giardia*, which may not hit until one to four weeks after ingestion. It will have you living in the bathroom, passing noxious rotten-egg gas, vomiting, and shivering with chills. Other parasites to worry about include E. coli and *Cryptosporidium*, both of which are harder to kill than *Giardia*.

For most people, the pleasures of hiking make carrying water a relatively minor price to pay to remain healthy. If you're tempted to drink "found water," do so only if you understand the risks involved. Better yet, hydrate prior to your hike, carry (and drink) 6 ounces of water for every mile you plan to hike, and hydrate after the hike.

CLOTHING

There is a wide variety of clothing from which to choose. Basically, use common sense and be prepared for anything. If all you have are cotton clothes when a sudden rainstorm comes along, you'll be miserable, especially in cooler weather. It's a good idea to carry along a light wool sweater or some type of synthetic apparel (polypropylene, Capilene, Thermax, etc.) as well as a hat.

Be aware of the weather forecast and its tendency to be wrong. Always carry raingear. Thunderstorms can come on suddenly in the summer. Keep in mind that rainy days are as much a part of nature as those idyllic ones you desire. Besides, rainy days really cut down on the crowds. With appropriate raingear, a normally crowded trail can be a wonderful place of solitude. Do, however, remain aware of the dangers of lightning strikes.

Footwear is another concern. Though tennis shoes may be appropriate for paved areas, many trails are rocky and rough; tennis shoes may not offer enough support. Water-proofed or not, boots should be your footwear of choice. Sport sandals are more popular than ever, but these leave much of your foot exposed, leaving you vulnerable to certain hazardous plants and thorns.

THE TEN ESSENTIALS

One of the first rules of hiking is to be prepared for anything. The simplest way to be prepared is to carry the "Ten Essentials." In addition to carrying the items listed below, you need to know how to use them, especially navigation items. Always consider worst-case scenarios like getting lost, hiking back in the dark, broken gear (for example, a broken hip strap on your pack or a plugged water filter), twisting an ankle, or a brutal thunderstorm. The items listed below don't cost a lot of money, don't take up much room in a pack, and don't weigh much, but they might just save your life.

> **Water: durable bottles, and water treatment like iodine or a filter**
> **Map: preferably a topo map and a trail map with a route description**
> **Compass: a high-quality compass**
> **First-aid kit: a good-quality kit including first-aid instructions**
> **Knife: a multitool device with pliers is best**
> **Light: flashlight or headlamp with extra bulbs and batteries**
> **Fire: windproof matches or lighter and fire starter**
> **Extra food: You should always have food in your pack when you've finished hiking.**
> **Extra clothes: rain protection, warm layers, gloves, warm hat**
> **Sun protection: sunglasses, lip balm, sunblock, sun hat**

FIRST-AID KIT

A typical first-aid kit may contain more items than you might think necessary. These are just the basics. Prepackaged kits in waterproof bags (Atwater Carey and Adventure Medical make a variety of kits) are available. Even though there are quite a few items listed here, they pack down into a small space:

Ace bandages or Spenco joint wraps

Antibiotic ointment (Neosporin or the generic equivalent)

Aspirin or acetaminophen

Band-Aids

Benadryl or the generic equivalent diphenhydramine (in case of allergic reactions)

Butterfly-closure bandages

Epinephrine in a prefilled syringe (for people known to have severe allergic reactions to such things as bee stings)

Gauze (one roll)

Gauze compress pads (a half dozen 4- x 4-inch pads)

Hydrogen peroxide or iodine

Insect repellent

Matches or pocket lighter

Moleskin/Spenco "Second Skin"

Sunscreen

Whistle (it's more effective in signaling rescuers than your voice)

HIKING WITH CHILDREN

No one is too young for a hike in the outdoors. Be mindful, though. Flat, short, and shaded trails are best with an infant. Toddlers who have not quite mastered walking can still tag along, riding on an adult's back in a child carrier. Use common sense to judge a child's capacity to hike a particular trail, and always count that the child will tire quickly and need to be carried.

When packing for the hike, remember the child's needs as well as your own. Make sure children are adequately clothed for the weather, have proper shoes, and are protected from the sun with sunscreen. Kids dehydrate quickly, so make sure you have plenty of fluid for everyone. To assist an adult with determining which trails are suitable for children, a list of hike recommendations for children is provided on page xxii.

Many of Wisconsin's state parks participate in the Junior Rangers/Wisconsin Explorers Program, an environmental education activity program for children and their parents. Activity booklets for Junior Rangers (grades K–3) or Wisconsin Explorers (grades 4 and up) are available at most park offices. When at least half of the activities in the booklet are completed, the child is awarded a patch and certificate available either from the park office or by mail. State parks also offer collectible cards for flora and fauna.

The outdoor store REI offers a Passport to Adventure for kids. You can pick up a passport and complete area hikes and bike rides to earn stamps and a certificate. The program is free and includes several hikes listed in this book.

GENERAL SAFETY

No doubt, potentially dangerous situations can occur outdoors, but as long as you use sound judgment and prepare yourself before hitting the trail, you'll be much safer in the woods than in most urban areas of the country. Here are a few tips to make your trip safer and easier.

- **Be careful at overlooks. While these areas may provide spectacular views, they are potentially hazardous. Stay back from the edge of outcrops and be absolutely sure of your footing; a misstep can mean a nasty and possibly fatal fall.**
- **Standing dead trees and storm-damaged living trees pose a real hazard to hikers and tent campers. These trees may have loose or broken limbs that could fall at any time. When choosing a spot to rest or a backcountry campsite, look up.**
- **Take along your brain. A cool, calculating mind is the single most important piece of equipment you'll ever need on the trail. Think before you act. Watch your step. Plan ahead. Avoiding accidents before they happen is the best recipe for a rewarding and relaxing hike.**
- **Ask questions. Park employees are there to help. It's a lot easier to gain advice beforehand and avoid a mishap away from civilization when it's too late to amend an error. Use your head out there, and treat the place as if it were your own backyard.**

ANIMAL AND PLANT HAZARDS

TICKS

Ticks like to hang out in the brush that grows along trails. Hot summer months seem to explode their numbers, but you should be tick-aware during all months of the year. Ticks, which are arthropods and not insects, need a host to feast on in order to reproduce. The ticks that light onto you while hiking will be very small, sometimes so tiny that you won't be able to spot them. Primarily of two varieties, deer ticks and dog ticks, both need a few hours of actual attachment before they can transmit any disease they may harbor. Ticks may settle in shoes, socks, and hats, and may take several hours to actually latch on. The best strategy is to visually check every half-hour or so while hiking, do a thorough check before you get in the car, and then, when you take a posthike shower, do an even more thorough check of your entire body. Ticks that haven't attached are easily removed, but not easily killed. If you pick off a tick in the woods, just toss it aside. If you find one on your body at home, dispatch it and then send it down the toilet. For ticks that have embedded, removal with tweezers is best.

MOSQUITOES

Although it's not a common occurrence, individuals can become infected with the West Nile virus by being bitten by an infected mosquito. Culex mosquitoes, the primary variety that can transmit West Nile virus to humans, thrive in urban rather than natural areas. They lay their eggs in stagnant water and can breed in any standing water that remains for more than five days. Most people infected with West Nile virus have no symptoms of illness, but some may become ill, usually 3 to 15 days after being bitten.

In the Madison area, the risk period runs from mid-June to early October, with August and September being the riskiest months. At this time of year—and anytime you expect mosquitoes to be buzzing around—you may want to wear protective clothing, such as long sleeves, long pants, and socks. Loose-fitting, light-colored clothing is best. Spray clothing with insect repellent. Remember to follow the instructions on the repellent and to take extra care with children.

CHIGGERS

Chiggers are parasitic mite larvae found on tall grass or other vegetation. They wait for passing hosts, attach themselves to a skin pore or hair follicle, and inject a digestive enzyme that ruptures the cells, causing red, itchy bumps which last for several days. Chiggers are too small to be seen with the naked eye. They are most commonly found in damp areas with a lot of vegetation, and on hosts they prefer to attach to skin under tight clothing, such as socks and underwear, or in concealed areas of the body, such as the groin and the armpits. One way to decrease the chance of chigger bites is to wear loose clothing when you're in the woods or other infested areas. You should also take a shower as soon as you get home from an outdoor expedition, to remove any chiggers before they attach to your skin. Keep the irritated area clean, and refrain from scratching. To relieve itching use a salve or cream that contains antihistamines (Caladryl or hydrocortisone salves are the most common). These will also help to prevent infection. If the welts continue to irritate you for more than a couple of weeks, they might be infected, and you should see a doctor.

EMERALD ASH BORER

This is a warning for anyone planning to build a campfire along the way or on an overnight Ice Age Trail hike perhaps. The emerald ash borer (*Agrilus planipennis*) is an exotic insect, native to Asia, that currently threatens ash trees in the Great Lakes region. The pest can be spread inadvertently in infested firewood, and most parks have strict rules about what wood you can bring into the park. By following some simple rules, you can help prevent the spread of these destructive insects. Purchase aged firewood near your campsite location; don't bring it from home. Many parks offer firewood at reasonable prices, and it is often available from private sellers just outside the parks. Firewood purchased at or near your destination should be used during your camping trip; don't take any to another destination. Buy wood that has no bark or loose bark (a sign the wood is very dry). This will reduce the chances of infestation while also making your fire easier to start.

SNAKES

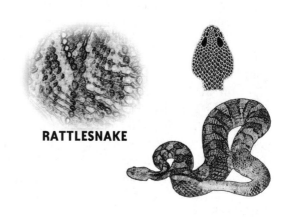

RATTLESNAKE

Generally speaking, snakes are not a concern in Wisconsin. There are 21 species, but only two are venomous—the Eastern Massasauga rattlesnake and the timber rattlesnake—and these are protected as endangered species. You are most likely to see small varieties of garter snakes. Although the chances of being bitten by a snake on one of the hikes in this book are practically nil, take proper caution. If you see a snake with a rattle, give it a wide berth.

POISON IVY/POISON OAK/POISON SUMAC

Recognizing poison ivy, oak, and sumac and avoiding contact with them is the most effective way to prevent the painful, itchy rashes associated with these plants. In southern Wisconsin, poison ivy ranges from a thick, tree-hugging vine to a shaded groundcover, three leaflets to a leaf; poison oak occurs as either a vine or shrub, with three leaflets as well; and poison sumac flourishes in swampland, each leaf containing 7 to 13 leaflets. Urushiol, the oil in the sap of these plants, is responsible for the

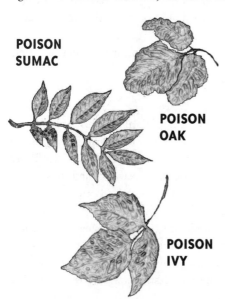

POISON SUMAC

POISON OAK

POISON IVY

rash. Usually within 12 to 14 hours of exposure (but sometimes much later), raised lines and/or blisters will appear, accompanied by a terrible itch. Refrain from scratching because bacteria under fingernails can cause infection and you will spread the rash to other parts of your body. Wash and dry the rash thoroughly, applying a calamine lotion or other product to help dry the rash. If itching or blistering is severe, seek medical attention. Remember that oil-contaminated clothes, pets, or hiking gear can easily cause an irritating rash on you or someone else, so wash not only any exposed parts of your body but also clothes, gear, and pets.

WILD PARSNIP

Wild parsnip, a member of the carrot family, possesses a long, thick taproot and commonly grows in sunny areas in fields and along roadsides. When conditions are right—usually in the plant's second summer—it sends up a single flower stalk two to four feet tall with hundreds of yellow flowers in flat-topped, umbrella-like clusters.

Wild parsnip can cause phyto-photo-dermatitis when the chemicals in the juices of the leaves, stems, and fruits react with ultraviolet light, causing burns to exposed skin. Once absorbed into the skin, the chemicals can be energized by ultraviolet light—even on a cloudy day—causing a burn similar to sunburn in appearance. The skin will redden within 24 to 48 hours and may be accompanied by blisters. A dark red or brown discoloration may also occur and can last as long as two years. Parsnip burns appear as streaks and long spots where a juicy leaf or stem dragged across the skin before exposure to the sun. The burning sensation lasts a day or two. Protective clothing and avoidance are your best protection.

TIPS FOR ENJOYING YOUR HIKE

Consider a few tips that will make your hike enjoyable and more rewarding:

- Take your time along the trails. Pace yourself for the longer hikes. The forests, fields, and wetlands of southern Wisconsin are filled with wonders both big and small. Don't rush past a tiny salamander to get to that overlook. Stop and smell the wildflowers. Peer into a clear stream for trout. Don't miss the trees for the forest. Shorter hikes allow you to stop and linger more than long hikes. Something about staring at the front end of a 10-mile trek naturally pushes you to speed up. That said, take close notice of the elevation maps that accompany each hike. If you see many ups and downs over large altitude changes, you'll obviously need more time. Inevitably you'll finish some of the "hike times" long before or after what is suggested. Nevertheless, leave yourself plenty of time for those moments when you simply feel like stopping and taking it all in.

- We can't always schedule our free time when we want, but try to hike during the week and avoid the traditional holidays if possible. Trails that are packed in the summer are often clear during the colder months. If you are hiking on a busy day, go early in the morning; it'll enhance your chances of seeing wildlife. The trails really clear out during rainy times; however, don't hike during a thunderstorm.

- Participate in some online wildlife observation counts. Cornell Lab of Ornithology operates ebird.org where you can log in for free and submit bird lists from your hikes or find out what's being seen at some of the area's birding hot spots. A similar count is being done for butterflies at www.wisconsinbutterflies.org/butterflies/sightings.

TOPO MAPS

The maps in this book have been produced with great care and, used with the hiking directions, will direct you to the trail and help you stay on course. However, you will find superior detail and valuable information in the United States Geological Survey's 7.5 minute series topographic maps. Topo maps are available online in many locations. A well-known free service is located at **www.terraserver.microsoft.com** and another free service with fast click-and-drag browsing is located at **www.topofinder .com**. You can view and print topos of the entire United States from these Web sites, and view aerial photographs of the same area at terraserver. Several online services such as **www.trails.com** charge annual fees for additional features such as shaded-relief, which makes the topography stand out more. If you expect to print out many topo maps each year, it might be worth paying for shaded-relief topo maps. The downside to USGS topos is that most of them are outdated, having been created 20 to 30 years ago. But they still provide excellent topographic detail.

Digital topographic map programs such as Delorme's TopoUSA enable you to review topo maps of the entire United States on your PC. Gathered while hiking with a GPS unit, you can also download GPS data onto the software and plot your own hikes.

If you're new to hiking, you might be wondering, "What's a topographic map?" In short, a topo indicates not only linear distance but elevation as well, using contour lines. Contour lines spread across the map like dozens of intricate spider webs. Each line represents a particular elevation, and at the base of each topo, a contour's interval designation is given. If the contour interval is 20 feet, then the distance between each contour line is 20 feet. Follow five contour lines up on the same map, and the elevation has increased by 100 feet.

Let's assume that the 7.5 minute series topo reads "Contour Interval 40 feet," that the short trail we'll be hiking is two inches in length on the map, and that it crosses five contour lines from beginning to end. What do we know? Well, because the linear scale of this series is 2,000 feet to the inch (roughly two and three-quarters inches representing 1 mile), we know our trail is approximately four-fifths of a mile long (2 inches are 2,000 feet). But we also know we'll be climbing or descending 200 vertical feet (five contour lines are 40 feet each) over that distance. And the elevation designations written on occasional contour lines will tell us if we're heading up or down.

In addition to the outdoor shops listed in the Appendix, you'll find topos at major universities and some public libraries, where you might try photocopying the ones you need to avoid the cost of buying them. But if you want your own and can't find them locally, visit the United States Geological Survey Web site at **topomaps.usgs.gov**.

TRAIL ETIQUETTE

Whether you're on a city, county, state, or national park trail, always remember that great care and resources (from nature as well as from your tax dollars) have gone into creating these trails. Treat the trail, wildlife, and fellow hikers with respect.

- **Hike on open trails only. Respect trail and road closures (ask if not sure), avoid possible trespassing on private land, and obtain all permits and authorization as required. Also, leave gates as you found them or as marked.**
- **Leave only footprints. Be sensitive to the ground beneath you. This also means staying on the existing trail and not blazing any new trails. Be sure to pack out what you pack in. No one likes to see the trash someone else has left behind.**
- **Never spook animals. An unannounced approach, a sudden movement, or a loud noise startles most animals. A surprised animal can be dangerous to you, to others, and to themselves. Give them plenty of space.**
- **Plan ahead. Know your equipment, your ability, and the area in which you are hiking—and prepare accordingly. Be self-sufficient at all times; carry necessary supplies for changes in weather or other conditions. A well-executed trip is a satisfaction to you and to others.**
- **Be courteous to other hikers, bikers, equestrians, and others you encounter on the trails.**

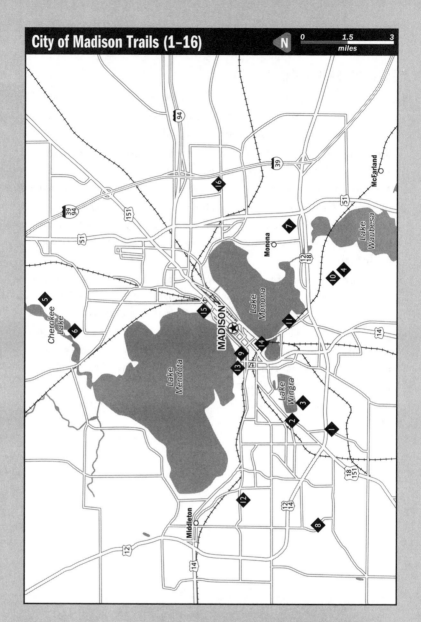

City of Madison Trails (1–16)

N

0   1.5   3
miles

MADISON

Lake Mendota

Lake Monona

Lake Wingra

Lake Waubesa

Cherokee Lake

Monona

Middleton

McFarland

CITY OF MADISON

01 ARBORETUM: Greene Prairie

KEY AT-A-GLANCE INFORMATION

LENGTH: 2.5 miles
CONFIGURATION: Loop
DIFFICULTY: Easy; some moderate
SCENERY: Mixed woods, prairie
EXPOSURE: Partly shaded, partly sun
TRAIL TRAFFIC: Light
TRAIL SURFACE: Packed dirt, crushed stone, exposed rocks and roots, a few narrow boardwalks
HIKING TIME: 1 hour
DRIVING DISTANCE: At the southeast corner of the intersection of Seminole Highway and the Beltline (US 12/18)
ACCESS: Trails are open 7 a.m.– 10 p.m.; parking dawn–dusk
MAPS: USGS Madison West; maps in the wooden box at the parking lot or at the visitor center across the highway (608) 263-7888
WHEELCHAIR ACCESSIBILITY: None
FACILITIES: None
SPECIAL COMMENTS: No pets allowed. Check park schedule for free guided tours on weekends. This portion of the park has many trail combinations, plus the Arboretum section on the north side of the lake and the central section of the park are listed herein as separate hikes (Arboretum: Wingra Marsh and Arboretum: Wingra Woods).

GPS Trailhead Coordinates

UTM Zone (WGS 84) 16T

Easting   0300949

Northing   4767506

Latitude   N 43° 02' 2.99"

Longitude   W 89° 26' 36.24"

IN BRIEF

Hike this southernmost portion of the Arboretum and explore oak savanna, pine forest, and one of the finest prairie restorations there is to see.

DESCRIPTION

The centerpiece of this portion of the 1,260-acre University of Wisconsin–Madison Arboretum is Greene Prairie, named for Henry Greene, a UW botanist who, during the 1940s and 1950s, did almost all of the restoration himself returning what was once farmland to its original role in the landscape. But the towering pines and oak savanna are no less impressive, and this hike offers a nice mix of all of them.

Take a map from the wooden box at the gate in the parking lot and then take the packed dirt trail to the left straight into the trees. This first segment takes you through Evjue Pine Forest parallel to the Beltline Highway down a lane carpeted with pine needles. The hum of tires will annoy some hikers, but the pine forest has a pleasant airiness to it and should not be missed. The rest of this hike is plotted to avoid the nearby urban world.

Directions ⟶

Follow the Beltline (US 12/18) west to the Seminole Highway exit. Go left on the overpass and through the four-way stop on the other side. The small gravel parking lot is immediately on your left at the corner. There is no exit from the Beltline here if you are going east. In this case, take the Todd Drive exit and take your first right to go back the opposite direction to the same Seminole Highway four-way stop. Turn left and immediately left again into the lot at the corner.

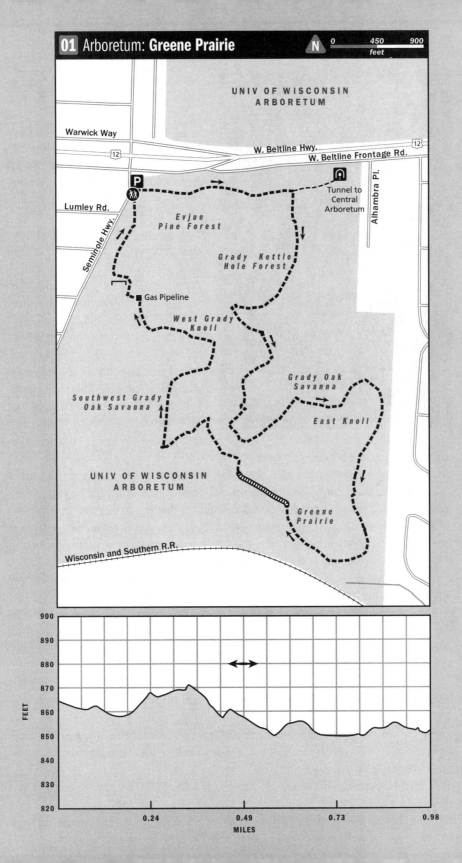

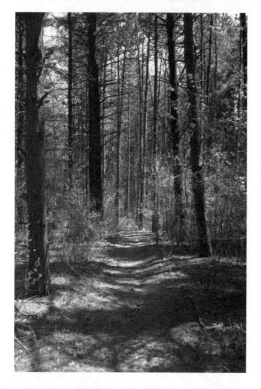

The trail through Evjue Pine Forest

At 200 feet you will pass the T2 trail marker and another 450 feet later, the T3 juncture. Both of these trails break to the right, heading deeper into the pines. Continue straight along here passing junction T4 300 feet farther on as well until you arrive at a clearing and trail junction T5, a total of a quarter mile from the trail entrance. To the left is a spur to the Beltline Highway, and straight across is the trail that will take you about 600 feet to T7 and a trail that goes under the highway through a tunnel. This is a good way to connect with another great hike, Arboretum Two, and the central portion of the park where the visitor center can be found.

By going right (south) at T5, you start to distance yourself from the traffic and avoid the trail along the edge of the Arboretum, which borders a residential neighborhood. On your left will be Old Field, a collection of mixed trees, and on your right the pines will eventually give way to oak and other deciduous trees after about 400 feet when you pass the U7 juncture and a trail that connects to the T3 and T4 paths back in the pine forest.

The trail here is a dirt access road. Another 700 feet brings you to the U4 juncture on your right and its trail all the way back to T3.

You will arrive at a crossroads outside the tree cover 300 feet later at U3. Go left on the crushed stone path and pass scattered trees in savanna as you cross West Grady Knoll. 300 feet on, there is a fork in the road. Take the trail that branches to the right at Y1 and to your right you will see prairie grass.

Less than 200 feet in, turn right at the Y2 juncture and just beyond that at Y3 go right again. This takes you off the wider ski trails and down a footpath just wide enough for your feet right through the tall grass and fragile vegetation. You are at the very center of the park, and this little patch of sunlight is a great place to find pasque flowers and bird's-foot violets in the spring. No matter how tempting, do not pick the flowers.

At the southern end of this 500-foot segment at Y4, the path rejoins the ski trail. Continue south by going straight here. The ground follows a gentle slope 200 feet under great oak trees. Pass juncture Y5, remaining on this trail as you explore Grady Oak Savanna. At the next juncture 500 feet later, Y6, continue straight across and hike 0.2 miles along the bottom of the slope of the savanna and just north of East Knoll, which will bring you out of the trees and to another access road trail at Y7. Go right here and observe how the trees spread out and the prairie grass starts moving in, a hint of what's to come. The road curves slightly to the west, and as you pass the Z4 juncture 800 feet later, stay straight and you will come to a path just 200 feet farther on that enters into the heart of Greene Prairie.

Held up as one of the finest examples of prairie restoration in the world, the prairie received a controlled burn in spring of 2007, which park administrators hope will protect that restoration. Urban development to the south has affected water runoff and unfortunately the park is now faced with losing the prairie to reed canary grass, an invasive species. This is the place to visit in spring when a wide variety of wildflowers bloom. But also during this time and in rainy periods, the trail can get soggy here and you might get your feet wet.

The trail does a 0.4-mile half loop through this southeastern corner of the park. When you come to Z6 at 0.3 miles, take the two-plank boardwalk to your left. This takes you back across the prairie and leaves you at the packed earth trail that re-enters the oak savanna through pussy willows. Go left here at Z1. To your left are quaking aspens. You pass through 500 feet of saplings before arriving at X4, heading left, and crossing 500 feet of the northernmost finger of Greene Prairie to arrive at the X5 juncture. If you go left you can hike all the way around the park edge around Southwest Grady Oak Savanna while passing along the western edge of the prairie that skirts Seminole Highway. Going straight takes you right across the savanna on a very rudimentary and sometimes very muddy trail. Instead, go right here with the prairie to your right and the oaks to your left.

When you arrive at X3, the next intersection 900 feet up the path, go left, and you are back into the sunshine. Take X2, 100 feet farther on, to the left, cutting back through the savanna. The trail is the dividing line between oaks on your left and pine on your right. The path goes up a medium grade 700 feet in. About 200 feet farther on, you will cross a gas pipeline that looks a lot like a trail in spring. Stay on the trail and follow it as it curves left.

About 200 feet west you will find a small clearing with tall grass on your right and a narrow footpath that enters it. Take this and, on the other side, find a bench on your right in the shade along the field's perimeter. The trail continues past and ducks back into the trees, soon arriving at juncture X1 and the trail that runs along the western edge of the park. Go right here along this access road trail, and you are more than 800 feet from your starting point at the parking lot.

NEARBY ACTIVITIES

Just 1 mile south of here on the right on Seminole Highway is a nicely paved bike trail at Dunn's Marsh. Continuing south to the next traffic light intersection to find McKee Road/County Road PD. Go right here to get to Star Cinema (608) 270-1414, featuring the area's only IMAX theater.

02 ARBORETUM: Wingra Marsh

KEY AT-A-GLANCE INFORMATION

LENGTH: 1.6 miles

CONFIGURATION: Out-and-back

DIFFICULTY: Easy

SCENERY: Mixed forest, marsh

EXPOSURE: Mostly shaded

TRAIL TRAFFIC: Moderate

TRAIL SURFACE: Mostly woodchip and packed dirt, some boardwalk and asphalt

HIKING TIME: 45 minutes

DRIVING DISTANCE: 1.7 miles west of Monroe and Regent Streets

ACCESS: Trails are open 7 a.m.–10 p.m., and parking is from dawn to dusk.

MAPS: USGS Madison West; park maps are inside wooden boxes at trail entrances.

WHEELCHAIR ACCESSIBILITY: None

FACILITIES: None

SPECIAL COMMENTS: Public tours and other programs take place on most weekends at the Arboretum. Contact the visitor center at (608) 263-7888. Pets are prohibited.

IN BRIEF

Step from the sidewalk in a popular west side neighborhood onto a trail through the marsh and forest along Lake Wingra's northwest shore.

DESCRIPTION

The Arboretum is made up of 1,200 acres of preserved land and, combined with Vilas Park, almost completely encompasses Lake Wingra. It all looks very pristine and natural, so it is hard to believe that this was all once farmland. Much of the land was purchased during the Great Depression, and with the help of Civilian Conservation Corps workers and ecologists such as Aldo Leopold, it was set on the path to become the astounding restoration of prairie, forests, and wetlands that we see today. This segment that curls around the northwestern shore of the lake is an easily accessible hike that never strays far from a busy street and yet offers as much natural beauty as the heart of the park.

The hike begins with a spring bubbling up from under a sandstone wall off Nakoma Road. There are a couple of benches along a mowed area right next to the parking lot where you can sit and watch waterfowl. The trail starts from the lot on an asphalt path shared

GPS Trailhead Coordinates

UTM Zone (WGS 84)   16T

Easting   0301545

Northing   4769295

Latitude   N 43° 03' 1.50"

Longitude   W 89° 26' 12.21"

Directions ———————→

Follow Monroe Street 1.7 miles west from where it intersects Regent Street downtown to where it splits into Odana Road and Nakoma Road. Take the curve left to Nakoma, and just half a block farther, you will find the parking lot on your left. The trail begins on the asphalt bike path from the parking lot.

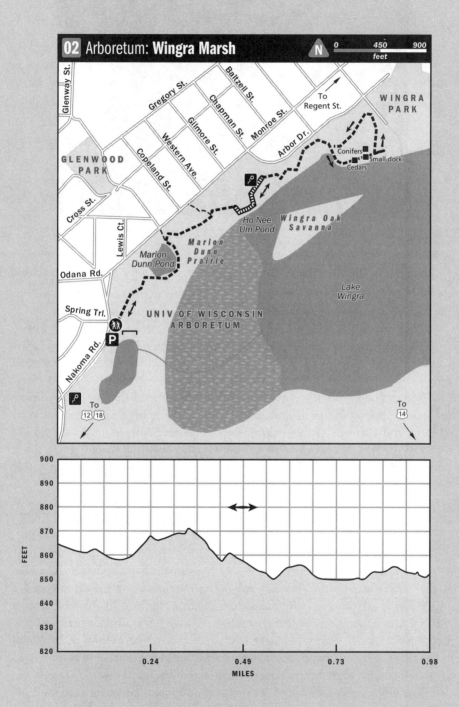

02 Arboretum: **Wingra Marsh**

N

0   450   900
feet

Glenway St.

Gregory St.

Baltzell St.

Chapman St.

Gilmore St.

Western Ave.

Monroe St.

Copeland St.

To
Regent St.

WINGRA
PARK

Arbor Dr.

Conifers

Cedars

Small dock

GLENWOOD
PARK

Cross St.

Lewis Ct.

Ho Nee
Um Pond

Wingra Oak
Savanna

Marion
Dunn Pond

Marion
Dunn
Prairie

Odana Rd.

Lake
Wingra

Spring Trl.

UNIV OF WISCONSIN
ARBORETUM

Nakoma Rd.

P

To
12 18

To
14

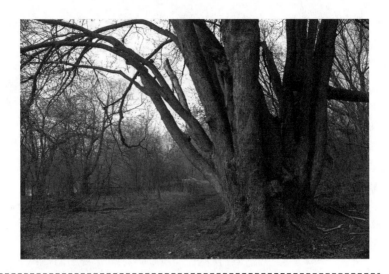

An oak just across the trail from Marion Dunn Marsh

by bicyclists, but only 250 feet in, a wood-chip footpath departs to the right into the forest. The underbrush is thick here, but 200 feet in, you arrive at the edge of the Marion Dunn Marsh and follow along the top of the earthen dike.

Look for turtles perched on rocks along the shore and expect a chorus of frogs. Another 200 feet farther, the land opens to Marion Dunn Prairie with a few scattered trees, some of them dead and barren, perfect for perching hawks and crows.

You can now see Lake Wingra to the south through the trees. The trail curls around this pocket of marsh and comes close to a busy three-way intersection on Monroe and Glenway streets, where there is another entry point to the trail at marker Q1. There in a wooden box you will also find trail maps for the entire Arboretum. It is also possible to park your car across the street and down one of the residential side streets.

Continue through the tall grass for another 100 feet and you are in the shade of the trees once again. You come to trail marker Q5 where another spur trail to the left connects to Monroe Street. Wildflowers are abundant here in the spring, especially bird's-foot violets.

The trail splits here at marker R2. Going straight bypasses a 350-foot loop to the marsh. Take the two-plank boardwalk to the right and follow it to the edge of the water, which is an inlet almost cut off from the rest of the lake. This is Ho Nee Um Pond and is almost guaranteed to have a few Canada geese or mallards lurking about. Still water stretches out to a long, narrow spit of land with the last line of trees between the marsh and the open lake. There are a lot of dead trees in this area. Keep an eye out for flickers and woodpeckers.

The loop passes the edge of the stagnant water and soon returns to the main trail at marker R3. Head right and 100 feet later, cross a spring. You can see the water bubbling up through the sand at the bottom. Water bugs play across the surface in the summer, and in the winter it is often still green with moss back here.

Another 100 feet later the trail crosses another spring large enough to become a creek. The boardwalk comes only to the edge of the water, and you must cross ten feet on stepping stones. Then the boardwalk resumes but ends just 50 feet beyond. Here the park opens to an area of regularly maintained grass. Stay right and look for the concrete culvert that crosses the trail. To your right is the edge of the open water again, with waterfowl hiding out and an abundance of dragonflies.

The wood-chip trail resumes nearby. The trail passes beneath a few maples and follows Arbor Drive. You cross a runoff channel 200 feet farther on and walk along the edge of Ho Nee Um Pond. Keep going another 200 feet and go right at the fork in the trail, staying inside the park. One hundred feet farther, the trail forks again. The path to the left is your return trail. Go right and follow the pond's edge 250 feet out to the point. A handful of spurs make the few steps to the water.

As the shoreline forces the trail to curve left, enter a patch of cedars, pass a small dock out into Lake Wingra on your right, and only 200 feet later, arrive at the far end of the trail and another entry point from Wingra Park.

The trail moves north from here through conifers as it makes a 0.2-mile loop through the woods. The corner of Arbor Road and Knickerbocker Street shows another entry point to the trail, but keep left as the tree cover becomes much thicker. Watch the trail for deer prints; it's not unknown for them to venture this far into the city. This trail brings you back to the fork where you went right at the pond's edge. Here you can follow the trail in reverse to return to the parking lot, exit to the street to take the sidewalk back, or go a block north to Monroe Street to restaurants and shops.

NEARBY ACTIVITIES

Monroe Street neighborhood has several nice restaurants and a Madison classic, Michael's Frozen Custard, is at the heart of it at 2531 Monroe Street (call [608] 231-3500). You can rent canoes at Wingra Canoe and Sailing Center (call [608] 233-5332), located in Wingra Park at the easternmost point of this trail.

03   ARBORETUM: Wingra Woods

KEY AT-A-GLANCE INFORMATION

LENGTH: 2.4 miles
CONFIGURATION: Loop
DIFFICULTY: Easy to moderate
SCENERY: Mixed woods, natural springs, ponds, Native American effigy mounds
EXPOSURE: Mostly shaded
TRAIL TRAFFIC: Moderate to light
TRAIL SURFACE: Packed dirt, a few narrow boardwalks, exposed rocks and roots
HIKING TIME: 1 hour
DRIVING DISTANCE: 2.8 miles from the intersection of Fish Hatchery Road and Park Street
ACCESS: Trails are open 7 a.m.–10 p.m., and parking is from dawn to dusk.
MAPS: USGS Madison West; maps in the wooden boxes at trailheads
WHEELCHAIR ACCESSIBILITY: None
FACILITIES: Restrooms at the nearby visitor center
SPECIAL COMMENTS: There are no pets allowed in the park. This central portion of the park has a wide variety of trail combinations, plus the Arboretum section on the north side of the lake and the southern third section of the park are listed herein as separate hikes (Arboretum One and Three).

IN BRIEF

Find the springs that feed Lake Wingra, visit the gardens, and explore the 1,200 acres of forest and prairie at the heart of the city.

DESCRIPTION

The University of Wisconsin's Arboretum is not your standard labeled garden. With more than 1,200 acres of restored wetlands, prairies, savannas, and woods, it is a remarkable ecological preserve in the heart of a city. Most of this land was purchased in the Great Depression, and the Civilian Conservation Corps did much of the initial work to set it up. Outside of Longenecker Gardens—which is a more traditional arboretum gathering more than 100 species of Wisconsin woody plants in 50 acres—the preserve looks simply like undeveloped landscape and gives little indication of the ongoing efforts of preservation and reclamation.

The trailhead is at the west end of the parking lot opposite the wooden sign and map box, which is at the head of another cutoff trail. Across the road to the south is the entrance to Longenecker Gardens where you'll find a bike rack and map box.

The trail passes over exposed rocks and tree roots or the same under leaves skirting

GPS Trailhead Coordinates

UTM Zone (WGS 84)   16T
Easting   0302250
Northing   4768731
Latitude   N 43° 02' 43.88"
Longitude   W 89° 25' 40.36"

Directions ——————→

Go south 0.5 miles on Fish Hatchery Road from where it begins at its intersection with Park Street. At the first traffic light, go right on Wingra Road 0.5 miles and turn left on Arboretum Drive. Follow this 1.8 miles along the lake and through the woods until you find the parking lot on your right across from Longenecker Gardens.

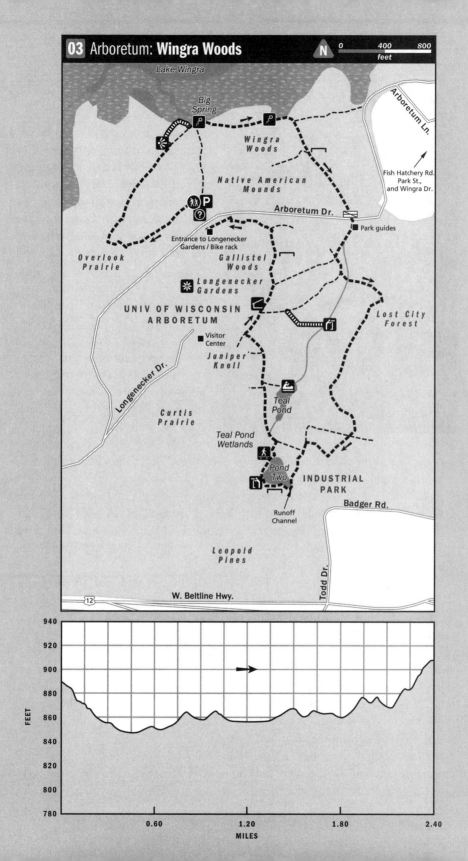

N

0   400   800
feet

Lake Wingra

Big
Spring

*Wingra
Woods*

*Native American
Mounds*

Arboretum Ln.

Fish Hatchery Rd.
Park St.,
and Wingra Dr.

P

Arboretum Dr.

Park guides

Entrance to Longenecker
Gardens / Bike rack

*Overlook
Prairie*

*Gallistel
Woods*

Longenecker
Gardens

**UNIV OF WISCONSIN
ARBORETUM**

*Lost City
Forest*

Visitor
Center

*Juniper
Knoll*

Longenecker Dr.

*Curtis
Prairie*

*Teal
Pond*

*Teal Pond
Wetlands*

*Pond
Two*

**INDUSTRIAL
PARK**

Runoff
Channel

Badger Rd.

*Leopold
Pines*

Todd Dr.

W. Beltline Hwy.

12

940
920
900
880
860
840
820
800
780

FEET

0.60   1.20   1.80   2.40

MILES

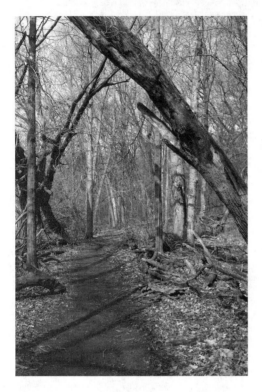

along the park road 700 feet before turning down through oak savanna with Overlook Prairie to your left. If you go left at trail marker M1, the path takes you along the prairie 700 feet and then back onto the Arboretum Drive. Go right here as the trail curves down the hill at a gentle grade as it gets closer to the lake. This is also a cross-country ski trail, and if you are hiking this in winter (which is a great hike) skiers have the right-of-way.

Expect a lot of fallen wood as you hike 0.2 miles to the lowest point of the trail. To the left are the springs that feed Lake Wingra. Also on your left is a two-plank boardwalk. Follow this into the marshy area to see the water up close. This 400-foot loop comes back to the trail you just left only 50 feet down the trail at M7.

Just beyond this is a stone platform with a railing and a bench. You can almost see the lake through the brush here. It remains green here just inside the water even in winter. To the right a cutoff trail leads back to the parking lot with a moderate grade. That trail cuts through some Native American effigy mounds.

Continue along the marsh's edge another 700 feet and find another large spring on your left. You encounter more rocks on the trail here and other smaller springs to the left before you head into some pines. At junction K4 go right. Going straight will take you out to Arboretum Drive. Uphill from K4 on a mild grade, cross gentle hills for 350 feet, and at the top find a bench at the K2 junction. To your right another trail cuts back to the parking lot, but stay the course to arrive at Arboretum Drive just another 700 feet across level terrain. At the gate here is a good place to lock up a bike if you want to jump on the trail in the middle. A crosswalk and a narrow twisting gate here keep out dogs and bikes. There is also another map box here.

Now you are entering Gallistel Woods. Four hundred feet from the road at the first junction (G5), go left, walk another 100 feet to another juncture (G4), and again go left to enter the Lost City Forest. In 1916 this was an ill-chosen development project, but nature had its way: the soggy substrata simply

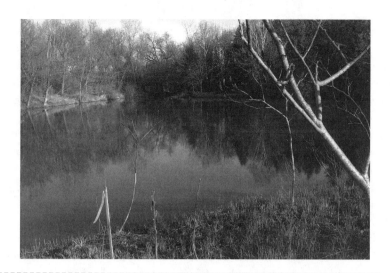

Teal Pond

swallowed up most of what was laid down on it, and so there are woods where there would have been suburbs. Go 130 feet past the G4 junction and cross a creek that drains all the way to the lake. This is the least-developed section of the trail, and though easy to follow, it can get muddy and the boardwalk does not go the entire length of the segment. Still this is nice and secluded, and you can observe a lot of wildlife through here. The trail heads south nearly 0.4 miles until it reaches junction L4, a four-way intersection, at a crushed-stone access lane.

Go straight across into a section of conifers and take the hiking-only trail. Meander 400 feet through the woods to rejoin the ski trail you just crossed. This brings you to L3 where you head south (left), though another trail heads west from here. About 300 feet past here, you can see an industrial park through the trees to your left and to the right you find the creatively named Pond Two (the second Teal Pond). Pass the trail to your right at L2 and continue past the pond's edge to L1 before turning right across a concrete runoff channel to circle the pond. The trail is well shaded here along the pond's south shore, and a bench 130 feet in offers a nice respite. Just past the observation platform on your right another 130 feet farther on, follow the trail right along the natural dike, passing through a stretch of sumac before arriving at a boardwalk that passes over the marshy terrain.

At the end of the boardwalk, turn left on an access road of crushed stone with a strip of grass down the middle to walk along the edge of Teal Pond Wetlands just beyond the brush to your left.

Go 500 feet up the trail to a marker that says F2 heads to the left, but this is incorrectly marked on the park's map and is just a western direction of the F3 juncture. Stay straight and find the F3 marker and trail just 40 feet later on your right, with a crushed-white-stone path to a canoe launch into Teal Pond.

Continue another 300 feet to the real F2, where a path to the left also sends you via Juniper Knoll to Curtis Prairie and Leopold Pines. There is much to see out in that direction, but the path chosen here keeps you from the noise of the Beltline Highway, which passes just south of this section of the Arboretum. At its southwesternmost point there is a tunnel under the highway to reach the southern portion of the park and the Arboretum Three hike.

Continue another 250 feet then turn right at F6. Walk 300 feet to come upon Gallistel Shelter House for skiers to the left. To the right is a spur trail that takes you to a nice boardwalk that nearly crosses Teal Pond and ends with a viewing platform. This area is open to the sun and full of cattails, frogs, and marsh birds. The boardwalk has a couple of observation benches along the way.

Return to the Gallistel Shelter and head right 250 feet where the trail starts to get a little steeper. Go left at juncture G1, which begins the steepest portion of the trail. It's about a 500-foot moderate-grade climb, and halfway up there is a bench if you need a rest or want to take in a nice patch of wildflowers in the spring.

On your right at the G6 juncture is a Native American mound. Take the trail left and 400 feet later, exit the woods. Pass through the gardens along the fence line to the right to find the exit, but this is a nice place to linger, especially in April and early May when all the trees are in bloom.

NEARBY ACTIVITIES

The Arboretum offers public tours and other activities on most weekends and in most weather. Go to **uwarboretum.org**, call (608) 263-7888, or check the seasonal map/brochures found in wooden boxes at park entrances to find out the schedule. The Vilas Zoo is located just across Lake Wingra in Vilas Park.

CAPITAL CITY STATE TRAIL: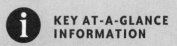
E-Way Segment

IN BRIEF

This popular multiuse trail on smooth asphalt takes you from the east side to the west side of Madison via wetlands, prairie, and a long greenway tucked into a residential area.

DESCRIPTION

From the entrance of Lake Farm Park, cross Lake Farm Road and start down the asphalt Capital City State Trail. The trail also goes north from here on the east side of the road, continuing all the way up along Lake Monona and eventually to the east side of Madison.

The trail starts out through prairie. At 0.3 miles you pass a park bench and some picnic tables just after that as the trail winds 0.2 miles through oak forest. Beyond that the prairie of the Nine Springs E-Way is to your right and chock-full of wildflowers including bergamot, coneflowers, Queen Anne's lace, and black-eyed Susans. A spur trail connects through the prairie to the Nine Springs E-Way trail, and this portion of the Capital City Trail is currently the return path for that hike, which begins just north of here. You might see deer and wild turkeys through these fields.

Agricultural fields begin on your left 0.3 miles from the forest, and you really seem far from the city. Continue 0.4 miles and

KEY AT-A-GLANCE INFORMATION

LENGTH: 8.0 miles one-way

CONFIGURATION: One way or out-and-back

DIFFICULTY: Easy

SCENERY: Prairie, mixed forest, marsh

EXPOSURE: Mostly sun

TRAIL TRAFFIC: Moderate

TRAIL SURFACE: Asphalt

HIKING TIME: 3–3.5 hours

DRIVING DISTANCE: 1.5 miles south of the Beltline Highway US 12/18 and South Towne Drive

ACCESS: Year-round

MAPS: USGS Madison West and Madison East; map boards at trailheads

WHEELCHAIR ACCESSIBILITY: Yes

FACILITIES: None on trail; restrooms and water at Lake Farm Park near trailhead and Nevin Fish Hatchery, just off the trail on Fish Hatchery Road

SPECIAL COMMENTS: Bicyclists must pay a state trail fee ($4 daily, $15 annual). Dogs allowed on a leash.

Directions

From the Beltline Highway (US 12/18), go south 0.8 miles on South Towne Drive (which becomes Raywood Road) to Moorland Road. Go left and drive 0.7 miles, even as the road bends right and becomes Lake Farm Road. This will bring you to the parking lot for Lake Farm Park/Centennial Springs State Park on your left and the trailhead on your right directly across from the park entrance.

GPS Trailhead Coordinates

UTM Zone (WGS 84)   16T

Easting   0308919

Northing   4766508

Latitude   N 43° 01' 38.02"

Longitude   W 89° 20' 43.10"

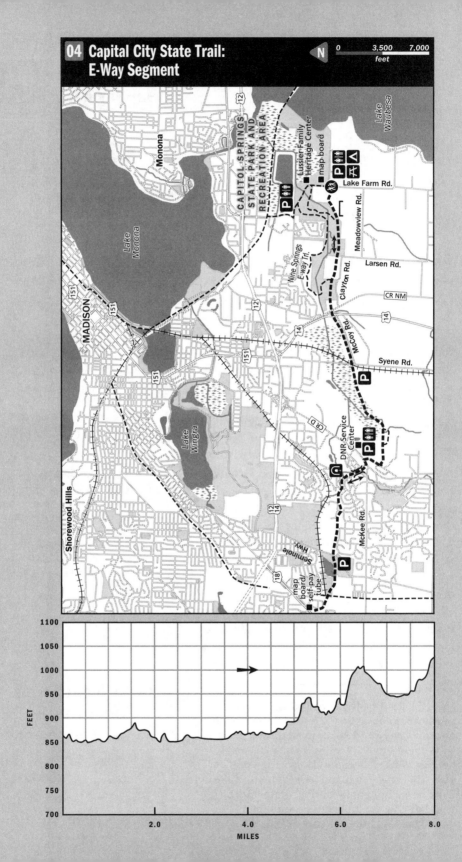

N

0   3,500   7,000
feet

Lake
Waubesa

Monona

CAPITOL SPRINGS STATE PARK AND RECREATION AREA

Lussier Family Heritage Center

map board

Lake Farm Rd.

Lake
Monona

Meadowview Rd.

MADISON

Nine Springs E-Way Trl.

Larsen Rd.

Clayton Rd.

CR NM

McCoy Rd.

Syene Rd.

Lake
Wingra

DNR Service Center

Shorewood Hills

Seminole Hwy

McKee Rd.

map board
self-pay
tube

FEET

1100
1050
1000
950
900
850
800
750
700

2.0   4.0   6.0   8.0

MILES

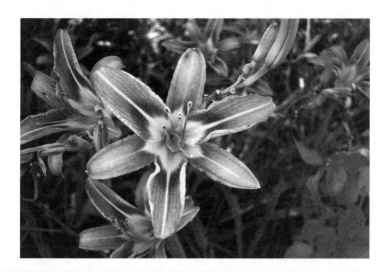

Lilies along the trail

pick up a bit of oak savanna on your left just before you come to the corner of Larsen Road and East Clayton Road. To your right an access road leads to a pump station behind a metal gate. Currently this is officially off limits. In the future there are hopes to get the right-of-way and use this corridor as a return trail for the Nine Springs E-Way trail.

The trail continues along Clayton Road with cropland to your right. At 0.3 miles the path climbs moderately as you approach a curve to the right that takes the path around the right side of a small ridge that separates it from the road for a short stretch. At the top of the hill, a trail goes to the right along a row of trees. This is where the Nine Springs E-Way trail first joins this trail on its return in the opposite direction. There is a bench at the top of the hill overlooking the fields to the right.

From the bench it's another 0.3 miles to County Road MM, with the trail following close to the edge of Clayton Road. At the next corner, cross MM and go right along the sidewalk, immediately crossing McCoy Road. Go left on the other side and cross the on-ramp to US 14, go under the overpass, and cross the ramp on the other side. The trail continues from here along McCoy Road.

The next 0.7 miles takes you along marshland to the right with a line of cottonwoods granting a bit of shade at times, but the trail is mostly exposed. Wildflowers line the trail. At 0.5 miles cross railroad tracks before reaching Syene Road 0.2 miles later.

Go straight across to a parking area on the right. The next 0.6 miles crosses through a bit of prairie and brush before heading into oak forest and public hunting grounds. There is no shade, however. Another 0.2 miles later, long-needle pines close in around the trail. You'll pass a bench just before the trail curves right with thick underbrush on either side. This is the most remote point on the trail.

From the bench at 0.2 miles, find a spur trail that rides parallel, an older version of the current trail. This loops off left through some prairie and crosses a small bridge before it rejoins the main trail again 800 feet farther on. Just past this the trail enter into woods for 0.1 mile, and then the path is open to the sky for the next 0.4 miles as it passes behind a school and climbs a hill up to Gunflint Trail. Follow this right to Glacier Valley Road. Take this to the right 0.3 miles through residences until it meets Fish Hatchery Road. To your right is the Nevin Fish Hatchery, which offers tours, restrooms, water, and park information during business hours. Take the sidewalk to the left 0.1 mile to cross Fish Hatchery Road at the traffic light at McKee Road.

The trail resumes on the other side going up a bit steeply to the top of a ridge and then bearing right away from the intersection and the busy roads as it descends into a corridor of forest with a certain secret garden quality to it.

Cross two bridges in the first 0.3 miles and then reach a short tunnel under Longford Terrace another 0.3 miles after that. It is quiet back here, but beware of bikers flying past around tight turns. A small creek trickles through around large rocks to your right, and the trail is mostly shaded by oaks.

Another 0.4 miles takes you across Edenberry Street through exposed terrain and finally into a mowed park area. This 0.3-mile stretch winds through the park slightly uphill and takes you to a wooded segment—the last 0.4 miles out to Seminole Highway, with condos to the right just outside the trees.

After crossing the busy street, the trail curves 0.3 miles through wildflowers, with a drainage area/wetlands to the right where you may see a lot of birds, especially during migration periods. Prairie is to your left as is a spur trail to the parking area for Dunn Marsh. This is another good trail entry point.

Enter a wooded area after this and continue 0.4 miles until you pass under a bridge, which is the future overpass for the Badger State Trail. Just past here an asphalt trail goes right. This is the Southwest Path, and the future connection to the Badger State Trail is just 0.1 mile to your right. Stay straight here, and the last 0.3 miles of the trail curve left past a pond on the right, then a playground, and finally another pond on the left before curling uphill to the end of the trail. There are no facilities there but a map board.

NEARBY ACTIVITIES

Lake Farm Unit at the head of the trail has some short trails in and around the marsh and the Lussier Family Heritage Center provides information about the history of the area. A great place for some homestyle Mexican food and great seviche is Juanita's Tacos not far from the trailhead on 2510 Rimrock Road. Call (608) 274-6231.

CHEROKEE MARSH NORTH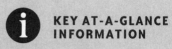

IN BRIEF

Find many species of birds along trails through prairie and boardwalks through the wetlands at this rich marsh along the Yahara River just north of Lake Mendota.

DESCRIPTION

Madison's famous chain of four lakes is the beneficiary of the Upper Yahara River, which, together with the Cherokee Marsh, drains the lands north of Lake Mendota. At 3,200 acres, the marsh is the largest wetland in Dane County.

Ten thousand years ago, the retreating glaciers created a lake here covering much more territory than the present day Mendota. The fine sediments left behind did not promote drainage, so the soil above them remained saturated, forming wetlands. With wetlands comes the partially decayed vegetable matter known as peat, which is up to ten feet thick in some places.

Nineteenth-century farmers couldn't use this land, so they did all they could to drain it. Perhaps all of the marsh would have been lost had the locals not put in a dam at the outlet of Lake Mendota in 1850, thus backing up water and making the areas we have today impossible to drain.

KEY AT-A-GLANCE INFORMATION

LENGTH: 2 miles

CONFIGURATION: Double loop

DIFFICULTY: Easy to moderate

SCENERY: Mixed forest, prairie, and wetlands

EXPOSURE: Mostly sun, with partial shade in the wooded stretch

TRAIL TRAFFIC: Light

TRAIL SURFACE: Crushed stone, packed dirt, grass, and boardwalks

HIKING TIME: 1 hour

DRIVING DISTANCE: 2 miles north on Sherman Avenue from where the Northport Drive intersection

ACCESS: Open 4 a.m.–1 hour after sunset

MAPS: USGS De Forest; posted on map board in parking lot

WHEELCHAIR ACCESSIBILITY: Restrooms and some trails

FACILITIES: Restrooms, picnic tables, bike rack, water fountain

SPECIAL COMMENTS: No dogs allowed. This is listed as a birding hot spot at Cornell University's www.ebird.org.

Directions

On the northeast side of Lake Mendota, North Sherman Avenue intersects Northport Drive (WI 113). Follow Sherman Avenue 2 miles north, passing Cherokee Country Club and ending right at the park entrance. Continue to the parking lot to find the trailhead. If the gates are closed, you can park outside them and follow a trail on the right that will take you straight north to the parking lot and trailhead.

GPS Trailhead Coordinates

UTM Zone (WGS 84)   16T

Easting   0307773.8

Northing   4782084.4

Latitude   N 43° 10' 1.51"

Longitude   W 89° 21' 53.05"

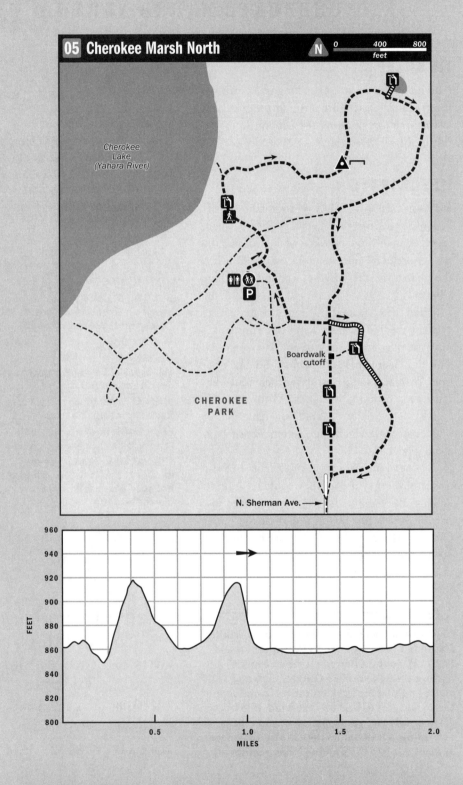

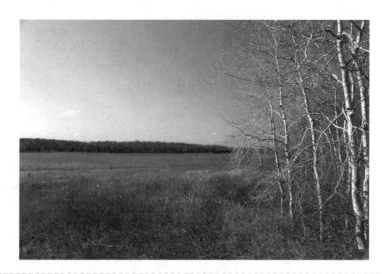

A widening of the Yahara River known as Cherokee Lake

If it's not one threat, it's another; more than 640 acres of the marsh eroded after that dam went in. The raised lake levels caused the buoyant peat to become floating bogs. Residential development in the 1960s caused a major tract of these bobbing sedge meadows to break free, creating the widened part of the Yahara known as Cherokee Lake. Wetland restoration efforts have gone a long way in returning the marsh to a healthier state, and what we have today is a rich environment for a variety of flora and fauna.

From the north end of the parking lot, go north on crushed rock, crossing an access road before entering the trees. The trail bends to the right, and then a branch heads out into the open on a mowed path. Pass this by and stay left inside the aspens. At the next four-way intersection 300 feet later, go straight across. The path to the left leads to other short trails through the woods and where the long boardwalk used to be. The path to the right is a cutoff that will skip the woods on the hill and the prairie beyond, taking you right back to the marshy area. Stay straight on the crushed-stone access road that slopes down on a couple of boardwalks out to viewing platforms over the marsh and the Yahara River. There was once an extensive boardwalk trail south of here, but unfortunately, a park manager decided to take it out, claiming environmental reasons.

Continue on down the access road, and 800 feet later, a trail rises up to the right. The access road continues down to the water's edge. The trail rises into the forest at a moderate grade.

Not long after cresting the hill just over 0.2 miles later, you come out of the forest to a bench overlooking a long slope of prairie that extends down to a pond in a small stand of woods. To the right is a cutoff trail that takes you back down and around back this hill and directly to the wetlands. Continue straight down the hill, taking the grassy trail to your left. Cross 0.2 miles of open meadow to a clump of trees at the bottom of the slope. Inside is a small pond with a boardwalk and platform that extends into the middle of it. Frogs and dragonflies are active here.

The trail then turns back up the hill another 0.2 miles and comes to the cutoff juncture still within sight of the bench at the top. Pass over the ridge and descend along the edge of the woods where the trail turns back into the shade for 200 feet before coming to a three-way intersection. Go left here, and the trail ventures out toward the marshy areas. Only 0.2 miles later, you hit another juncture. To the right cuts back to the parking lot, but go straight for your return trail. Go left onto the boardwalk, which meanders into the marsh to a raised viewing platform 400 feet in. Listen for sandhill cranes here. The added height of the platform should give you better odds of spotting one and several other species of birds.

Just past the platform, a cutoff trail takes you back out of the marsh, but continue straight for another 400 feet to reach the end of the planks. When the trail leaves the boardwalk, expect to have some tricky going if there has been any amount of rainfall. Waterproof footwear or sandals are your best bet here, though during dry periods, you generally have little to worry about.

Follow the trail in a long loop south that cuts through prairie before returning to less spongy terrain and slightly higher ground at 0.2 miles. At the first juncture, find a trail heading left to the park gates. Continuing, however, go right, heading back north. Along this crushed-rock trail, you come across two viewing platforms leaning into the marsh to the left. However, they are not raised like the previous one. This return segment of the loop takes you a quarter mile back to the entrance to the boardwalk (you pass the boardwalk cutoff trail first). Go left here 300 feet to where another exit takes you to the southern end of the parking lot, but stay on the trail and go right across the prairie for another 600 feet, bringing you back to the forest trail near where you started the hike. Head left 100 feet, taking another left to exit to the parking lot.

This park is excellent for bird-watching, and you can expect to see plenty of waterfowl, herons, and cranes. In April you will find many migratory species. Share your observations at Cornell University's **www.ebird.org,** where you can also see what others are seeing and when.

NEARBY ACTIVITIES

The Madison Mallards are a college-level summer baseball team playing at Warner Park near North Sherman Avenue and Northport Drive. Find out when there's a home game by going to **www.mallardsbaseball.com** or calling (608) 246-4277.

CHEROKEE MARSH SOUTH 06

IN BRIEF

Cross open fields and wetlands and hike up and down small hills in oak forest as you find viewpoints along this trail through the lower portion of Cherokee Marsh along the Yahara River.

DESCRIPTION

The damming of Lake Mendota kept Cherokee Marsh from being drained for agriculture in the late 19th century, but it wasn't just the pioneers that dealt with land management. Native Americans once set fires to maintain the open fields. The marsh area remains important as it filters out excess fertilizer from upland runoff, helping to keep the lakes cleaner.

The park is the focus of wetland, prairie, and oak savanna restoration projects, and many species of birds, such as the marsh hawk and the short-eared owl, benefit from these efforts. This is the lower portion of the marsh closest to where the Yahara River, which runs through it, empties into Lake Mendota.

Directions ⟶

Follow WI 113 (First Street) north from where it meets US 151 (East Washington Avenue). At the first traffic light, go right where it becomes East Johnson Street, but then follow the curve with Pennsylvania Avenue a block later. It becomes Packers Avenue 0.4 miles from there without leaving the main road, and finally it becomes Northport Road as you stay on this. Just be careful to follow the WI 113 signs. A total of 4 miles from US 151 at School Road, go right for three quarters of a mile. The park entrance is a small lot on your left. Pass through a gate here set back 50 feet from the road, and continue down a gravel road 0.4 miles to the parking lot. The trailhead is to the left.

KEY AT-A-GLANCE INFORMATION

LENGTH: 3 miles

CONFIGURATION: Out-and-back with interconnected loops

DIFFICULTY: Easy to moderate

SCENERY: Mixed forest, prairie, and wetlands, river views

EXPOSURE: Shaded and sunny portions

TRAIL TRAFFIC: Light

TRAIL SURFACE: Packed dirt, some crushed stone

HIKING TIME: 1.5–2 hours

DRIVING DISTANCE: 0.75 miles north of Northport Drive (WI 113) and School Road

ACCESS: 4 a.m.–dusk

MAPS: USGS Waunakee

WHEELCHAIR ACCESSIBILITY: None

FACILITIES: None

SPECIAL COMMENTS: Bring bug spray. Portions of this trail can be soggy, especially if there has been rain, so plan your footwear accordingly. Dogs are not allowed.

GPS Trailhead Coordinates

UTM Zone (WGS 84)   16T

Easting   0306218

Northing   4780600

Latitude   N 43° 09' 11.99"

Longitude   W 89° 23' 0.00"

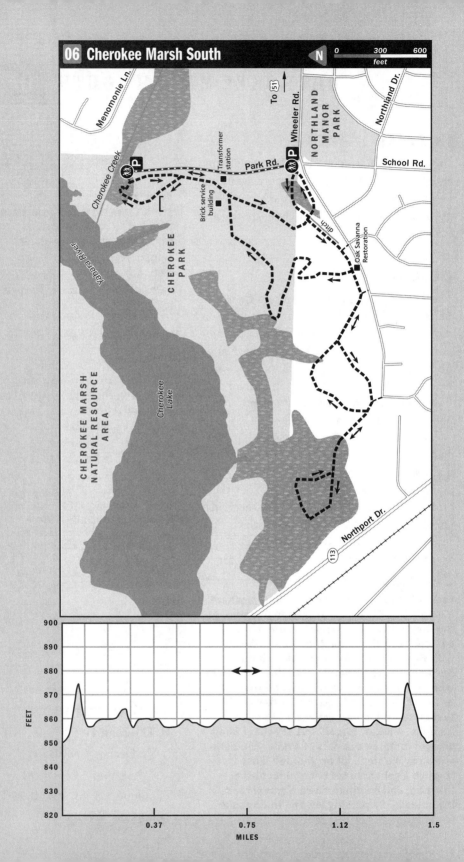

N

0   300   600
feet

Menomonie Ln.

To 51

Wheeler Rd.

Northland Dr.

NORTHLAND MANOR PARK

School Rd.

Cherokee Creek

P

Transformer station

Park Rd.

P

Brick service building

ditch

Oak Savanna Restoration

CHEROKEE PARK

Yahara River

CHEROKEE MARSH NATURAL RESOURCE AREA

Cherokee Lake

Northport Dr.

113

900
890
880
870
860
850
840
830
820

FEET

0.37   0.75   1.12   1.5
MILES

If the gates in front of the park entry road are closed, you can still park there and pick up the trail at a point to the left of the gate. The gravel parking lot at the end of the entry road has a small dock on Cherokee Creek that feeds into the Yahara River to the west. Look for the trailhead next to a cottonwood to the left as you enter the lot where you'll find a small sign that says CONSERVATION PARK and a wire across the entry.

Step around or duck under the wire to find the grassy trail splitting left and right. Head left away from the creek. The trail goes up gently, and in summer the grass may be higher than your head. As you gain a little altitude on the hill, you get an overview of the cattails to the left across the entry road. To the right, the ridge is still higher than you, so you don't see the river beyond the other side.

At 550 feet from the trailhead, find a wooden post where the trail goes right up the hill or down to left. You can see water in the distance from here to the right. Go left down to some invasive buckthorn bushes and find a marshy area to the right where you might come across cranes and herons on their spindly legs searching for a meal. The path follows along the edge of the entry road for another 500 feet where you arrive at a transformer station. Cut stumps are graying in the sun to your right in more soggy terrain. The deadwood makes a nice home for shelf fungi. Beyond this you enter into a maintained area around a brick service building, and the trail seems to disappear. Staying in front of the building, follow a direct line across the lot to arrive at the other side and pick up the cut-grass trail again.

The trail shows some sandy spots, and in summer you see many ant mounds along the way. Two hundred feet from the brick building, enter the woods through a stand of cottonwoods and pussy willows. Trail grass can get long here, but it is generally maintained. Here is one of the segments of the trail that affords a bit of shade. The trail can get soggy and even muddy back here. At the first trail juncture 400 feet into the trees, go left through a small clearing. The low area to the left shows fallen trees and marsh. At the next intersection, go left as you cross over a ditch full of stagnant water and, needless to say, mosquitoes in season. Go straight across the next juncture following the trail to the edge of the park where it turns left. Telephone wires/power lines mark the street to the right and thick brush separates you from a residential neighborhood. Follow along about 500 feet and you'll come to a short trail to the right which leads to the outside parking lot. Instead, continue left here around the loop another 500 feet as the trail descends gently. Go right at the juncture and take an immediate left, entering a wide clearing. The brush and the ditch pass along the left, and on your right, a gash in the woods is wide open to the sky. Come out of this section of the trail 500 feet later at cedar chips and an oak savanna restoration area. To your left is an exit trail 50 feet to Wheeler Road. Street parking and entry here are also possible.

Halfway across the 600-foot section of oak plantings, pass a wooden post and a trail to the right up a hill into woods. The southernmost section of the trail

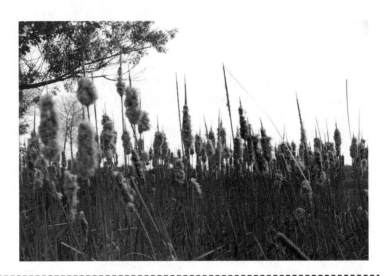

Cattails at the edge of the marsh

is a loop from here, and this is your return route. So keep straight along here to the end where your trail goes right at another juncture where you can also exit to Wheeler Road to the left. The trail is uneven with the natural shape of the ground.

This garden to your left was cleared of box elders in 2007 in order to make way for some oak saplings. Previously the taller and faster-growing box elders were edging out the oaks, causing them to grow into the road in search of sunlight. The buckthorn and honeysuckle understory was also cleared. Fifteen oaks have been planted here, and over time it will look less like a garden as the understory overpowers the cedar chips.

Following the trail right away from the road, you immediately pass a big boulder to the right and see dead trees standing out of brush in a marshy area. Lots of cottonwoods stand here as you pass through deeper into marsh 500 feet to the first juncture. Go left; the straight path is your return from the big loop.

Pass through some shrubs and then cross prairie marsh, with grasses undulating in wind and the occasional mourning doves bursting from hiding as you pass. To the left is the residential street over the tall grasses, and you can hear the highway in the distance.

A trail goes left out to Wheeler Road, and as you continue on another 100 feet, you pass a post marking your return trail to the right. Go straight here where the trail shows a bit of crushed rock. The road is firm and crosses through marsh on both sides until you arrive 300 feet later at the edge of more woods. In the wetlands tall gray trunks stand like columns to the left and red-winged blackbirds keep up a constant chatter. This is the closest point to WI 113, and the hum of wheels can distract, yet it is surprising how much animal activity you find here. You are likely to spot deer among the oaks. At the first trail juncture,

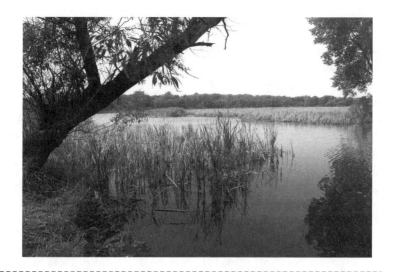

Cherokee Creek joins the Yahara River

go left; the right is the return path. The trail takes you on a 0.3-mile loop back to this point with oak leaves covering tree roots along the path. You may find some unofficial side trails into the underbrush, but stay on the main trail to complete the loop and then head back out into the marsh until you come once again to the wooden post.

Go left here, and the trail dips down to its lowest and marshiest point. This whole segment is going to give you soakers in rainy periods, but higher ground comes in 350 feet or so. This affords a view of the water far ahead and the rising opposite bank of the river. But the view is short-lived as brush envelops you 200 feet farther on and the trail rejoins the return to the oak savanna 600 feet after that. Once you reach the savanna again, go left to that wooden post and break left into the woods. Look for raspberries on the left side of the path here in July. The trail goes uphill on crushed rock. When you crest the small hill, you walk along the top before the path curls left and descends again through the dip between this hill and the next. Just beyond the trees to the left is standing water. At the top of the next hill, the path doubles back. Head down again, then up again, and once again you double back making a 900-foot *S*-trail through the oaks.

Exit the woods at a post with a broken piece of chain on the left. The trail goes right and left. Go left into the sun with trees along your left and grassy fields with milkweed and Indian paintbrush to the right. The path rises sharply and crests the hill and you are granted a view back across marshy area toward the highway where you've just been. The curve brings you around the end of this field to head back the other direction, this time with the trees to your left and the grasses to your right. Pass through some oaks and some young aspens to the right. To the left is a narrow stretch of trees that marks the edge of the higher ground and the marsh beyond. This loop brings you back within sight of the brick building. Return to the path in front of the structure and follow it back toward the parking lot until you pass the marshy area and come to the hill. At the wooden post, go left 250 feet up the hill to the top where you find a bench on your right with a great view of the marsh to your left.

Head downhill from here along the top of the small ridge taking in great views of the marsh. The path follows a curve to the right along the edge of some oaks, and you come your closest to the open water, though it is still a few hundred feet beyond the cattails. The last curve brings you around to the back of this ridge and the exit back to the trailhead and parking lot. Before you leave, check out the short mud trail right along the edge of the creek, left of the dock, which is popular for fishing and is a nice little foray into the cattails 100 feet from the parking lot.

NEARBY ACTIVITIES

Cherokee Marsh North offers more hiking with a boardwalk and another view of the Yahara Watershed. Warner Park is at Sherman Avenue and WI 113 (Northport Drive) where you can catch a Madison Mallards baseball game during the summer. Check out their schedule online at **www.mallardsbaseball.com** or call (608) 246-4277.

EDNA TAYLOR CONSERVATION PARK
(with Aldo Leopold Nature Center and Woodland Park)

07

IN BRIEF

The frogs take up the chorus and the birds have the melody at this symphonic wetland and forest nature preserve that abuts the Aldo Leopold Nature Center and Woodland Park, popular for school field trips and a goldmine for bird-watchers within the city.

DESCRIPTION

A glacial drumlin runs right down the middle of this park, and the trail rides its back. Edna Taylor was a teacher and dairy farmer who sold 37 of her 98 acres to Madison to help create this 56-acre conservation park. Sadly, she didn't live to see the completion of it.

The trail begins at the corner of the lot at a giant memorial stone dedicated to Edna Taylor. There are no facilities here except a trash can. The dirt and grass trail starts across prairie and savanna along the low ridge left by the last of the retreating glaciers. Grass will grow high on either side, and this path is set between marshland on either side. This 1,000-foot length is unshaded. Cattails abound, and you can expect to see waterfowl (Canada geese and mallards are abundant), cranes, and herons. Flitting along the tops of the cattails are the usual redwing and tricolor blackbirds and the occasional kingbird (a black bird whose breast and the tip of its tail are white).

KEY AT-A-GLANCE INFORMATION

LENGTH: 3.1 miles (plus 0.5-mile extra loop)

CONFIGURATION: Out-and-back with 3 loops

DIFFICULTY: Easy

SCENERY: Wetlands, oak forest, savanna, ponds, interpretive trail

EXPOSURE: Half and half

TRAIL TRAFFIC: Light to moderate

TRAIL SURFACE: Packed dirt, grass, crushed stone, boardwalk

HIKING TIME: 1.5 hours

DRIVING DISTANCE: 1 mile from the Beltline Highway (US 12/18) and Monona Drive

ACCESS: 4 a.m.–1 hour after sunset

MAPS: USGS Madison East; artistic maps on map boards near Aldo Leopold Nature Center

WHEELCHAIR ACCESSIBILITY: Yes, in most places. Wear gloves—there are a lot of bird droppings in Aldo Leopold.

FACILITIES: Restrooms and water at park office during business hours

SPECIAL COMMENTS: No dogs allowed. Report park bird sightings at ebird.org.

Directions

From the Beltline Highway (US 12/18), go north on Monona Drive 0.6 miles and take a right on Femrite Drive. The parking lot for Edna Taylor is on the left 0.4 miles from Monona Drive. The trailhead is at the lot. (The entry to Aldo Leopold Nature Center is also on the left just 800 feet from Monona Drive.)

GPS Trailhead Coordinates

UTM Zone (WGS 84)   16T

Easting   0311311

Northing   4769171

Latitude   N 43° 03' 6.45"

Longitude   W 89° 19' 0.75"

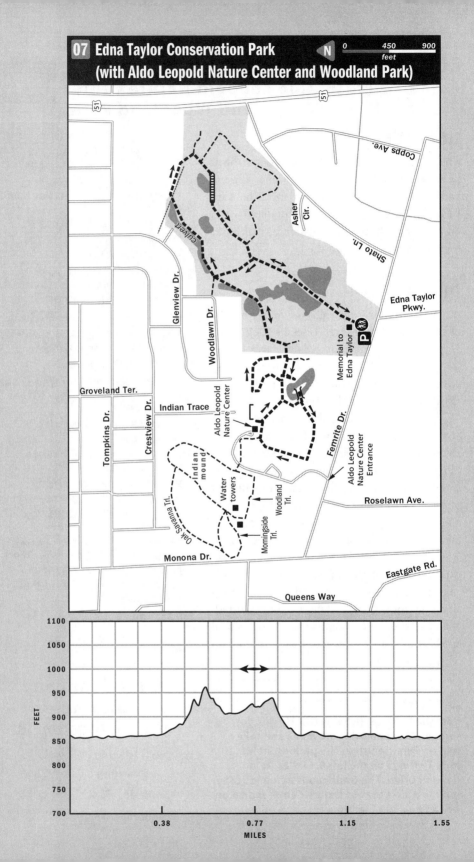

07 **Edna Taylor Conservation Park**
(with Aldo Leopold Nature Center and Woodland Park)

N

0   450   900
feet

US 51

Copps Ave.

Asher Cir.

Shato Ln.

Edna Taylor Pkwy.

Culvert

Glenview Dr.

Woodlawn Dr.

Memorial to Edna Taylor

P

Groveland Ter.

Crestview Dr.

Tompkins Dr.

Indian Trace

Aldo Leopold Nature Center

Fenrite Dr.

Aldo Leopold Nature Center Entrance

Indian mound

Oak Savanna Trl.

Water towers

Woodland Trl.

Morningside Trl.

Roselawn Ave.

Monona Dr.

Eastgate Rd.

Queens Way

FEET			
1100			
1050			
1000			
950			
900			
850			
800			
750			
700			

0.38   0.77   1.15   1.55

MILES

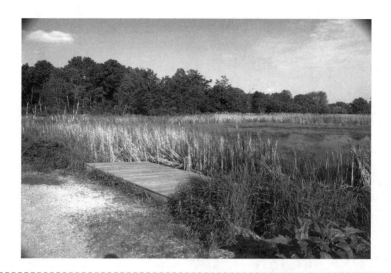

An observation platform at the water's edge—great for spying water fowl

At the other end of the pond, the brush closes in around the trail with some oaks to your left. You might find raspberries here in July but the park policy is no picking. Pass into the shade beyond this where there's an enormous oak to your left. A patch of prairie to your right has a stunning array of wildflowers. The trail forks, and you need to go left; your return path brings you back here from the right. Pass into a very shaded oak forest with a crushed-rock path. Four hundred feet later the trail opens up, and the sides slope into marshland. Cross a culvert here to find cottonwoods to the left and willows to the right. At the trail juncture, go left. This takes you along a long pond on the right with lily pads and blue-flag iris. The trail to the right exits the park in a residential neighborhood. Concrete blocks in the trail keep a low point from getting too muddy. Cattails stand on either side of you. To your right, a big cottonwood stands right before the next pond. Now you have water on either side of you. There are viewing platforms on either side leaning out into either pond.

As the trail continues into smaller willows, pass under another oak. Then the trail opens to the sky as brush closes around you. The surface is packed dirt with roots and occasional rocks. You come out into a field as you exit Edna Taylor Park and enter Aldo Leopold Park through a line of evergreens. Signs make you aware of the change of parks.

Before you is a large pond with an island in the middle. Typically you will find hordes of Canada geese here, and if you come in spring, you'll see the tiny chicks. Geese can actually get aggressive, especially with young children who aren't much taller than the largest goose neck! The pond fills with tadpoles during this time as well, and not long after, the place comes alive with frog calls.

Use the wooden platforms along the edge of the pond to have closer looks at the water and to spot birds. Across the field you can see the water towers of the

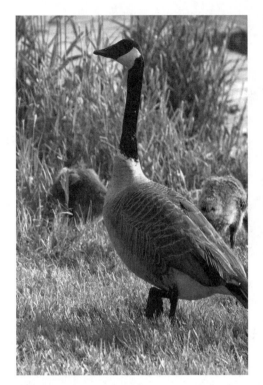

Town of Monona inside Woodland Park. To continue on the trail, keep the pond to your left and follow the shoreline. You'll see the bridge to the island, and you might take a few moments to cross over and have a look around.

On the west side of the pond, trails go in many directions through the prairie and vary with park cutting. They provide access to plants in the middle of the fields and an educational trail that runs throughout Aldo Leopold Park. The trail leaves the water and passes along the park edge to the south. There are apartments beyond the line of mostly pine trees on your left.

The trail bends right near a stand of black walnut trees and passes along the prairie to a large mowed area with a picnic table and a wooden shed with a brick chimney to the left. Keep straight and come to a sign on the right welcoming you to Aldo Leopold Park. Here there is a turnaround right next to the nature center. A map box holds brochures and nature passports and includes information in Spanish. The nature center has restrooms, water, and park guides during business hours.

Continue along the left side of the road heading north past the turnaround and find another trailhead. Go left here aa it cuts through the trees and brush, crosses the park entry road, and comes to a post marked WOODLAND TRAIL. Go left here through mowed grass on an unmarked path parallel to the road until you reach a map board that shows the layout of the Woodland Park trails. Go right, and the trail takes you into the woods and up the hill. You pass between the water towers and come to a trail juncture. Go left here on Morningside Trail. The trail loops out to Monona Drive, but rather than take the loop back, come around the bend and take a left down the Oak Savanna Trail. This will bring you around the edge of the park reconnecting at the Woodland Trail where you can see two Native American mounds. Keep going left and follow the short curve of the trail back around into the mowed area and follow that until it comes once again to the wooden post where you started. Retrace your steps across the road and back to the turnaround where you rejoin the trail in Aldo Leopold Park.

From where you come back to the trail, go left and take the trail directly back to the pond. Go left and watch as you walk along the pond for a trail that cuts left across the prairie. Follow it to the park edge where you pick up shade beneath the line of trees. Go right along the trail that curves back into the open in a small oak savanna where you will find a informational sign regarding the savanna. Continue to the entrance of Edna Taylor Park, and go left following your steps back through the ponds.

Beyond the ponds lies the trail to the left out of the park and the trail to the right from whence you came at the beginning of the hike. The next portion of the trail seems the most remote. Stay straight, don't duck back into the woods. Instead follow another crushed-stone path with a long pond to your left. You have willows along this path and some cottonwoods to the right. Follow it 800 feet to the end of the pond, where there's a large culvert on the left. Just beyond that the trail appears to end at a chain-link fence. From this gate enter the back of the playground at Glendale Elementary School. Go right along the fence until the end of the mowed area and the trail resumes going into thick woods on a packed dirt trail.

The trail goes right at the next juncture before an enormous cottonwood. The left trail goes 0.3 miles up and over a hill but bypasses the upcoming board-walk. It is also the end of an optional loop that would take you back through again what you are about to see.

Going right you come to a narrow clearing on your left that runs to the top of the hill. Stay straight on the trail and come to a 250-foot boardwalk right through cattails as high as six to eight feet above the boardwalk in some places. Open pond is about 20 feet off to your right. On the other side, the boardwalk extends onto dry land ending at a packed dirt trail full of rocks and roots. Oak trees tower over the low-lying underbrush.

The trail reaches another juncture as it comes into the open. Go right and follow the trail back to the original drumlin trail where you go left back to the lot. If you go left here, you can take an additional 0.5 miles up and across a hill starting in oak savanna and then into thicker forest until it curves back down the hill and sends you back through the boardwalk section again.

Note: Kids will enjoy the nature passport available at the box at the turn-around outside the Aldo Leopold Nature Center. Some may want to start their hikes from here instead, but regardless, hikers with children definitely will want to pick up the passport before starting.

NEARBY ACTIVITIES

The City of Monona has a public swimming pool at 1011 Nichols Road, no more than a ten-minute drive from here. Call (608) 222-3098 for more information.

08 ELVER PARK

KEY AT-A-GLANCE INFORMATION

LENGTH: 3.4 miles

CONFIGURATION: Figure eight

DIFFICULTY: Easy to moderate

SCENERY: Prairie, mixed forest, ponds, city skyline

EXPOSURE: Half and half

TRAIL TRAFFIC: Light

TRAIL SURFACE: Mowed grass, packed dirt, some asphalt

HIKING TIME: 1.5 hours

DRIVING DISTANCE: 1.1 miles south of The Beltline Highway (US 12/14)

ACCESS: 4 a.m.–10 p.m. year-round

MAPS: USGS Middleton; map board in ballpark parking lot

WHEELCHAIR ACCESSIBILITY: Limited to a few paths around the open center of the park

FACILITIES: Restrooms, water, playground, shelter, picnic area

SPECIAL COMMENTS: An outstanding disc-golf course offers an alternative trail starting from the southeast corner of the ice-rink depression on the south side of the park. Dogs are allowed on leashes below the sledding hill from March 15 to November 15 only.

IN BRIEF

Follow a prairie loop atop a hill overlooking Madison and then explore the woods where an excellent disc-golf course is tucked in among the trees.

DESCRIPTION

At 227 acres, this is the largest of Madison's community parks, and it seems there is always something going on here. Beginning from the first parking lot, look for the smaller pavilion closer to the park entrance. An asphalt path passes a playground and some tennis courts beyond the pavilion. Follow this as it leads you out toward the soccer field. At 0.15 miles the asphalt curves toward the street and a crosswalk. Leave the path here and follow the edge of the cut grass as it curves behind the end of the soccer field and heads toward the bottom of the hill just 250 feet away. The trail becomes a wide mowed path and begins up the slope with trees and brush on either side until you reach the beginnings of prairie toward the top. It's 0.2 miles from the bottom to a trail juncture at the top. There are nice views of Madison behind you. Red-tailed hawks frequent this field, as well as many songbirds. Going right will take you across the center of the prairie, but go straight. Three hundred feet

GPS Trailhead Coordinates

UTM Zone (WGS 84) 16T

Easting 0296121

Northing 4768101

Latitude N 43° 02' 17.65"

Longitude W 89° 30' 10.15"

Directions →

From The Beltline Highway (US 12/14), take the Gammon Road exit. Go left on Gammon Road/McKenna Boulevard 1.1 miles to the park entrance on the left. Park in the first lot on the left. The trailhead is at the southeastern corner of the lot near the smaller of two pavilions.

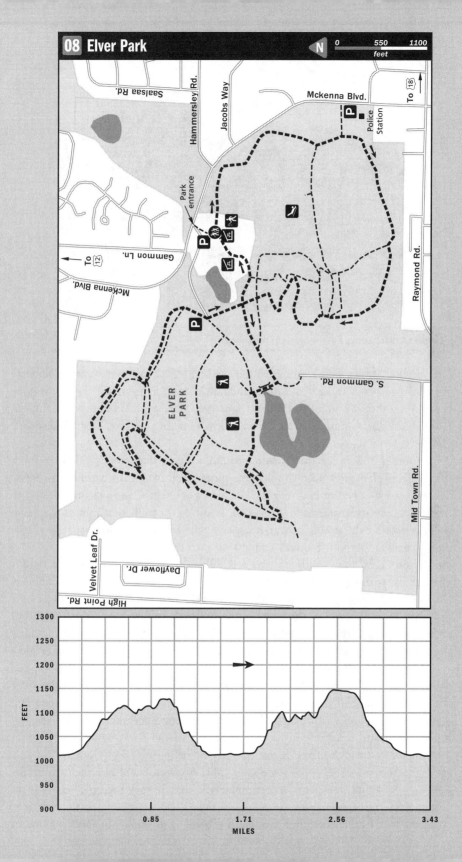

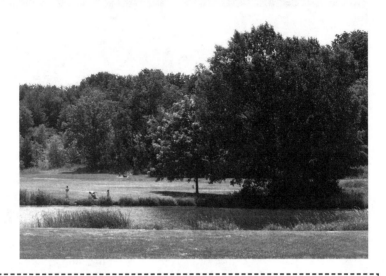

Children fish in the pond at the center of the park.

later on the left is a spur trail out to the road and the local police station. Stay on the trail as it bends right with brush gradually closing in around it. From the spur trail it's another 0.3 miles to the next juncture. Here a trail comes down the hill from your right. Continue straight and follow two fairways of the park's disc-golf course.

Another 0.2 miles brings you around a bend that slopes down a short distance and then rises up through some pines. A clearing runs from left to right, and you see a concrete pad (a golf "tee") to your left. Continue into the pines beyond the clearing and follow this trail passing two trails that join at the same point on your right, and finally arriving at a place where the wide path goes right and a narrow footpath plunges straight on into the forest. Take this and find a packed-dirt path that winds its way 0.3 miles down the hill, passing around a chain halfway down. If you are lucky, you may see an owl through here. (This is the most undeveloped segment of the park, and you can bypass it, if you prefer a groomed trail. Go right at the entry to the footpath and loop into the forest, and then follow the 17th-hole fairway to its end, then go left to head down the hill.)

From the bottom of the hill from either trail, go straight a bit farther until you come to the asphalt path and then follow that to the left. From the mapped trail, it is 0.2 miles to another juncture that goes right and crosses a bridge over the water to the ball diamonds. To your left here is a nice bit of wetlands and a good place to find visiting birds during the migration periods. Go left along the asphalt path and it takes you to the north half of the park, which will make a 1.6-mile loop through mixed forest back to the ballpark parking lot.

Into the woods 200 feet, the trail splits in two. These are one-way trails, coming and going, for skiers. For simplicity's sake, always take the left branch. Uphill 0.15 miles later, there is a spur footpath exiting the park to your left. Another 150 feet farther and around the bend, you come to another fork in

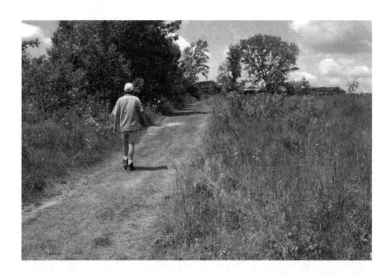

A prairie walk at Elven's highest point

the trail. Stay left and it's 0.25 miles to the next juncture, where you will find the parallel trail coming back to the right, and two trails that lead directly right and would take you out toward the ballparks again. Just ahead is another fork; stay left and hike 0.25 miles to the next multispoke juncture. Again there's the parallel path behind you from the right, two paths that go slightly to the right ahead, and two more that go left. Take the trail to the left, which takes you on a 0.5-mile loop that will reconnect to the forward paths. Halfway up this loop is another meeting point of these parallel trails. Stay left once more. At the end of the 0.5-mile loop, go left and it's 0.2 miles more to exit the woods into the mowed area along the ballpark parking lot. You can follow the park road from here back to the other lot, or cross the lot and go to the corner of the nearest of the ball diamonds. From the beginning of the asphalt path, leave the asphalt and go on the grass trail toward the woods, passing the pond on your left and reaching another asphalt path. Follow this left back to the smaller pavilion and the parking lot.

This park is quite popular for its variety of activities. In the winter there is ice skating as well as skiing, and the sledding hill is the best in town. Runners in training use that hill for an intense workout. This is also the site of the Fourth of July fireworks. Madison Metro bus routes 50 and 58 serve the park.

NEARBY ACTIVITIES

Vitense Golfland at 5501 West Beltline Highway at Whitney Way can be reached by taking Schroeder Road heading east from Gammon Road (halfway back to the Beltline Highway from Elver Park). Here you'll find indoor/outdoor minigolf, batting cages, a driving range, and a par 3 golf course. Call (608) 271-1411 for more information or go to **www.vitense.com.**

09 MADISON CAPITOL AND DOWNTOWN

**KEY AT-A-GLANCE
INFORMATION**

LENGTH: 3.0 miles

CONFIGURATION: Loop

DIFFICULTY: Easy

**SCENERY: Historical buildings,
downtown shops, the Capitol, views
of Lakes Mendota and Monona**

EXPOSURE: Mostly sun

TRAIL TRAFFIC: Moderate to heavy

TRAIL SURFACE: Sidewalks

HIKING TIME: 1 hour

**DRIVING DISTANCE: 0.5 miles from
the Capitol Square**

ACCESS: Year-round

MAPS: USGS Madison West

WHEELCHAIR ACCESSIBILITY: Yes

**FACILITIES: In shops and
restaurants along the route**

**SPECIAL COMMENTS: This area is
busiest on Saturday mornings,
especially during Wisconsin Badger
football games and the Farmers'
Market.**

IN BRIEF

Stroll the eclectic downtown area, visit the majestic Capitol, climb Mansion Hill, and take in the lakeshores on both sides of the isthmus.

DESCRIPTION

Starting from the corner of Lake Street, begin up State Street toward the Capitol. Just about every style of ethnic food can be found in the next seven blocks (0.5 miles) from the classic Wisconsin State Street Brats to more exotic fare such as Nepalese, Turkish, and African. Clothing, music, books, a bike shop, and an assortment of gift shops and boutiques make this a nice option to the usual mall-variety stores. Street musicians, university students, (and a few panhandlers, unfortunately) are ubiquitous and add to the vibe that is quintessentially Madison.

You pass State Street Brats on your right halfway up the first block. Cross Gilman Street and in the next block to your left across the street is Lisa Link Peace Park where a historical marker remembers Madison's role in the antiwar movement in the 1960s and 1970s. Continue toward the Capitol and pass Sacred Feather, a fine hat store and one of the only freestanding houses along here. You'll cross the one-way, traffic-heavy Gorham Street and

GPS Trailhead Coordinates

UTM Zone (WGS 84) 16T

Easting 0304826

Northing 4771906

Latitude N 43° 04' 29.11"

Longitude W 89° 23' 50.62"

Directions

From the Capitol Square, go northeast 0.2 miles (three blocks) on Wisconsin Avenue to Gorham Street. Go left and follow Gorham 0.4 miles as it crosses State Street and bends right, becoming University Avenue. Two blocks later, turn right on Lake Street and park in the parking ramp half a block down on the right. The hike begins another half block beyond at the corner of Lake and State streets.

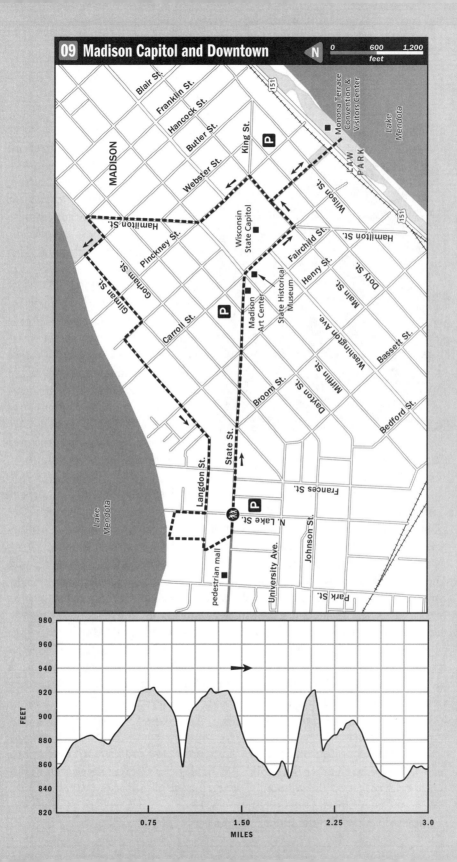

N

0   600   1,200
feet

MADISON

Blair St.

Franklin St.

Hancock St.

Butler St.

Webster St.

King St.

151

Monona Terrace
Convention &
Visitors Center

Lake
Mendota

LAW PARK

Wilson St.

Hamilton St.

Pinckney St.

Wisconsin
State Capitol

Hamilton St.

151

Gilman St.

Gorham St.

Carroll St.

Madison
Art Center

State Historical
Museum

Fairchild St.

Henry St.

Main St.

Doty St.

Washington Ave.

Bassett St.

Mifflin St.

Dayton St.

Broom St.

Bedford St.

State St.

Langdon St.

Frances St.

N. Lake St.

Johnson St.

Park St.

Lake
Mendota

University Ave.

pedestrian mall

FEET

980

960

940

920

900

880

860

840

820

0.75   1.50   2.25   3.0

MILES

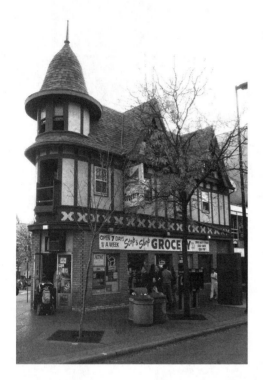

another block later Johnson Street heading the opposite direction. Henry Street crosses this intersection as well. Cross Johnson Street and then Henry Street to stay on State Street. At this corner, find the towering glass corner of the Madison Museum of Contemporary Art (closed Mondays, check the **mmoca.org** or call [608] 257-0158 for hours and exhibit information). There is a somewhat upscale rooftop terrace restaurant and bar. The view of State Street makes it worth a visit. The museum is part of the Overture Center for the Arts complex, which runs along the entire next block. Look for the old facades of two of the previous structures that once stood here—most notably the Civic Center; they were worked into the new building.

Across the street is the Orpheum Theatre, which brings in a mix of independent and big-name films as well as several concerts throughout the year. The lobby restaurant has a somewhat classy and yet casual atmosphere and offers great meals.

In the last block of State Street before you reach the Capitol Square, find The House of Wisconsin Cheese, which offers an outstanding assortment of Wisconsin's finest product along with many other delectable gift ideas and souvenirs. At the top corner of State Street are three museums: The State Historical Museum, the Wisconsin Veteran's Museum, and the Madison Children's Museum.

Cross the street to get to the Capitol at the corner of Mifflin and Carroll streets. The Capitol is open to the public, free daily tours are available, and from Memorial Day through October you can climb to the observation deck for great views of the city in all directions. Hours are Monday through Friday 8 a.m. to 6 p.m. and 8 a.m. to 4 p.m. on weekends and holidays. Call (608) 266-0382 for more information.

Go right along Carroll Street to Main Street, and head left. Halfway along the block is Martin Luther King (MLK) Jr. Boulevard. Go right here and follow it two blocks to get to the Monona Terrace. Based on a design by Frank Lloyd Wright, the convention center's rooftop terrace offers views of Lake Monona and occasional live music in the summer months.

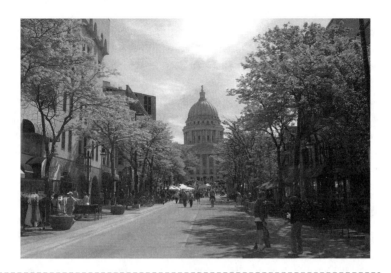

The view of the Capitol from State Street

Return along MLK Jr. Boulevard to the Capitol and continue around the square, going right on Main Street to Pinckney Street. Go left here and follow it to Mifflin Street. Cross Pinckney to the right and then Mifflin to the left and take the angling Hamilton Street right and down the hill from the Capitol. You will walk three blocks (0.25 miles) to Gorham and cross to James Madison Park. This park along the shore of Lake Mendota offers canoe and sailboat rentals and is often alive with ultimate Frisbee games and sunbathers.

Go left and pass the 1863 Gates of Heaven synagogue, a sandstone and brick structure brought here from West Washington Avenue to be preserved. At Butler Street, go right one block and then left, climbing Gilman Street into what is known as the Mansion Hill District. Have a look at some fine houses from some of the wealthiest of the 19th century Madisonians. After two blocks, go right on Wisconsin Avenue and come to the Edgewater Hotel. Go left on Langdon Street and begin passing more rather large houses. Many of these are Greek fraternity or sorority houses. The Greek system began at the University of Wisconsin in 1857, and many of the chapter houses you see now were built in part as an answer to the housing problem before the advent of residence halls.

At the intersection of Carroll and Langdon streets is a historical marker in honor of Frank Lloyd Wright and his relationship with the Madison area. You can follow Carroll Street to the lakeside where steps lead you down for a view of the water. Continuing down Langdon Street, follow the street's bend to the right and then continue two more blocks to Lake Street. Go right one short block to the end of the street and follow the lakeside promenade to the left, which will take you to the University's Memorial Union Terrace. This is an excellent place to watch the sunset from the various tables and docks. Food and drink are available outdoors in season and live musical acts are regularly scheduled on Thursday, Friday, and Saturday evenings. These events move indoors by late fall.

Heading away from the lakeside, cross through the parking lot with the Union to your right. On your left is an enormous redbrick building that looks more like a fortress. This is the 1893 Red Gym which was once home to UW basketball and various other events.

Cross Langdon Street at the crosswalk in front of the Memorial Union and take the angle walk through Library Mall that passes the central fountain. Just beyond that is a concrete speaker's pulpit. Going left there will take you between the Memorial Library and University Bookstore and returns you to your starting point at State and Lake streets.

NEARBY ACTIVITIES

This is the heart of the Mad City and activities are too numerous to list. The Dane County Farmers' Market on the Capitol Square on Saturday mornings from April through October is a Madison social event as much as a time to get local produce, cheese, meat, and baked goods. Another market is held off the square on Martin Luther King Jr. Boulevard on Wednesday mornings. Check out **www. visitmadison.com** for a calendar for other downtown events such as Maxwell Street Days and Art Fair on the Square.

NINE SPRINGS E-WAY TRAIL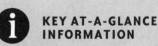

IN BRIEF

Prairie and marsh along Spring Creek just south of Madison's Beltline Highway are home to wild turkeys, deer, and a variety of birds and wildflowers. Enter a world that seems much farther from the city than it is.

DESCRIPTION

The Nine Springs E-Way Trail is a 5.4-mile-long green corridor along the south side of Madison. Laid out in 1970, it includes wetlands, farmland, and prairie, and is an important part of the area's hopes for sustainable urban development and natural resource preservation. It includes part of the Capital City State Trail and Lake Farm Park and abuts Capital Springs Centennial State Park and Recreation Area.

At the gravel parking lot, you'll find an accessible pit toilet, a self-pay tube, and a map board to the left of the trailhead. A larger kiosk is near the entrance to the parking lot with more information about the greater park.

Pass through a metal gate and come to a T intersection. Go left to explore the first loop, which amounts to a 0.6-mile hike through prairie and to the highest point on the trail where you have a modest view of the e-way and the surrounding city. In summer you pass

KEY AT-A-GLANCE INFORMATION

LENGTH: 5.4 miles

CONFIGURATION: A small loop within a large loop and a short out-and-back

DIFFICULTY: Easy

SCENERY: Prairie, wetlands, creek, some forest

EXPOSURE: Mostly sun

TRAIL TRAFFIC: Light but moderate along the Capital City Trail segment

TRAIL SURFACE: Uneven cut grass, mowed paths, dirt, bridges, and boardwalk

HIKING TIME: 2–2.5 hours

DRIVING DISTANCE: 1.1 miles from the Beltline Highway (US 12/18) and the South Towne Drive exit

ACCESS: 5 a.m.–10 p.m. year-round

MAPS: USGS Madison East; at kiosk at trailhead

WHEELCHAIR ACCESSIBILITY: Only the viewing platform and boardwalk

FACILITIES: Accessible pit toilet, picnic tables

SPECIAL COMMENTS: Hiking is not allowed when trails are maintained for skiing. Wild parsnip is common and shouldn't be touched (see Animal and Plant Hazards, page 8). There are daily fees for dogs ($3) and cross-country skiers ($5).

Directions

Exit the Beltline Highway (US 12/18) at South Towne Drive and go south. This becomes Raywood Road. Go left 0.8 miles later on Moorland Road, continuing 0.3 miles to the trail parking lot on your right. The trailhead is at the southwesterly end of the lot.

GPS Trailhead Coordinates

UTM Zone (WGS 84)   16T

Easting   0308626

Northing   4766930

Latitude   N 43° 01' 51.44"

Longitude   W 89° 20' 56.53"

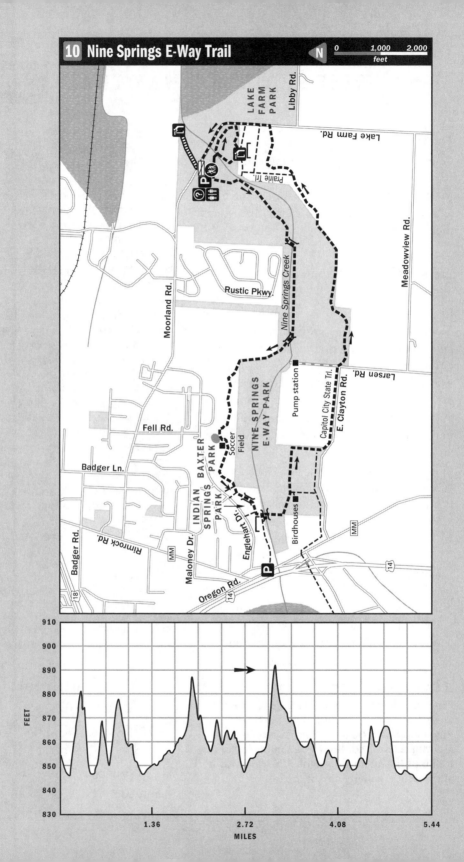

N

0   1,000   2,000
         feet

LAKE
FARM
PARK

Libby Rd.

Lake Farm Rd.

Prairie Trl.

Meadowview Rd.

Nine Springs Creek

Rustic Pkwy.

Moorland Rd.

NINE
SPRINGS
E-WAY
PARK

Pump station

Capitol City State Trl.

Larsen Rd.

E. Clayton Rd.

Fell Rd.

Soccer
Field

INDIAN
BAXTER
SPRINGS
PARK

Badger Ln.

Birdhouses

MM

Badger Rd.

Rimrock Rd.

Maloney Dr.

Englehart Dr.

MM

18

Oregon Rd.

74

14

FEET

910
900
890
880
870
860
850
840
830

1.36   2.72   4.08   5.44

MILES

through rather tall grass, and the flowers throughout are impressive. Cross Spring Creek on a wooden bridge with railings. To the left you can see the road. Go left on the other side of the bridge starting uphill through false sunflowers, yellow coneflowers, bergamot, and Queen Anne's lace. The trail follows the edge of a gentle hill. As it makes the curve, pass apple trees on the left and a short trail out to Lake Farm Road. You can cross over to the Lussier Family Heritage Center and Lake Farm Park. The apple trees, of course, are beautiful in spring. Continue right and climb the hill on a moderate grade. At the top you have a very nice view of the surrounding land all the way to the highway and of the marsh to the east. There are only a couple trees near here; the rest is prairie laden with wildflowers.

Continue over the hump and find a bench and two wooden platforms as well as a memorial plaque for Bud Morton, a champion for the e-way, who called it Mother Nature's Bedroom. The trail that goes left from this clearing takes you 400 feet down to a dead end at the creek edge, or just before that you can take a 0.2-mile trail south to the paved Capital City State Trail. Explore if you wish; otherwise go right from the bench and down the hill back to the bridge, and take the right branch from the trailhead.

The trail goes to the north edge of the e-way and heads west along the trees, which, later in the day, shade the trail. You have prairie to your left, but occasionally you pass in and out of clumps of trees and brush as you walk parallel to the creek. The trail is nicely cut grass, unlike some of the field grass on the prairie loop, which is bristly and can be difficult to walk on, especially with sandals. After 0.5 miles you come to a bridge over the creek.

Go right on the other side through high grass on a trail that goes straight along the creek. There is an abundance of birds here, from blackbirds to waterfowl. To the right beyond the marshy area, you can see a trailer court. At 0.4 miles you reach a large bridge over the creek. If you continue straight, you enter an area with a brick building governed by Madison Metropolitan Sewerage District. The park has been trying to negotiate an easement for hikers to pass along the gravel road that connects this area to the Capital City State Trail at the intersection of Larsen Road and Clayton Road. If this happens then you are looking at your return path for this hike. Some hikers pass through here anyway, but technically it is not allowed.

Cross the big bridge to your right and follow the path to the left into more prairie. Go under power lines as the trail puts prairie to your left and farmland to the right. From the bridge to the woods beyond the prairie is 0.4 miles, and you pass a line of box elders and a small clearing before the trees take over in earnest with shagbark hickory. The trail here is dirt, with twigs, sticks, roots, and mossy patches. Five hundred feet in, you find a bench on the right facing the trees. Another 500 feet brings you to another grassy trail out in the open, where you will find two ponds full of cattails. The trail goes around either side of the first one and then the second larger one as well, with a path that crosses between them. To the right of the second pond is a path out of the park to a residential

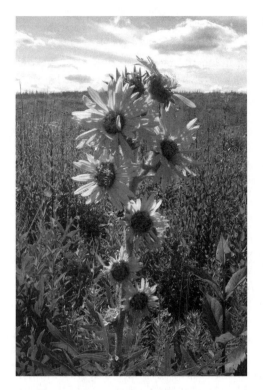

A compass plant

neighborhood. Go to the end of these two ponds to behind the goal of a soccer field in Baxter Park. Go left here as the trail slips back into the woods to the left of the soccer pitch and passes a lot of dead wood in a wet area before finding tall cottonwoods. The trail continues left into the woods with houses along the perimeter to the right.

Now oaks enter the mix, smaller at first and then some larger ones. Much of the trail is cedar chip through here as it leads you into the area known as Indian Springs. Trails spur to the right out toward the neighborhood, and 800 feet into the woods, there's a bench on the right at the head of one of these trails. Stay left and cross an 8-foot plank bridge over a ditch. Stay left once again as you pass a spur trail and come to a bench on the right overlooking a pond. This is a fine place to spy some local wildlife coming for a drink.

To your left the trail goes around the pond, passing a clearing mowed to the creek's edge on your left. Come around the pond and arrive at a bridge to the left and a trail that leads straight out of the park to a turnaround at Anderberg Drive. That's a good place to park and then come right to this pond.

Cross the narrow railed bridge to the left and go left through the field along the creek to some trees where the trail heads right. Cross a field 400 feet and then go left (east). A spur trail at 500 feet doubles back and takes you along some birdhouses. Keep going straight 0.2 miles instead. To your right a trail will go between two private agricultural fields along a row of tall trees. Follow it right (south) 600 feet to the Capital City State Trail. This is asphalt and you should go left here following the multiuse trail 0.4 miles to the gravel road that goes left from the Larsen Road and Clayton Road intersection. Once the easement is granted, you can cross back to that bridge and go east back to the trailhead, retracing your steps. Until then continue on this path 0.9 miles to the prairie trail on the left back into the e-way or 1.2 miles to Lake Farm Road to walk left 0.4 miles to the parking lot.

Be sure to check out the boardwalk into the marsh opposite the parking lot. A raised viewing platform 900 feet out gives nice views of waterfowl and eventually will be part of a more complete boardwalk trail.

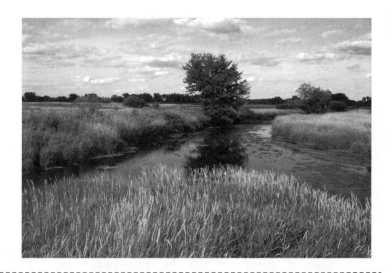

A view of wetlands from the end of the boardwalk

NEARBY ACTIVITIES

Check out a little hole-in-the-wall *taqueria* on Rimrock Road in the strip mall next to the Citgo station. Juanita's Tacos offers great no-frills Mexican tacos but is exceptional for seafood, especially seviche. Stop in at 2510 Rimrock Road or call (608) 274-6231. Capital Springs State Recreation Park offers more trails through the marsh just across the street from the trailhead as well as access to Lake Waubesa. The Capital City State Trail runs along the southern border of this trail and crosses the city to connect to other multiuse paths.

11 OLIN-TURVILLE PARK/ TURVILLE POINT

KEY AT-A-GLANCE INFORMATION

LENGTH: 2 miles

CONFIGURATION: Loop within a loop

DIFFICULTY: Easy

SCENERY: Mixed forest, Lake Monona, the Capitol, a small prairie

EXPOSURE: Mostly shaded

TRAIL TRAFFIC: Light

TRAIL SURFACE: Packed dirt, stones, and tree roots, some mowed paths

HIKING TIME: 0.75–1 hour

DRIVING DISTANCE: 1.2 miles from John Nolen Drive and the Beltline Highway (US 12/18)

ACCESS: 4 a.m.–1 hour after sunset

MAPS: USGS Madison East

WHEELCHAIR ACCESSIBILITY: None

FACILITIES: Restrooms, water, shelter, picnic area

SPECIAL COMMENTS: No dogs allowed. This trail is good for runners who like a little challenge. The loops through the oak savanna and prairie are best, and some may not prefer the occasional roots along the other trails.

GPS Trailhead Coordinates

UTM Zone (WGS 84) 16T

Easting 0306589

Northing 4769511

Latitude N 43° 03' 13.17"

Longitude W 89° 22' 29.73"

IN BRIEF

Venture out to Turville Point jutting into Lake Monona, take a tour through the woods and a bit of prairie, and have a picnic with a view of the Capitol.

DESCRIPTION

From the trailhead start straight for the woods to a grassy trail into oak savanna. Through the trees to the left is Lake Monona. Pick up a packed-dirt trail and come to a sign that reads CONSERVATION PARK-TURVILLE POINT. Pass through a gate and at the first trail juncture, go left on a dirt footpath. Brush thickens into the savanna as you go. Just 200 feet along the trail, a spur trail breaks left from the main trail. Take it to the water's edge where basswoods dangle their leaves into the lake. The trail is uneven here with tree roots and strewn branches and twigs. This spur lasts only 0.1 mile before curving to the right and rejoining the main path again. There isn't much difference in length, but being closer to the lake is nicer.

Go left at the connection; the trail curves gently toward the lake again as it heads downhill. The trail is roughly maintained; a mower

Directions

From the Beltline Highway (US 12/18) go north on John Nolen Drive 0.7 miles to the Olin Avenue intersection. Go right on Olin Turville Court as it runs parallel to John Nolen Drive. Follow this 0.25 miles to the park entrance and go right. Follow the park road 0.25 miles and stay right as it takes a turn around the pavilion at the top of the hill. To the southeast of the pavilion along the road is a small perpendicular parking area. The trail is at the lakeside corner of the lot.

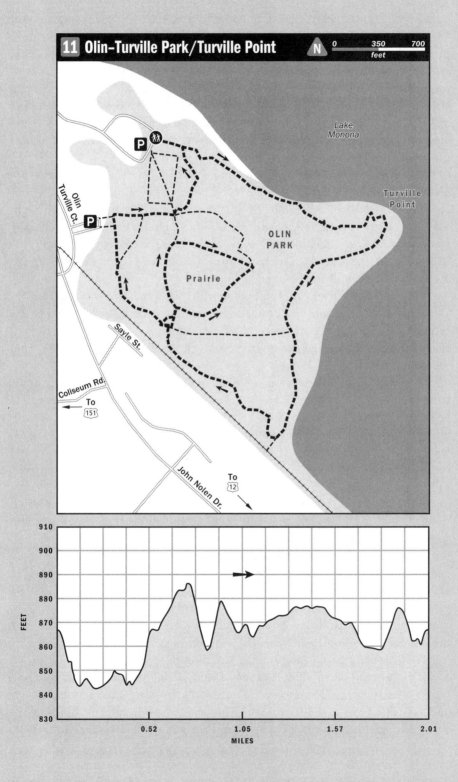

puts a wide cut through the brush on either side of the path, and it is not grassy. Pass a narrow footpath spur trail to the right at 200 feet. Then the trail bends to the right into a hollow. Heading slightly uphill, the path breaks from the lake on crushed rock and then descends again. You can see water through the trees both on the left and right as you head out onto Turville Point. The trail breaks left at a right angle and heads straight toward water where it curls around the edge of the point. There have been reports of osprey and bald eagles out here and you get a view of sky as you round the point. Cattails grow along the lake edge and a short spur trail goes out onto the rocks at the very tip of the point.

From the rocks to the next spur trail is 0.25 miles. The trail heads south along the point with the lake on the left. The earth is typically damp as it runs close to the waterline and even below it at times. You can hear the Beltline Highway (US 12/18) from here. The path bends right and heads easily uphill and away from water. As you climb, the land slopes to the left. The tree coverage is primarily black walnuts. Crest the hill at the cutoff path that bears right. Stay left through a small dip in the trail and up another slope.

Where the trail levels off, you find views out over the lake in spring and fall. Descend on the other side on a crushed-rock surface with occasional wood beams to prevent erosion. The path skirts the lakeshore one more time. During the hot summers, the lake can get quite green and the smell might deter some from the area.

The trail passes along the water's edge again after 0.15 miles and then heads to the right away from water. Pass a spur trail to the left out to a commercial zone outside the park. The trail continues gently uphill for 0.2 miles through a scattering of acorns, walnuts, and hickory nuts. You can expect a nice selection of woodland wildflowers along here. The trail forks at 0.2 miles, the left trail continuing on the outer loop. Go right here and cross a woodland trail coming from your right (that previous cutoff path from the lakeside) and then step into a large clearing in the middle of the conservation park. This is a prairie restoration in progress. Go left and follow the 0.4-mile looping trail through native grasses and wildflowers around the clearing back to this point again. If you want to shorten this hike, continue out the other side of the prairie and take a trail past a chain and then cross straight through the oak savanna to the parking area. Otherwise when you finish the prairie loop and come back to the trail juncture where you entered it, go right as you head back into the woods. The trail will follow along the top of a ridge that drops about 20 feet down on your left and looks out over the railroad tracks and John Nolen Drive beyond that.

At 0.1 mile from the juncture, the trail turns to the right away from the edge and starts to head downhill as it bends around the hill that the prairie is resting on. An alternative trail heads to the right up along the edge of the prairie. Stay left and pass a trail exit to a different parking lot to the left just before you arrive at a T at a concrete access road. Go uphill to the right with oak savanna to the left.

At 0.1 mile many trails intersect. Just to your left is that chain, beyond which is the oak savanna between you and the parking lot. This is an option with trails going along the perimeter in either direction or at an angle right over the gentle hill. A trail to the right takes you out into the prairie loop, and another trail goes straight through the woods parallel to the prairie trail. Look for a trail on your left that passes between the two wooden posts of a gate in the conservation park fence. The narrow footpath skirts to the right of the oak savanna and passes 0.1 mile through the woods back to the first trail juncture on this hike. The path to the left takes you back out of the park and across the lawn to the parking lot.

NEARBY ACTIVITIES

The Capital City Trail follows an asphalt path from the north end of the park 1.1 miles across Monona Bay and along the lakeshore. This takes you to the Monona Terrace Community and Convention Center (**www.mononaterrace.com**) which is based on a design by Frank Lloyd Wright.

12 OWEN CONSERVATION PARK

KEY AT-A-GLANCE INFORMATION

LENGTH: 1.5 miles

CONFIGURATION: Loop

DIFFICULTY: Easy, with some moderate

SCENERY: Mixed woods, prairie, city skyline overlook

EXPOSURE: Shaded and sun

TRAIL TRAFFIC: Light

TRAIL SURFACE: Packed dirt, grass, wood chip

HIKING TIME: 1 hour

DRIVING DISTANCE: 1.1 miles west of University Avenue and Whitney Way

ACCESS: 4 a.m.–1 hour after sunset

MAPS: USGS Madison West; on map board

WHEELCHAIR ACCESSIBILITY: None

FACILITIES: Restrooms, drinking fountain

SPECIAL COMMENTS: No dogs or bikes allowed. Trails are groomed for skiing in winter. Listed at ebird.org as a birding hot spot. Madison Metro bus routes 8 and 15 serve the park.

IN BRIEF

One of Madison's best-kept secrets, the prairie here offers an overlook to the city that shows only a fraction of the buildings and gives the illusion that there is nothing around you but forest.

DESCRIPTION

Just the fact that this used to be a farm should give you an idea of how much Madison has grown over the years. On a hilltop overlooking Madison's west side, this 93-acre park was once the summer retreat of former University Professor Edward T. Owen. He called it Torwald. A professor of French, Owen feared that reckless urban development would spoil the natural beauty of Madison. With colleagues John Olin and Edward Hammersley, he donated land for a 12-mile pleasure drive on the west side. Today, prairie and oak savanna have reclaimed the park. Coneflowers, goldenrod, bluestem, and many other prairie flowers and grasses create a sea of waving colors in the growing season. Various entry paths from all sides give a neighborhood-park accessibility to the place, but the tall trees around its perimeter give the illusion that much of the surrounding world is undeveloped.

GPS Trailhead Coordinates

UTM Zone (WGS 84) 16T

Easting 0297475

Northing 4771913

Latitude N 43° 04' 22.42"

Longitude W 89° 29' 15.36"

Directions

From its intersection with University Avenue on the west side, follow Whitney Way south 0.2 miles to Old Middleton Road. Go right (west) 0.6 miles to Old Sauk Road. Turn left and at 0.4 miles the park entrance is on your left. Follow the park road to the parking lot. The trailhead is to the right of the lot entry in the northwest corner of the lot.

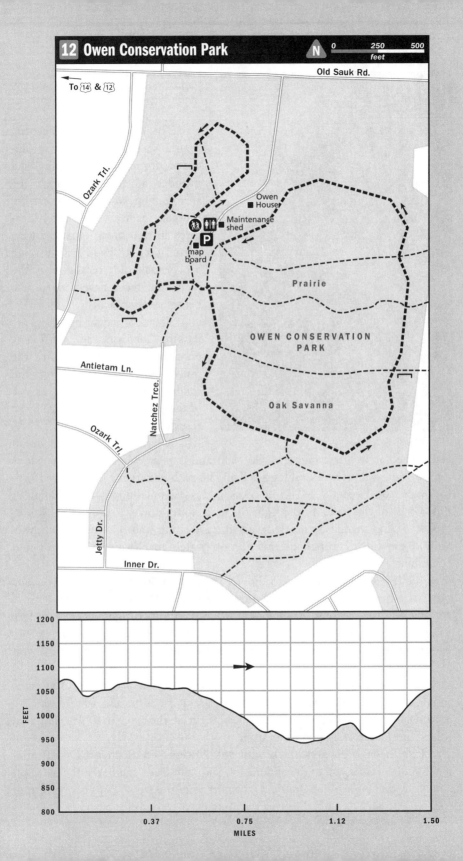

N

0   250   500
feet

Old Sauk Rd.

To 14 & 12

Ozark Trl.

Owen
House

Maintenance
shed

P

map
board

Prairie

OWEN CONSERVATION
PARK

Oak Savanna

Antietam Ln.

Natchez Trce.

Ozark Trl.

Jetty Dr.

Inner Dr.

1200
1150
1100
1050
1000
950
900
850
800

FEET

0.37   0.75   1.12   1.50
MILES

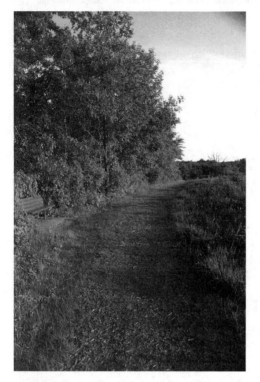

A bench overlooking the prairie

The loop around the central prairie is a common evening promenade for locals, but this hike includes a segment through the surrounding woods on a narrow footpath as well. The forest features an assortment of wildflowers more suited to shade and a varying topography that recalls what the west side must have looked like before development.

There is a map board in the parking lot with an aerial-view photograph of the park with the trails highlighted. Look for the trailhead in the northwest corner of the parking lot to the left of the restrooms.

A grassy trail heads uphill and immediately hits a juncture. Go right and pass a padlocked wooden door into a stone wall that resembles a cellar. The path is narrow, just wide enough for one's feet. Expect a lot of tree roots as this 0.2-mile loop rounds the hill in this corner of the park. To the right the land slopes down. It rises above you to the left and is shaded by maples. Pass along a stone wall on your left midway around the hill. Throughout this section watch for Virginia broadleaf and columbine.

You'll reach a cutoff trail to the left back to the lot but go right here. The trail passes another stone wall and a trailside bench. The path rises steeply from here with a few log steps. At the next fork in the trail, go right. There are more wood beams laid here in the trail, so watch for them because grasses start to lean over the already narrow trail, sometimes preventing you from seeing where you are stepping.

At the next juncture, stay left. Right takes you out of the park. You come to another park bench where the trail begins to rise a bit and wildflowers are prominent. The trail curves left but head right at the next trail. The left trail returns in the direction you came from.

Pass through an area thick with wildflowers and reach a four-way trail juncture. Left takes you to the parking lot, and right leads you out of the park. Go straight and enter into the prairie. Once in the prairie, wood chips cover the trail to the right, which eventually gives way to mowed grass. Trails crisscross the open prairie to the left. The view here is amazing with only the tallest landmarks puncturing the green of Madison.

Pass a trail on your left, continuing on an easy grade to the bottom of the hill with the trees to your right. As you come to oak savanna, the trail bends left to cross the southern end of the park.

The forest on your right draws back about 100 feet. A lone oak stands in the middle of the field. As you cross the field, you come into the shade again of another oak tree. A trail goes right where you can find some small loops through the trees and three exit trails to the surrounding residential areas.

Brush thickens on the left blocking the field to the north from view in green seasons. The canopy over the trail opens to the sky just as the trail starts its turn north up the opposite side of the prairie/savanna center. The trail takes you through open and shaded patches. There is a bench at the trail that cuts back across the savanna and another trail goes right into the trees and out to residences. You'll find a similar trail juncture 300 feet from here and another 300 feet beyond that, which would take you left to the parking lot.

Keep going straight and uphill. Grasses can grow taller than six feet here. The trail makes an easy 0.3-mile semicircle along the edge of the forest, taking you across the northern portion of the prairie. There is a lot of intervening brush to your left. As the trail heads west and starts to bend south for the return, you see that where you are walking is lower than the hump of the central prairie. The land slopes down to the right into the forest. You reach the edge of the park road where a gate offers an entry point to the trail that is before the parking lot, which is nice if you enter the park walking.

At the next trail juncture, a branch goes to the parking lot to the right. You can observe a row of trees to your left that goes directly across the prairie dividing it with another alternative trail.

Trilliums and wild geraniums are abundant in the spring. Be aware that the park often administers springtime burns as part of the efforts to restore the prairie by eliminating invasive plants. You can call the Madison Parks Division at (608) 266-4711 to find out if there was a burn.

NEARBY ACTIVITIES

In 1890 two of Owen's children died during a diphtheria epidemic. Two boulders on Regent Street, just west of the Speedway Road and Highland Avenue intersection, commemorate them and mark Owen Drive, a pleasure drive Professor Owen donated to the city in their names. Take a bit of the pleasure drive by following Regent Street west from here, where it becomes Owen Drive as it passes through Hoyt Park to connect with Mineral Point Road.

13 PICNIC POINT

KEY AT-A-GLANCE INFORMATION

LENGTH: 8 miles

CONFIGURATION: Two-way out-and-back

DIFFICULTY: Easy, but moderate west of Picnic Point

SCENERY: Lake Mendota, mixed forest, and views of the Capitol and the university

EXPOSURE: Mostly shaded, with some open stretches

TRAIL TRAFFIC: Heavy along campus, moderate toward the point, light beyond the point

TRAIL SURFACE: Crushed rock, packed dirt, some asphalt

HIKING TIME: 2.5–3 hours

DRIVING DISTANCE: From University Avenue and Park Street, go north 2 blocks to reach the trailhead.

ACCESS: The preserve opens at sunrise and closes at 10 p.m.

MAPS: USGS Madison West; interactive and printable maps are online at lakeshorepreserve.wisc.edu.

WHEELCHAIR ACCESSIBILITY: From the trailhead to Picnic Point but not the trail segment beyond

FACILITIES: Restrooms on the trail and back at the Memorial Union

SPECIAL COMMENTS: Dogs allowed on leashes; bicycles limited to designated areas

IN BRIEF

Stroll along the shores of Lake Mendota, see the university, and find the best view of the Capitol from across the water.

DESCRIPTION

There is perhaps no more famous strolling destination in Madison than Picnic Point. This narrow peninsula into Lake Mendota is a magnet for nature lovers, joggers, and the hopelessly romantic. The trail runs the length of the University of Wisconsin–Madison's Lakeshore Nature Preserve, which protects this beautiful portion of Lake Mendota from development, preserving it for both ecological and environmental study and pure aesthetics.

Also referred to as the Lakeshore Path, it has two parts: the more popular eastern portion, the Howard Temin Lakeshore Path, which runs from the university to Picnic Point, and the Lake Mendota Lakeshore Path, which starts at Picnic Point and heads west. The latter is open only to foot traffic while the former is shared with bicyclists in many places. Altogether it makes the most beloved walk in the city, enjoyed by residents, students, and visitors alike.

The trailhead is located just past the docks at the terrace behind the Memorial Union at

GPS Trailhead Coordinates

UTM Zone (WGS 84) 16T

Easting 0304364

Northing 4772194

Latitude N 43° 04' 38.02"

Longitude W 89° 24' 11.37"

Directions

From University Avenue downtown turn right onto Lake Street and park in the ramp on your right. Walk to the end of Lake Street and follow it left past the Memorial Union Terrace to reach the trailhead.

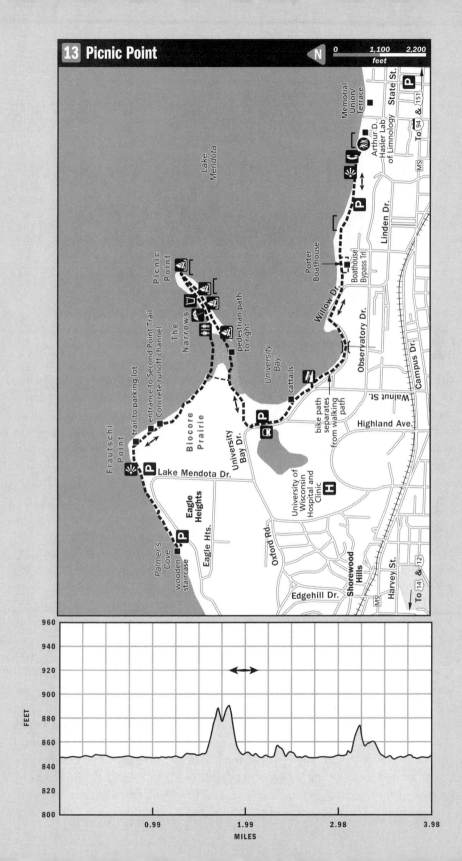

N

0   1,100   2,200
feet

Lake
Mendota

Memorial
Union/
Terrace

Arthur D.
Hasler Lab
of Limnology

State St.

To 94 & 151

MS

Linden Dr.

Picnic
Point

Porter
Boathouse

Boathouse
Bypass Trl.

Willow Dr.

Observatory Dr.

Campus Dr.

The Narrows

pedestrian path
to right

University
Bay

cattails

entrance to Second Point Trail

Concrete runoff channel

trail to parking lot

Walnut St.

bike path
separates
from walking
path

Highland Ave.

Frautschi
Point

Biocore Prairie

University Bay Dr.

Lake Mendota Dr.

Eagle
Heights

Eagle Hts.

Oxford Rd.

University of
Wisconsin Hospital and
Clinic

H

Shorewood
Hills

Harvey St.

MS

To 14 & 12

Palmer's
Cove

wooden
staircase

Edgehill Dr.

960
940
920
900
880
860
840
820
800

FEET

0.99   1.99   2.98   3.98

MILES

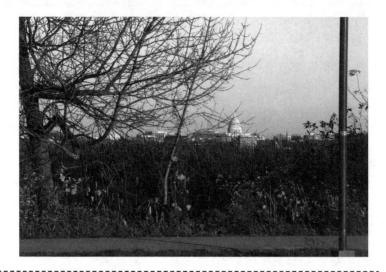

A view of the Capitol from University Bay

the University of Wisconsin. Look for a gravel path right behind the Arthur D. Hasler Lab of Limnology. The trail here shows high traffic as many students, joggers, and bicyclists pass through here.

Just over 100 feet in on your right is a park bench and a good lookout point out over the water to your halfway point and the trail's namesake, as well as a staircase down from campus to your left. The trail skirts the lake's edge 5 to 15 feet above the water level throughout this section, offering plenty of shade and views out onto the water.

In another 500 feet pass another trail coming down from the left via Muir Woods. Just past this is an emergency phone and an access road coming down the hill also on your left. On your right side is a viewing platform under a weeping willow; trail users sometimes lock their bikes here. Beyond here, 900 feet on the left and up a few stairs, is one of the university permit-only parking lots.

Once you pass this, the trail opens up to the lawn behind some dormitories. Students lounge here studying, sunbathing in between trees, or simply escaping for a moment.

The building coming up on your left is Porter Boathouse where the UW crew teams keep their boats. When they are moving shells in and out of the boathouse, gates close on the path and all trail traffic is diverted around the back of the building for that short stretch.

An asphalt bike path joins the trail and the hiking trail runs alongside it until Lot 126 on your right about 1,300 feet past the boathouse. This lot requires a permit from Monday through Friday from 7 a.m. to 4:30 p.m. Cross the entrance to the lot and look for the hiking trail as it descends to the right and becomes a narrow path of packed dirt running at a level five feet lower than the bike trail. This is Willow Creek Woods, and the trail runs 500 feet through it before rising up to join the bike path again and cross the bridge over the creek itself. After this, foot traffic stays right, and the bikes have their own separate strip of asphalt. Exposure from here is partly shaded as the trail passes beneath one willow or basswood tree after another until you reach a boat landing 0.25 miles away. Beyond this there is no shade until you enter the gates of Picnic Point another 0.4 miles beyond that.

Throughout this stretch University Bay is on your right. Red-winged blackbirds bob atop cattails, over which is a view of the Capital. Painted turtles cross from here to Class of 1918 Marsh inland to your left. This segment from the bridge to the stone gate is a good place to see migratory birds in season. In fact the marsh across the street has its own little loop trail popular with birders. Beyond all this to your left is the sprawling University Hospital.

Lot 129, just outside the entrance to the point, has a three-hour limit and is closed after 10 p.m. This is a good starting point for anyone looking to cut out the busiest portion of the trail close to the university. The bus stop here is served by the free route 80 bus, which runs from Eagle Heights to the Memorial Union.

The entrance to the Picnic Point section of the preserve is through a gate in a stone wall next to the parking lot, where there is also a map of the entire park. Just inside the gate, a trail cuts left to Eagle Heights, but follow the trail to the right along the eastern shore of the point. Short paths through the trees and underbrush on your right grant clear views across the lake.

The clearing shows mowed lawn to the left, a nice spot for picnics or taking a break in the sun. This lawn tapers and ends where the trail again enters the trees about 800 feet from the park entrance. Just past this is a cutoff trail to the left, which leads directly to the next segment of the trail and bypasses the point itself.

Continuing on, an area under the trees opens up to accommodate two fire pits to your right.

Look for stacks of free firewood along the path. The park provides this out of protection from the emerald ash borer, an invasive insect species that travels with firewood from outside a region.

A small beach 0.2 miles later on your left is The Narrows, the thinnest point on the peninsula. Just past here the trail splits from the main. Follow along to the right on a packed-dirt path for another 0.2 miles until it brings you to Picnic Point. There are three more fire pits along this stretch and a water pump on your left just 200 feet past the beach. The fountain portion of this water pump (known as a "bubbler" as drinking fountains are often called in Wisconsin) is specially designed with a reservoir so that it doesn't require you to keep pumping to take a sip.

The point is another small clearing, and there are side paths down to the water's edge that will give you better views of the city after the leaves have come in during spring. The point also has a fire pit and a bench with a view; however, in summer the view is mostly obscured by foliage.

As you return look for the narrow trail to the right, which follows the western side of the peninsula and looks down over the slope to the water a bit before rejoining the main trail again at The Narrows and the beach. Stay right here and again veer west down another narrow path. Restrooms with pit toilets are 200 feet down on your left. Just beyond this look for the two largest trees, a pair of basswoods out on the point.

This segment is really quite different from the rest of the trail, and many visitors to the point have never even explored it. The trail becomes a mix of packed dirt and sand, and the city seems very far away. You enter a marshy area where the noise of the frogs overpowers the volume of the birds. Six hundred feet beyond this is an abandoned shelter house and the other end of the cutoff trail you passed heading out to the point. Stay right here.

The trail becomes more challenging past this point, rising and falling and given over to exposed roots and rocks. It breaks from the shore and heads inland to Biocore Prairie, the result of a restoration project in 1997. The trail skirts along the corner before ducking back into the woods.

About 200 feet in, cross an old concrete water channel with a gate. Just beyond this is the entrance to Second Point Trail. Stay right along the shoreline. Another trail branching off to the left 400 feet beyond this would take you to the parking lot or deeper into North Shore Woods.

Coming up on your right is a scenic viewpoint to the lake at Frautschi Point. From here pass through Tent Colony Woods, where from 1912 to 1962 as many as 300 graduate students would set up wall tents and live with their families for the summer. When you reach the parking lot 0.5 miles past the point, look for a wooden staircase down to the right to Raymer's Cove. Go here to get down to the water's edge and see the sandstone cliffs. This is particularly nice at sunset.

If you are too tired to do the return trip, the free route 80 bus stops at Eagle Heights across Lake Mendota Drive from the parking lot. It will take you all the way back to the Memorial Union. This lot is also a nice starting point for an out-and-back hike, or you can arrive here by bus and take the trail one way to downtown.

NEARBY ACTIVITIES

The Memorial Union attracts not just students but Madisonians of all ages to take in the views, enjoy a drink or burger on the lovely lakeside terrace, and listen to live music on weekends in seasonable weather. Try some of the University of Wisconsin's very own ice cream inside. The Capitol is a ten-minute walk from here up State Street, the city's liveliest strip of shops, coffee shops, and restaurants.

SOUTHWEST PATH

IN BRIEF

Join hikers, bikers, skaters—many of whom may be commuters—on a paved former rail bed where it passes through the heart of Madison, past Camp Randall, and then enters a corridor of shade trees and private gardens on the near west side.

DESCRIPTION

Also known as the Southwest Commuter Path, this nicely paved and heavily traveled trail clearly serves more than just recreational purposes. It follows a path right along the downtown corridor just south of the University of Wisconsin, and is the quickest bikeable route from the Capital City Trail along Lake Monona to the end of that trail and on to the Military Ridge State Trail. Bikers can have a snicker at rush-hour traffic, which typically cannot get from downtown to the near-west side as quickly or efficiently. On Badger game days this is a straight shot to Camp Randall Stadium from either end of the trail. And if you are merely out for a pleasure ride, the railroad corridor heading southwest from the stadium is rich with shade trees and flower gardens.

Brittingham Park has a bike rack, picnic tables, and portable toilets. The shore here

KEY AT-A-GLANCE INFORMATION

LENGTH: 9 miles (4.5 one way)
CONFIGURATION: Out-and-back/one way
DIFFICULTY: Easy
SCENERY: Urban, shade trees, prairie flowers
EXPOSURE: Mostly sun with a partly shaded portion west of the stadium
TRAIL TRAFFIC: Moderate to heavy
TRAIL SURFACE: Asphalt
HIKING TIME: 2–4 hours
DRIVING DISTANCE: 0.3 miles southeast of West Washington Avenue and Regent Street
ACCESS: Open year-round
MAPS: USGS Madison West; www.ci.madison.wi.us
WHEELCHAIR ACCESSIBILITY: Yes
FACILITIES: Other than portable toilets at Brittingham Park and a couple of water fountains, there are few on-trail facilities, but you are never far from local restaurants and bars until after you pass Camp Randall stadium. There are drinking fountains at Glenway Street and at the endpoint of the hike.
SPECIAL COMMENTS: The trail is plowed during the winter. There are numerous road crossings throughout the trail. This is a multiuse path, so be aware of bicyclists and in-line skaters.

Directions

There are many places to access the trail throughout its length with on-street parking never far away. The trailhead is on North Shore Drive 0.3 miles west from where it intersects with John Nolen Drive. Park in the lot next to the Brittingham Boathouse on the shore of Monona Bay. The trailhead is to the west of the boathouse where a double-wide crosswalk spans North Shore Drive and heads northwest alongside the railroad tracks.

GPS Trailhead Coordinates

UTM Zone (WGS 84) 16T
Easting   0305414
Northing   4770756
Latitude   N 43° 03' 52.41"
Longitude   W 89° 23' 23.18"

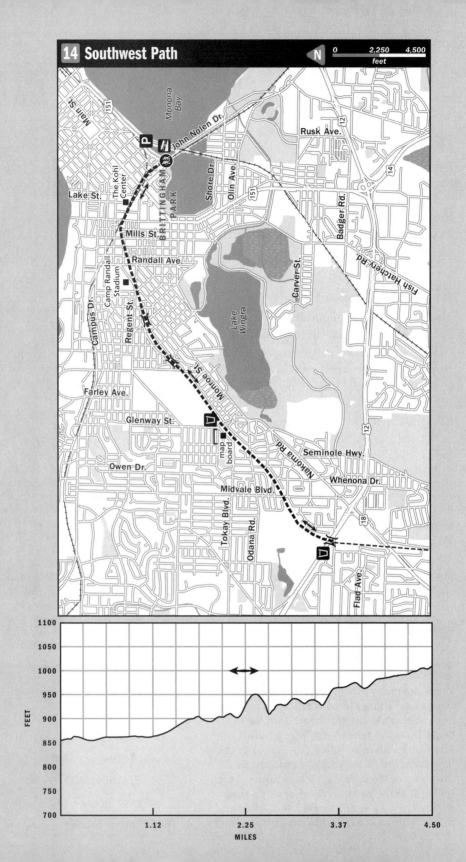

Spooner Street Bridge over the trail

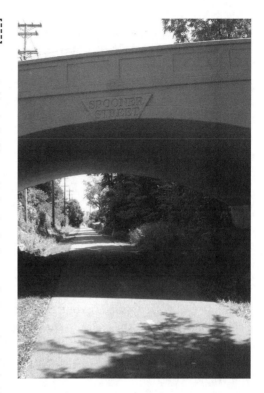

along Monona Bay is popular with local anglers. From the parking lot east of Brittingham boathouse on North Shore Drive, follow the asphalt Brittingham Park Path west (keeping Monona Bay to your left) past the boathouse to the Southwest Path trailhead. (Heading the other direction, this path connects across John Nolen Drive to the Capital City Trail along Lake Monona.)

Cross North Shore Drive and take the Southwest Path along the right side of the railroad tracks. Cross Wilson Street a block later and then at Doty Street, the path crosses left over the tracks and continues on that side. The next street is Main Street and then the sometimes very busy West Washington Avenue. If traffic is too much, go left and cross at the lights at Regent Street and come back along the other side of the street. Looking up Washington Street, you can see the Capitol at the top of the hill. (You can actually see the dome from several other hiking trails, some of them many miles distant from Madison.)

The trail continues here passing Williamson Bicycle Works and Fitness in the old Madison depot to your right. A Milwaukee Road passenger train still on an old section of tracks houses Global Express, a shop selling fairly traded handicrafts from around the world.

On the right just past here is the Kohl Center, an arena for concerts and home of the University of Wisconsin's men's and women's basketball and ice hockey.

A pedestrian bridge crosses over Park Street. The rails to your right are still used for trains carrying coal to one of the city's coal-burning power plants across Mill Street 0.2 miles from the Park Street overpass. At this point the trail is again even with the surrounding neighborhoods. This means street crossings. You'll cross Spring Street at an angle, hit the sidewalk on the other side for 40 feet, and then cross Charter Street. Still alongside tracks, cross Orchard Street and pass a large satellite dish on your left. One block later is Randall Avenue. Across the street and to your right is The Stadium Bar which is quite popular during sporting events.

By now you can see the 80,000-seat Camp Randall Stadium, named for a Civil War–era Union Army base that once occupied the site. The camp itself was named for Wisconsin governor Alexander Randall who rallied volunteers for the war.

The asphalt trail ends at a busy intersection. Cross Monroe to your right at the light and then cross Regent to your left from the tiny concrete island. The trail resumes on concrete and crosses Crazylegs Lane and Breese Terrace in the space of less than 300 feet.

The asphalt resumes here, and there is a trail map to the left side of the trail. If you're looking for a place to eat, here's a good place to leave the trail. Go left to Monroe Street to Mickey's Dairy Bar to your left serving hearty breakfasts (legendary in Madison) until 2:30 p.m. (Be warned they are cash only!) New Orleans Take-Out is a fine choice next door. Farther up the street heading away from the stadium are a couple of coffee shops and the quality sit-down Mediterranean eatery The Dardenelles.

Back on the trail the rail bed is burrowed through the rise and fall of the neighborhoods and the yards will be higher than the path. The abundance of trees on the left side partly shades your way. Pass under the concrete Spooner Street Bridge 800 feet from the trail map and a metal bridge just beyond that. You can see gardens and some trees along the right side of the trail. Just past the bridge, ramps lead up to Fox and Prospect avenues to your left and Prospect Avenue to your right.

Along the trail a lot of wildflowers have been planted and property owners take obvious pride in their portion of the trailside. Tall black walnut trees provide shade as you approach another crossing at Edgewood Avenue and again at Commonwealth Avenue. You can walk to the left 0.3 miles to Monroe Street to find several more restaurants and the Laurel Tavern, as well as Wingra Park on the Wingra lakeshore (see also Arboretum: Wingra Marsh).

From Commonwealth Avenue pass a prairie garden on the right, cross a small bridge with wooden railings, and begin down a 0.6-mile corridor straight to Glenway Street. The ramp up and to the right to Virginia Terrace is your last exit before Glenway Street. The rail bed here is higher than the rooftops of some of the old two-story houses down to your left. A gully to your right follows the trail and separates it from a line of trees. Beyond the modest woods are a cemetery and a golf course.

On the other side of Glenway Street is a map board, a bench, and a drinking fountain. The neighborhood association sometimes posts notes about what's blooming on the trail, and there is an overview trail map of the City of Madison. Just past here to the left is a small park and playground nearly hidden in the trees. On the right side of the trail, look for cup plants in midsummer. Private gardens abound.

Dudgeon Prairie, 0.4 miles later, is a patch of flowers to the left before you cross busy Odana Road and enter Westmoreland Neighborhood. Find a picnic table here on the left. The next section takes you 0.5 miles to Midvale Boulevard.

Halfway there is a sign offering the story of Nakoma Neighborhood, a 1915 urban development that followed the contours of the land. Before this the native Ho-Chunk tribe made camps here.

Across Midvale Boulevard is Midvale Heights Neighborhood. At the right of the trail are two statues of bison and a stone circle with a sundial at the center. Shade trees remain to the left, but residences are much farther off to the right than before, and soon forest takes over as the trail runs along the southern edge of another golf course.

The path follows a long slow railway left turn which brings you 0.5 miles to a fork. Left will take you out to Hammersley Road (the portion on the north side of the Beltline Highway [US 12/18]) or you can take the bridge over it. This is the busiest thoroughfare in town, and you can be thankful you're not in traffic. On the other side of the bridge, the trail curls right and down to a bench and drinking fountain before it continues its descending curve back under the bridge leaving you at the crossing of Hammersley Road.

The Southwest Path actually continues another mile from here, passing between warehouses and under US 151/Verona Road until it connects with the southwestern end of the Capital City State Trail. But this makes a good turn-around point. There is no parking lot here, but some of the residential side streets allow for it.

NEARBY ACTIVITIES

Some of the neighborhoods, such as Dudgeon-Monroe (**www.dmna.org**) and Nakoma (**www.mynakoma.org**), offer walking tours with downloadable maps and information. Monroe Street—near the stadium and again off the trail at Commonwealth Avenue—offers a variety of shops, restaurants, and bars.

15 TENNEY PARK TO SCHENK'S CORNERS

KEY AT-A-GLANCE INFORMATION

LENGTH: 3.9 miles

CONFIGURATION: Misshapen lollipop

DIFFICULTY: Easy

SCENERY: Two lakes, river, locks, residential neighborhoods

EXPOSURE: Mixed

TRAIL TRAFFIC: Moderate

TRAIL SURFACE: Asphalt, concrete, some grass, and dirt

HIKING TIME: 1.5–2 hours

DRIVING DISTANCE: 1.7 miles from the Capitol Square

ACCESS: Park portions are open 5 a.m.–10 p.m.

MAPS: USGS Madison East; www.visitmadison.com

WHEELCHAIR ACCESSIBILITY: Yes

FACILITIES: Restrooms, water, picnic areas, playgrounds, changing rooms, lighted tennis courts, boat landings at Tenney Park; several restaurants and bars in the Atwood-Schenk's Corners area

SPECIAL COMMENTS: Dogs not allowed in Tenney Park

IN BRIEF

Follow the Yahara River from the locks at Lake Mendota to its outlet into Lake Monona and then stop in for a drink or a bite to eat in one of Madison's long-standing neighborhoods.

DESCRIPTION

From the parking lot, cross Sherman Avenue to the corner of Marston Avenue. Follow the asphalt path to the left as it passes through some trees. Halfway down the block, the trail goes right and crosses a 1929 stone bridge over the Tenney Park lagoon. It is photogenic any time of the year, but especially when the lily pads are out. On the other side is a bench where the path continues through the park. The first trail juncture leads left over another bridge to a parking lot, but stay right. At the next juncture another trail goes right to another bridge. Again stay straight, and the path takes you to a metal bridge over the water leading left nearly on the other side of the block-long park.

At the end of the bridge, go left through the parking lot until you come to the Yahara Parkway Bike Path to the right as it goes south along the Yahara River. There is an observation platform at the water's edge. Facing south, you'll see a ramp going right up to

GPS Trailhead Coordinates

UTM Zone (WGS 84)   16T

Easting   0306933

Northing   4773841

Latitude   N 43° 05' 33.72"

Longitude   W 89° 22' 19.91"

Directions

From the Capitol Square, go east on East Washington 1.2 miles to Baldwin Street. Go left 0.5 miles to Sherman Avenue and turn right. The parking lot is on your left one block later. The trailhead begins at the parking lot entrance.

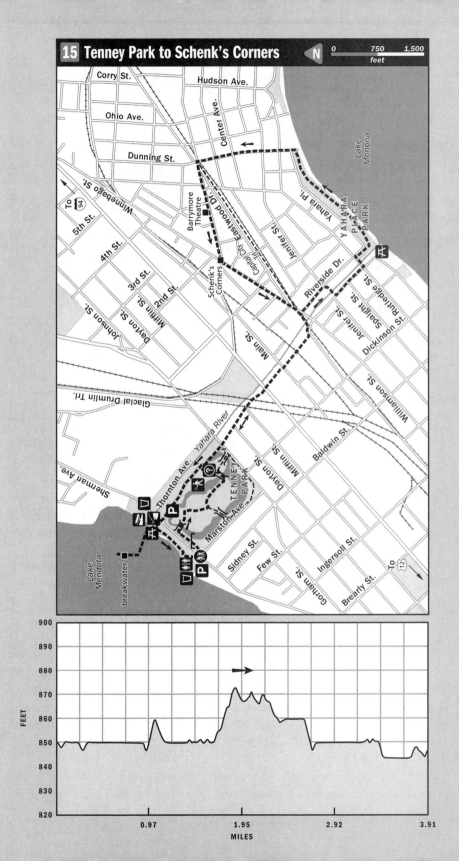

N

0	750	1,500

feet

Corry St.

Hudson Ave.

Ohio Ave.

Center Ave.

Lake Monona

Dunning St.

To 94

5th St.

Winnebago St.

Barrymore Theatre

Capital City Eastwood Dr.

Janifer St.

YAHARA PLACE PARK

Yahara Pl.

4th St.

3rd St.

2nd St.

Mifflin St.

Dayton St.

Johnson St.

Schenk's Corners

Main St.

Riverside Dr.

Janifer St.

Spaight St.

Rutledge St.

Dickinson St.

Glacial Drumlin Trl.

Yahara River

Williamson St.

Baldwin St.

Sherman Ave.

Thornton Ave.

TENNEY PARK

Marston Ave.

Mifflin St.

Dayton St.

Sidney St.

Few St.

Ingersoll St.

To 12

Lake Mendota

breakwater

Gorham St.

Brearly St.

FEET			
900			
890			
880			
870			
860			
850			
840			
830			
820			

0.97	1.95	2.92	3.91

MILES

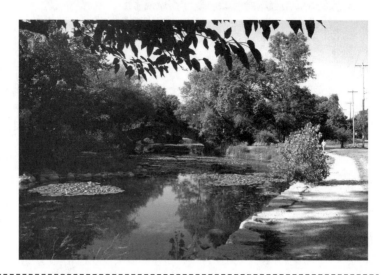

The lagoon at Tenney Park

Johnson Street; stay on the trail and follow it through the short tunnel under the street (this is lighted at night). On the other side, the trail resumes along the river, and at 0.1 mile, you will cross railroad tracks. The rail bed is no longer operational and a metal bridge goes left over the water. A future trail may run through here. At 0.1 mile pass under Washington Avenue (with exits up to the street and a bus stop for bus routes 6, 14, 15, 27, 29, 56, and 57). This is Steensland Bridge named for a Norwegian counsel and former Madison resident Halle Steensland. It was originally built in 1904. It was replaced in 2006 with the current construction, which is in the Prairie School style of architecture. At night it is well lit and quite attractive. The path beneath is very wide, but stay aware of bicyclists.

One block later cross Main Street and half a block later some railroad tracks. It's another half block to a cul-de-sac at Thornton Avenue and Williamson Street. The Capital City Trail crosses from left to right on an asphalt path. At the corner to your right is Mickey's Irish-style pub, which has a weekly night of free bluegrass music. Call (608) 251-9964.

Go left from the cul-de-sac on the Capital City Trail, and it takes you across the Yahara River on an old metal railroad bridge. Come to traffic lights at Williamson Street. Cross here (there is a button to force the change of lights) and head down Riverside Drive on the sidewalk in a residential neighborhood to Jenifer Street. Cross the river back the other way on the bridge and go left down Thornton Avenue another block to Rutledge Street to a bench and some prairie flowers.

The mouth of the Yahara River where it empties into Lake Monona is just beyond, and you can find a picnic table there and a small green space, but nothing more. Cross the bridge at Rutledge Street. (You could have just stayed

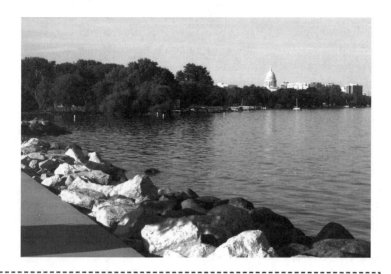

The breakwater near the locks—an excellent place to watch the sun set

on Riverside Drive, of course, but I am a fan of crossing bridges.) On the other side, a dirt trail goes down to the right into Yahara Place Park. The footpath follows 0.4 miles of the shore of Lake Monona with cottonwoods and willows for shade. There is a playground here as well as picnic tables and rocks along the shore that make nice meditative perches. This is a wonderful spot in the morning when the sun is rising. Or find something to do along the hike for the rest of the day and come back, because the end of the trail is the perfect spot for a sunset.

At the end of the park, come to Dunning Street. Take this left five blocks (0.3 miles) to Atwood Avenue. At the corner on the right is the Harmony Bar, which has a good bar menu featuring excellent pizza. The recipe for the dough is akin to a state secret.

Cross the busy Atwood Avenue and go left. This is the Atwood-Schenk's Corners neighborhood. Coming up on your left is Monty's Blue Plate Diner, a Madison classic for breakfast. On your right is the Barrymore Theatre. Built in 1929 as the Eastwood, it was the third movie theater in Madison. Today it brings in nearly 100 live music concerts.

There are various small restaurants along this four-block stretch, and the neighborhood hosts a festival every July. You will come to Schenk's Corners where Atwood meets Winnebago Street. The former Schenk General Store building at 2009 Winnebago Street, now home to Schenk Huegel Co., once sold everything from groceries and housewares to cigars and clothing. Wonders Pub, right across the street, has a good fish fry on Fridays and is a beer connoisseur's tavern. A weekly "neighborhood appreciation night" features some impressive cheap bar eats.

Cross Winnebago at the traffic light and go left on the other side, passing before Chase Bank and following Winnebago Street back to Williamson Street to the traffic lights to pick up the Capital City Trail once again. Go back over the bridge and retrace your steps along the Yahara River to Tenney Park.

When you come back through the tunnel under Johnson Street, follow the park road straight out to Sherman Avenue and cross the street to the entry road to the locks. If you go right across the bridge on Sherman Avenue, there is a boat landing on the north side of the street. Just above it to the east (right) are several park benches perfect for a chat or sunset. You can also watch boats pass through the locks from the bridge.

The hike continues across Sherman Avenue, passing the locks office where you can find water, restrooms, and a picnic table. There is a wheelchair-accessible ramp to a fishing platform. Originally there was an earthen dam on this spot where a gristmill, sawmill, and brewery once operated. Locks were built to replace it in 1896. These were replaced in 1959. The water level in Lake Mendota is five feet higher than that of Lake Monona.

Go around the lock building to the left and find the breakwater. You can follow this out to its point. Rocks line the concrete sidewalk, and benches are spaced out evenly along its length. This is a good place to watch Rhythm and Booms fireworks around the Fourth of July if you don't want to brave the crowds at Warner Park. The view of the Capitol and the university is perfect, and the sun sets over the lake from here.

Coming back from the point, go right (west) along the shore of Lake Mendota and a crushed-rock trail takes you past the small beach area to the parking lot. A massive willow split down the middle still grows in all directions on a small point to your right and offers another fine place to take a break. There are restrooms in the changing house, and there's a drinking fountain at the entrance to the lot. Bus routes 2 and 27 stop here.

NEARBY ACTIVITIES

This side of town is neighborhood-proud. Yahara Place Park is the site of Marquette Neighborhood Waterfront Festival in June. Atwood-Schenk's Corners neighborhood festival is in July. Just west of this hike are La Fete de Marquette around July 14, the Orton Park Festival in August, and the Willy Street Festival in September. Check **www.madison.com** for an events calendar.

TOM GEORGE GREENWAY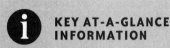

IN BRIEF

This chain of three small neighborhood parks is more of a secret garden. The narrow stretch of green space on either side of Cottage Grove Road is a nice short hike that begs you to linger amid oaks and wildflowers.

DESCRIPTION

This place seems like a best-kept secret, and here I am blowing its cover. The hike actually traverses three separate parks, but you wouldn't know it. Elvehjem Sanctuary to the south was named for Conrad A. Elvehjem. Born in nearby McFarland, he was a renowned UW professor and biochemist who first identified and discovered the importance of the vitamin niacin Heritage Prairie Conservation Park to the north is another neighborhood park featuring a prairie remnant on a rocky hill. Tom George Greenway, named for a former alderperson who used a lot of his own funds to beautify the Cottage Grove Boulevard, connects the two parks with a trail.

This can all be a little confusing, depending on the entrance you take. I recommend the trailhead on the north side of Cottage Grove Road and then doing two out-and-backs from this central point. Alternative entrances can be found at Heritage

KEY AT-A-GLANCE INFORMATION

LENGTH: 2.2 miles

CONFIGURATION: Double out-and-back

DIFFICULTY: Easy to moderate

SCENERY: Mixed forest, highway overlook, prairie

EXPOSURE: Mostly shaded

TRAIL TRAFFIC: Light

TRAIL SURFACE: Packed dirt

HIKING TIME: 1 hour

DRIVING DISTANCE: 1 mile east of US 51 on County Road BB

ACCESS: 4 a.m.–1 hour after sunset

MAPS: USGS Madison East

WHEELCHAIR ACCESSIBILITY: None

FACILITIES: None on the trail, but Elvehjem Park has a shelter and restrooms

SPECIAL COMMENTS: Dogs not allowed.

Directions ——————————➤

From US 51 (Stoughton Road) take County Road BB (Cottage Grove Road) east one mile. Parking is on the street at the trailhead near a large wooden sign that says TOM GEORGE GREENWAY. Park on the westbound side of the street. The trailhead is 70 feet to the right of the sign.

GPS Trailhead Coordinates

UTM Zone (WGS 84)   16T

Easting   0313455

Northing   4772754

Latitude   N 43° 05' 4.42"

Longitude W 89° 17' 30.37"

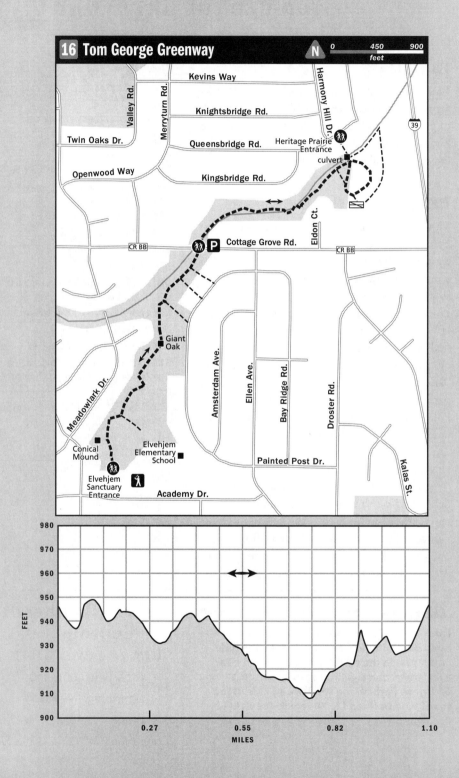

Prairie on Queensbridge Road or the Elvehjem Sanctuary on Academy Road at the south end.

A grassy trail descends off the edge of the sidewalk where you'd hardly suspect to find a hiking trail. Mixed forest surrounds you, and tall grass stands along the intermittent water to your left where a storm runoff, concrete culvert emerges from under Cottage Grove Road. Large rocks have been placed here to stop erosion at the opening. Residences are just a stone's throw to either side of this corridor of green space, and 300 feet in, the path becomes packed dirt. Expect songbirds, butterflies, and wildflowers throughout the park, and the occasional coyote scat is evidence of bigger visitors. At the opposite side of the first small clearing, cross a culvert and follow the trail back into woods.

Brush closes in around you. Highway noise from Interstate 94 rises in the distance. Soon the terrain to your left slopes up a bit, and tall cottonwoods fill out the canopy. The trail widens as you pass a storm drain to your right. Cross over another culvert and through some more trees before the trail opens to the sky with tall grass on either side and pines lining the path. A trail leads up to the right through sumac, a potential cutoff for your return path. Keep going past this to a fork in the trail. Left will take you across the ditch to your left and out of the park to Queensbridge Road, where a sign marks the trail as the entry to Heritage Prairie Conservation Park. This is an alternative starting point with on-street parking. The path to the right splits as well. The right branch is your return path, and the left trail goes into the woods where the canopy reaches over you but doesn't quite block out the sky. This trail goes up the hill becoming crushed stone in a few places. At the top you find medium-size oaks, and then the trail curves to the right. Beyond the brush to your left is the highway.

Come to another fork in the trail with a metal fence post to the right. To the left is a spur trail that leads to an opening in the park fence and a view of the highway and the Cottage Grove Road police station. The trail to the right goes down the hill, steeply passing through bushes as it makes its way back to where you started the climb up the hill. The aforementioned cutoff trail is to your left as you descend, and you can opt for that, which is a bit steeper. At the bottom you can retrace your steps to Cottage Grove Road for the second half of this hike.

However, there is more to explore here if you are willing—though the trail isn't always clear. If you go to the left-leading path toward the park exit on Queensbridge Road, you might see a faint trail through the grass that follows along the right side of the ditch heading toward the highway. This follows a wider loop of about 0.2 miles up that hill to your right. As you follow the shrinking ditch on your left, watch for a much clearer path about 300 feet from the juncture. This will lead to the right up the hill through a clump of aspens as you approach the curve at the top. The trail goes up a bit more and widens out. To your right the earth drops away into a small gully with some exposed rocks in the understory. The highway is again to your left, and you are on the outside of the fence at the crest of the grassy ridge. Go to the right along the fence to find that

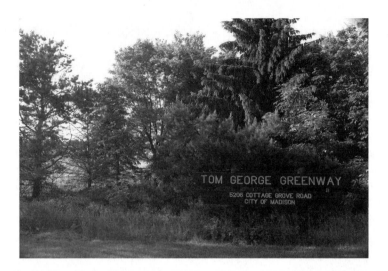

The trailhead at Cottage Grove Road

gate that leads you back into the park and follows the return path down the hill once again.

Retrace your steps to Cottage Grove Road. Cross the street to the south side and enter the woods there on the western side of the storm sewer. Once again the trail quickly draws you from a well-manicured residential neighborhood and a busy street into an unexpected tangle of woods.

Now you are heading south, and it is quieter without Interstate 94 nearby. Spur trails to either side lead to backyards. The trail surface shows more tree roots and is more rugged. The character of the terrain is different. You will see more basswoods and some black walnuts as well as red oaks. This side seems more like a ravine and a thicker forest. The area is suitable for tree houses and children's forts (you may find one), and with more fallen wood, fungi hunters will have more to see than wildflower fans. The canopy is thick.

Come to an intersection where the trail to the left heads uphill and exits the park on the sidewalk on Painted Post Drive with crushed rock about halfway up. Stay right. Sandy patches appear in the trail. The trail rises moderately through dirt, sand, tree roots, and some dead-leaf cover, and then passes around a giant oak tree. Watch for a trail to the left up to an elementary school where there are picnic tables in a mowed park. Other little footpaths lead right to more backyards.

Come to a T-intersection. The left trail heads up to that school; go right down the hill a bit until the main trail bends left again so that it continues through the middle of the forest. Come to a large rock that marks a trail to a conical mound. The mound was constructed by a hunting and gathering culture around 400 A.D. and was used to mark where they met to bury their dead. You can follow this spur trail right just 20 feet, but there is little sign of the mound itself.

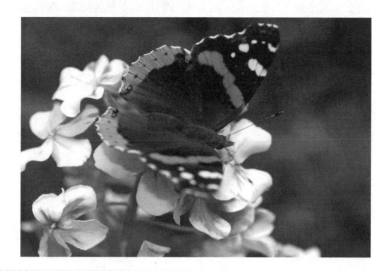

Butterflies and wildflowers are common along the trail.

Continuing along the main path, pass a post to the right that reads ELVEHJEM SANCTUARY CONSERVATION PARK. One hundred feet after this, the trail enters a mowed park area with a ball diamond and Elvehjem Elementary School to the left. The trail sign is set back into the woods and not easily seen if you choose to start your hike from this park on Academy Drive to the west of the school. Elvehjem Park has a shelter and restrooms. Retrace your steps back to Cottage Grove Road or you can walk east toward the school to pick up Ellen Avenue and follow it north to Cottage Grove Road.

NEARBY ACTIVITIES

Stop in at Culver's for the custard of the day or a famous "butter burger" on Cottage Grove Road just before you return to US 51 (Stoughton Road). In mid-May nearby Heritage Sanctuary on 600 Meadowlark Drive is awash with trilliums and a short walk from the entrance to Heritage Prairie.

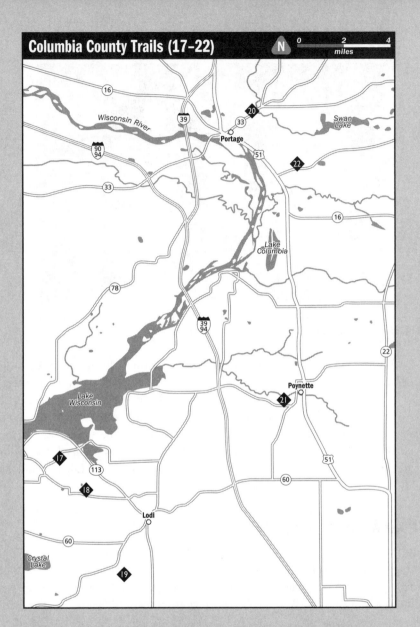

Columbia County Trails (17–22)

N

0   2   4
miles

16

Wisconsin River

39

20

33

Swan Lake

90 94

Portage

33

51

22

16

78

Lake Columbia

39 94

22

Poynette

21

Lake Wisconsin

51

17

113

60

18

Lodi

60

Crystal Lake

19

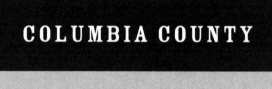

COLUMBIA COUNTY

17   GIBRALTAR ROCK STATE NATURAL AREA

KEY AT-A-GLANCE INFORMATION

LENGTH: 1.4 miles

CONFIGURATION: Out-and-back with a loop

DIFFICULTY: Moderate to strenuous

SCENERY: Mixed forest, cliffs towering over rolling farmland

EXPOSURE: Mostly shaded

TRAIL TRAFFIC: Light

TRAIL SURFACE: Old asphalt, exposed rock, packed dirt

HIKING TIME: 30 minutes

DRIVING DISTANCE: 1.2 miles from the intersection of WI 113 and County Road V

ACCESS: Always open, year-round

MAPS: USGS Lodi

WHEELCHAIR ACCESSIBILITY: None

FACILITIES: None

SPECIAL COMMENTS: Rock climbing, though popular in the past, is currently prohibited. Pets must be on a leash.

IN BRIEF

The climb to this extraordinary lookout over the Wisconsin River valley will take your breath away in more ways than one.

DESCRIPTION

This region of Wisconsin is really a geologist's dream. From the sandstone of the Cambrian period to the carving work of the glaciers there is a whole glossary of land features. Gibraltar Rock is a sandstone bluff that rises up out of the earth like a fallen asteroid, and if you aren't ready to exert yourself a bit, this might not be your first hiking choice. Gibraltar Rock is an outlier from the Black River Escarpment. At one time it must have been attached and then became isolated by erosion. There are others in the area, but this is the highest.

A preservation group called Friends of Our Native Landscape made this park their first project. A famous landscape architect by the name of Jens Jensen led the call to protect this area after the group formed in Madison in 1920. When the land became available in 1927, he and his colleagues, forward thinkers from Madison and the University of Wisconsin, took action and acquired the deed. The preserved area was

GPS Trailhead Coordinates

UTM Zone (WGS 84)   16T

Easting   0289259

Northing   4802806

Latitude   N 43° 20' 54.78"

Longitude   W 89° 36' 0.75"

Directions ——————→

From Lodi, go north on WI 113 4 miles, then west on County Road V 1 mile, then south (left) on the gravel Park Road 0.2 miles to reach the parking lot.

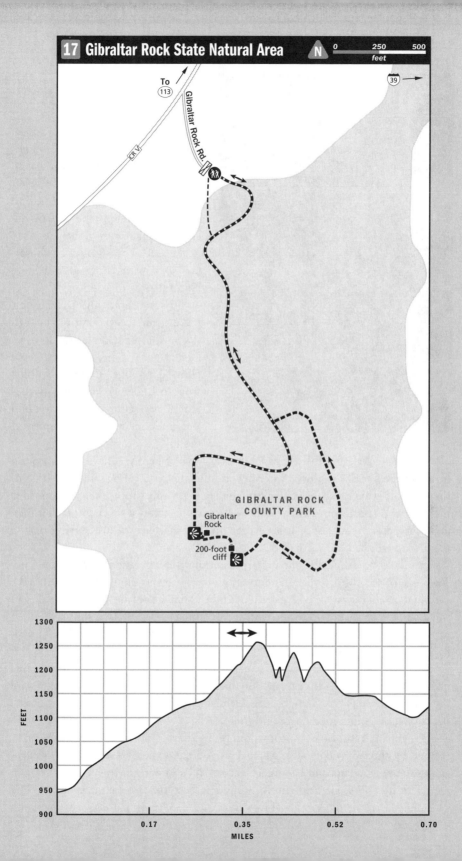

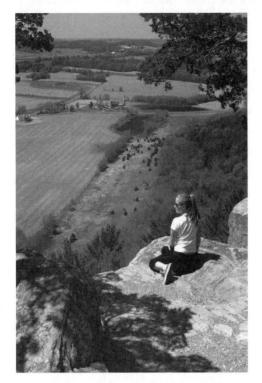

first known as Richmond Park in honor of a pioneer couple James and Emma Richmond, who along with other families, had first homesteaded nearby. You can find a stone marker at the top of the cliff commemorating the preservation group. The 35 acres of Gibraltar Rock were designated a State Natural Area in 1969.

As you enter the parking lot, there is an access road to the left. It's hard to imagine traffic up here, but at one time, vehicles were allowed passage. Efforts to put a stop to underage drinking parties led the park administrators to build the gate you see at the bottom of the hill.

The hike starts up the old asphalt access road where you have to go around or under the bar of the closed gate. Beyond this the road follows a steep climb to the summit. If you want a little extra challenge on this short hike, you can take the narrow dirt path directly from the lot, which is merely a short cutoff that then joins the access road just a little farther on. But the burn of just staying on the main road will be plenty for most.

At the top of the bluff, the underbrush thins out a bit and the views open up. The edge of the cliff is breezy, and those given to vertigo should be warned. Take care here as there is a lot of loose sand, and the flat stones are less level than you think. In recent years two locals who were familiar with the location have fallen to their deaths. Climbing down to lower ledges is not advisable, and in fact all rock climbing is prohibited.

To the south is a sheer 200-foot cliff overlooking a large bog and scenic valley. On a clear day you can see for miles into the Wisconsin River valley and the hazy blue hills of Baraboo. The farmland spreads out before you with the occasional patch of woods here and there.

Migrating raptors are not uncommon as they come here to catch thermals formed by the warm cliff face. Most days you can expect to see turkey vultures riding the up currents and having a look at who's looking at them.

The first lookout area on your right is best for just taking it all in—the sweeping horizon, the circling birds, and the geometric patterns of farmland.

Another 200 feet east is another prime lookout point, and this one offers a fine view of the cliff itself where it juts out from the rest of the bluff and shows off its layered colors of sandstone. This is a good photo angle. The plant life along the cliff is mostly ferns, columbine, and cliff goldenrod. Wildflowers populate the grassy areas set beneath pines, towering red oaks, and cedars.

Most visitors will come for the vista and then just head back down the hill. But the trail beyond, though not as dramatic as the cliffs, offers a moderate challenge and rich plant life. The trail descends over roots and rocks and around a few sizeable boulders, a bit challenging at the beginning but becoming less so after the first 300 feet. From here the trail is still narrow as it passes through thicker undergrowth and tall red oak and basswood. You can expect to have to climb over fallen timber that shows a variety of fungi for the mushroom enthusiasts. You can also find bird's-foot violets and pasque flowers here in the spring.

From the cliff down the slope and back around to the access road is just less than 0.3 miles and leaves you already a third of the way back down that access road to the parking lot.

Gibraltar Rock is a good place to come in late September and early October when the leaves are turning. The views of the colors below are stunning.

NEARBY ACTIVITIES

The Ice Age Park and Trail Foundation has an office in nearby Lodi where you can get maps and more information about the trails (218 S. Main Street, Lodi, [608] 592-1433). Lodi Coffee Roasters roasts its own as the name suggests. Stop in for a good cup of Joe and wireless Internet access at 107 South Main Street, Lodi ([608] 592-3325; www.lodicoffee.com).

18   ICE AGE TRAIL: Groves-Pertzborn Segment

KEY AT-A-GLANCE INFORMATION

LENGTH: 2.6 miles

CONFIGURATION: Out-and-back

DIFFICULTY: Moderate to strenuous

SCENERY: Forest, ravine, some prairie

EXPOSURE: Mostly shaded

TRAIL TRAFFIC: Light

TRAIL SURFACE: Rough dirt path

HIKING TIME: 1–1.5 hours

DRIVING DISTANCE: 7.4 miles west from the Interstate 39 and WI 60 intersection

ACCESS: Year-round except during the gun hunting season in November

MAPS: USGS Lodi; *Ice Age Trail Companion Atlas*

WHEELCHAIR ACCESSIBILITY: None

FACILITIES: None

SPECIAL COMMENTS: Beware of poison ivy. This is a good place to pick berries.

GPS Trailhead Coordinates

UTM Zone (WGS 84)   16T

Easting   0290843

Northing   4800596

Latitude   N 43° 29' 44.83"

Longitude   W 89° 34' 47.41"

IN BRIEF

Take a trek through a ravine that lies between two rounded hills set right along the edge of the unglaciated "driftless zone."

DESCRIPTION

The Ice Age Trail is the result of a lot of work by a lot of people. Ray Zillmer, a Milwaukee lawyer, came up with the concept and founded the Ice Age Park and Trail Foundation in 1958. The plan was to make a park not measured in acres but in miles—a serpentine hiking path that would follow the terminal moraine from the last advance of glaciers into Wisconsin. This is the line where the massive sheets of ice stopped advancing and from where they eventually retreated.

Senator Gaylord Nelson and Congressman Henry Reuss were instrumental in establishing the trail as a national scientific reserve in 1964, and in the 1980s it was designated as both a state and national scenic trail.

Trails are low impact. Nothing is paved, and they are minimally maintained so as to preserve the natural look of the area. Often you can feel as if you are the first person on the trail in a very long time, and it's only the yellow squares posted intermittently on trees and occasional trail posts that reassure you that you are on the right path.

Directions ⟶

From the intersection of WI 60 and WI 113 in the town of Lodi, go north 1.2 miles to County Road J. Head left 1.9 miles to find the parking area for the Ice Age Trail on your left just before the intersection of County Road J and Lovering Road. The trailhead is at the parking lot to the left of the trail kiosk.

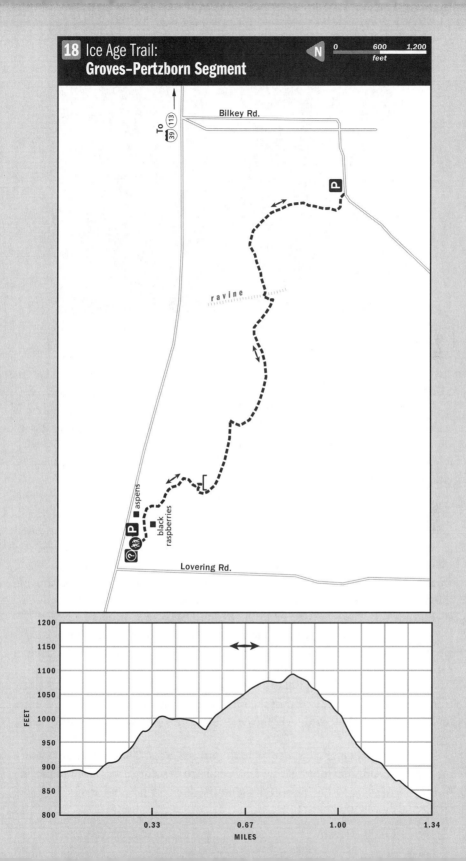

18 Ice Age Trail: Groves–Pertzborn Segment

N

0   600   1,200
feet

Bilkey Rd.

To 39 113

P

ravine

aspens

P

black raspberries

?

Lovering Rd.

FEET

1200
1150
1100
1050
1000
950
900
850
800

0.33   0.67   1.00   1.34

MILES

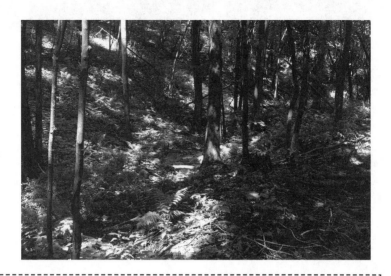

A ravine along the trail

You can thank the myriad volunteers and landowners that helped make this 1,000-mile trail possible. The section you are hiking, in fact, is private property.

Before hiking the trail, check the kiosk for trail news or warnings. There is a map and also information on identifying poison ivy. There is enough of it here to warrant posting this warning, so take a moment to make sure you know what it looks like. Wild parsnip can also be found here and is far less infamous than the ivy, but arguably much worse.

The trailhead is 30 feet off to the left of the kiosk as you face it. The trail is narrow, and you can expect tree roots and uneven dirt surface. It curves left and 300 feet down the trail, you enter a rather thick stand of aspens. Aspens often clump like this because, unlike seed-producing trees, they actually spread via shoots from the root system. These colonies are considered one single entity and a particularly large colony of aspens in Colorado is alleged to be the largest living thing on the planet. They are aggressive but native to Wisconsin. Their white or silverfish trunks create a contrast in the darker forest for a nice visual effect.

Throughout this stretch find black raspberries (known locally as black caps) along the trail. They are a bit less sweet than raspberries and usually are ripe as early as late June on into mid-July.

The trail continues uphill on a moderate grade. There's a bench 0.3 miles from the trailhead. At the crest of the hill, only another 300 feet from here, enter into a small meadow with wildflowers. To your right are agricultural fields, typically cornfields.

Cross this open area and enter back into the trees. There's a large boulder on your left, and soon after that the trail begins to descend just a bit. In the spring this is a good place to find jack-in-the-pulpit and may apple, and several fern species populate the understory.

The climb resumes 500 feet past the boulder. In another 0.2 miles, cross a private access road that comes up the hill from your left and leads to the crops 100 feet to your right. Continue across another 400 feet and come to a grassy area to the right. The trail continues past, heading through another stand of aspens.

Climb only a bit more and then come over the ridge and look down into a marvelous ravine. May apples are in abundance here. The *Ice Age Trail Companion* compares this to a rain forest, and truly there is something of the ravine that does give the feeling you are not in Wisconsin. Woods with thick brush often close in around you and give the impression you could be anywhere. When a space opens up like this under the canopy of oaks and basswoods without a lot of intervening brush, and the landscape folds with a crease between two ridges, it certainly does leave an impression. Watch for owls, and if you are really lucky, you might see a Cooper's hawk that has been spotted around here.

Follow the trail as it switches back and forth, taking you down into the bottom of the ravine on a moderate grade and then follow an easterly trail up the opposite side. The slope is not so steep that it should be a concern for falling.

Cross the next ridge and begin your descent to the end of the trail. When you come upon some old power lines, you are actually halfway down the hill. The path shows sandy spots as you pass some cedar. The canopy is thinned out, and you have only partial shade. This is another nice area for picking black caps. Beware: they do stain your hands a bit.

The ground is soft and spongy beneath your feet as burrowing creatures such as moles are common. As the trail dips into a gully, head left and come up on the other side to Bilkey Road opposite a tree farm.

You could drop off another vehicle here to do this one way, but the distance is short and the times I've been here, I've seen enough wildlife to make a second pass worth it.

NEARBY ACTIVITIES

Cross the Wisconsin River on the only free ferry in Wisconsin. The Merrimac Ferry operates 24 hours a day taking cars, bicycles, and pedestrians from the eastern bank at Okee to the western side at Merrimac. On the other side check out the geological wonder that is Parfrey's Glen at the head of the Ice Age Trail segment that connects the site to Devil's Lake State Park.

19 ICE AGE TRAIL: Lodi Marsh Segment

KEY AT-A-GLANCE INFORMATION

LENGTH: 7.8 miles

CONFIGURATION: A loop and an out-and-back

DIFFICULTY: Moderate

SCENERY: Prairie, mixed forest, and bluffs

EXPOSURE: Half and half

TRAIL TRAFFIC: Light

TRAIL SURFACE: Cut grass paths, narrow packed-dirt trails

HIKING TIME: 3 hours

DRIVING DISTANCE: 24 miles from Interstate 39 and US 151

ACCESS: Year-round

MAPS: USGS Lodi; *Ice Age Trail Companion Atlas*

WHEELCHAIR ACCESSIBILITY: None

FACILITIES: None

SPECIAL COMMENTS: Dogs allowed on leashes from May 1 through July 31. The northernmost portion of the trail is closed during the nine-day deer-hunting season at the end of November. There is an alternative trail exit at Riddle Road. The marsh loop has a corresponding nature trail guide in a box at the trailhead.

GPS Trailhead Coordinates

UTM Zone (WGS 84) 16T

Easting 0293342

Northing 4795282

Latitude N 43° 16' 55.22"

Longitude W 89° 32' 49.37"

IN BRIEF

Follow a guided nature loop across a hilltop prairie overlooking the marsh, then climb a bluff through forest and restored prairie with views of rolling farmland.

DESCRIPTION

Lodi Marsh and its springs surround the upper 2 miles of Spring Creek. These are breeding grounds for several species of birds, including great blue herons, sandhill cranes, willow and alder flycatchers, and blue-winged warblers. If you are into moths—and who isn't?—this is a moth-rich environment, several of which are found only in wetlands. Some rare species include the silphium borer moth, Newman's brocade, and the ottoe skipper. On the south side of the marsh is a 240-foot knob hill partly covered with dry-mesic forest composed primarily of red oak, sugar maple, and basswood. The south slope, however, is prairie.

This segment of the Ice Age Trail has two parts. The first is a 1.5-mile lollipop out through the knob-hill prairie that borders the wetlands west of the trailhead parking lot. The second stretch is one way or out-and-back heading east from the marsh trailhead and lot

Directions ———————————→

From where it intersects with US 151, take I-39 north from Madison 16 miles to Exit 119-Lodi/Arlington. The exit loops, and you go right (west) 4.4 miles on WI 60 to reach Lodi. From the intersection of WI 60 and 113 (Main Street and Portage Street) in Lodi, take WI 60 west 0.6 miles. Turn left on Riddle Road, also known as Lodi-Springfield Road. There is a kiosk 3 miles from here on the right side of the road and an area for parking right at the trailhead.

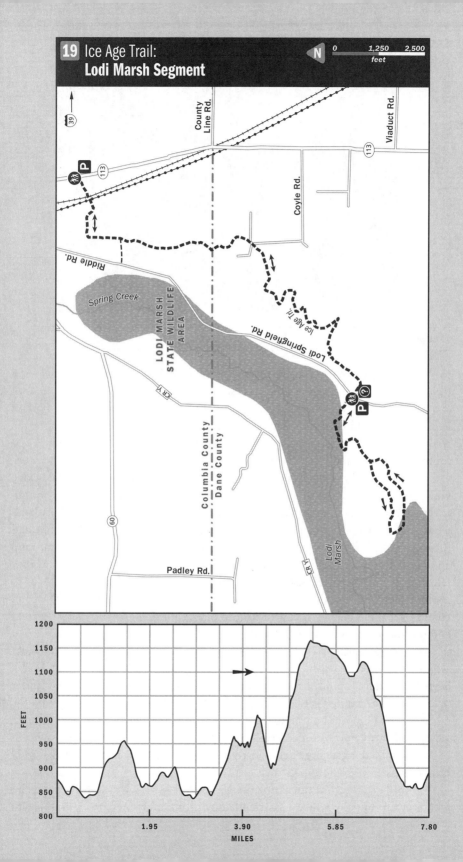

County Line Rd.

Viaduct Rd.

113

Coyle Rd.

113

39

P

Riddle Rd.

Spring Creek

LODI MARSH STATE WILDLIFE AREA

Lodi Springfield Rd.

Ice Age Trl.

P ?

C.R.Y

Columbia County
Dane County

60

Padley Rd.

C.R.Y

Lodi Marsh

1200
1150
1100
1050
1000
950
900
850
800

FEET

1.95   3.90   5.85   7.80
MILES

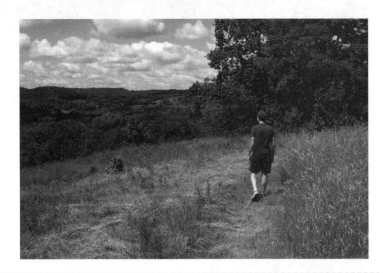

The prairie loop

to WI 113 just south of Lodi. At the little turnaround-cum-parking lot, there is a trail kiosk and a map box that occasionally has maps and the nature trail companion in it. From the lot, head west descending into prairie. You'll find an abundance of wild bergamot, but beware of the wild parsnip that leans into the trail at times. If the trail has recently been mowed and you're not wearing closed footwear, there is a higher risk of getting exposed to the parsnip juices.

At 0.15 miles you enter into oak savanna. The trail then passes along a ridge with a steep slope down to the right where you can see flowing water. The trail curves left 0.2 miles later and enters a clearing. Far to the left is rolling farmland. Continue another 0.2 miles to the fork for the loop. Go right up the hill and through partial shade for 0.3 miles where the trail descends to the turnaround another 0.1 mile later. The trail comes back 0.4 miles to an access road that runs left to right. Stay right. Look for the trail post with the yellow swatch on it to avoid taking intermittent maintenance or prairie restoration paths. The trail climbs over the hump to the north to reconnect with the inbound stem. Go right and return to the parking lot.

From the parking circle, cross Lodi-Springfield Road and find the next segment of the trail to the right. This is the trailhead for the East Lodi Marsh Segment. It starts uphill through prairie and then heads into mixed forest after 0.25 miles. The canopy is thick here, and the packed dirt path curves around the crown of the bluff until a trail marker leads right at 0.1 mile with a view out to a valley and farmland. The path re-enters the trees, mostly aspens, and switches back downhill along a gorge before arriving at a bridge 0.35 miles away. A second bridge is just several steps past that.

From here the trail opens to the sky for the next 1.1 mile before you hit woods again. Initially you are surrounded by brush, and you climb a grassy path uphill, offering more views of farmland in the distance. The path winds through open prairie then, offering an easy climb higher and higher on the hill. Follow the posts across the field when the path is not clear as may be the case after a restorative prairie burn. On the opposite end is a farmhouse and barn; the trail heads toward them. Pass behind a row of trees to enter another field. The trail goes right at a trail sign with brush on either side, and then heads downhill to a bench on the left with a trail sign and mileage to Lodi: 2 miles. You're actually only 1 mile from the parking lot at the end of this segment, however.

Most of this stretch is downhill through oak-hickory forest with some exposed rock in the surrounding terrain. The trail is a narrow, packed-dirt footpath with tree roots and scattered rocks and becoming rockier and steeper as you go. At 0.5 miles you come to a spur trail to the left. This takes you 0.15 miles out to Riddle Road. This exit trail must be used during deer season at the end of November when the last portion of this trail is closed.

Just past the exit trail is an ATV trail crossing left to right, and this is where you see the hunting warning. Past here follow a 0.15-mile narrow corridor of trees and brush surrounded by agricultural fields. At the end the trail heads to the right into the sun and borders the fields as it heads east. Watch for trail posts. As you pass through a break in the trees, there will be one ahead and to the right. This will lead you to a crushed-rock road to the left; don't go right. You'll pass under a viaduct at 0.2 miles and then continue up the road to the parking lot 0.1 mile from there. Pass through a gate and go left to the lot. Lodi is 0.4 miles north of here on WI 113. The Ice Age Trail does continue into town on sidewalks and paths. It will eventually connect to the Groves-Pertzborn Segment on the other side of town.

NEARBY ACTIVITIES

On Main Street in downtown Lodi you can find Suzy the Duck. Spring Creek passes under the street here and waterfowl frequent the area. You can feed them with food from a nearby vending machine. Suzy is the nickname for whichever duck happens to build its nest in a small stone basket here. Look for cafes, coffee shops, and a bakery along Main Street.

20 ICE AGE TRAIL: Marquette Segment

KEY AT-A-GLANCE INFORMATION

LENGTH: 10.2 miles

CONFIGURATION: Out-and-back

DIFFICULTY: Easy

SCENERY: Fox River, prairie, oak forest

EXPOSURE: Mostly sunny

TRAIL TRAFFIC: Light

TRAIL SURFACE: Uneven dirt and grass footpath, wooden bridges

HIKING TIME: 4 hours

DRIVING DISTANCE: 32.7 miles from the juncture of US 151 and Interstate 39

ACCESS: Year-round (see Special Comments)

MAPS: USGS Portage; *Ice Age Trail Companion Atlas*

WHEELCHAIR ACCESSIBILITY: None

FACILITIES: None

SPECIAL COMMENTS: Posted park hours in the City of Portage are 8 a.m. to 10 p.m., but for the Ice Age Trail this merely governs the two southern parking lots. If you plan on parking overnight or quite early in the morning, simply call Portage Parks and Recreation at (608) 742-2178 and let them know.

IN BRIEF

This trail follows the winding path of the Fox River through prairie, forest, and wetlands. It's a walk in the sun along the embankment of a once-important river route.

DESCRIPTION

The trail starts along the Portage Canal, which connects the Fox River with the Wisconsin River, and thus the Great Lakes with the Mississippi River. You can trim almost a mile off the one-way distance of this hike by driving to the second parking lot at the end of Agency House Road on the west side of the canal.

There is a map box that may offer maps from time to time and a kiosk and two benches. From the lot at the trailhead, enter mixed forest with abundant maple on a packed-dirt path. One hundred feet into the woods, a bridge crosses to the left over the canal. You can walk the grassy roadside north on the other side of the water if you prefer. Otherwise, continue on this forested path 0.8 miles to another pedestrian bridge that passes over a small dam just before where the Portage Canal meets the Fox River. At the other side, go right on an asphalt path 200 feet through the second trail parking lot. There are two more benches here

GPS Trailhead Coordinates

UTM Zone (WGS 84) 16T

Easting 0302755

Northing 4824778

Latitude N 43° 32' 59.59"

Longitude W 89° 26' 30.42"

Directions

From its intersection with US 151, take I-39 north 29.5 miles. Take Exit 87 to WI 33 and continue 3.2 miles, passing Albert Street, crossing the Portage Canal and taking a left onto a gravel road that runs parallel with WI 33 for 400 feet back in the direction you came. This is the parking lot for the Ice Age Trail, and a sign marks it as such. The trailhead is at the lot, close to the canal.

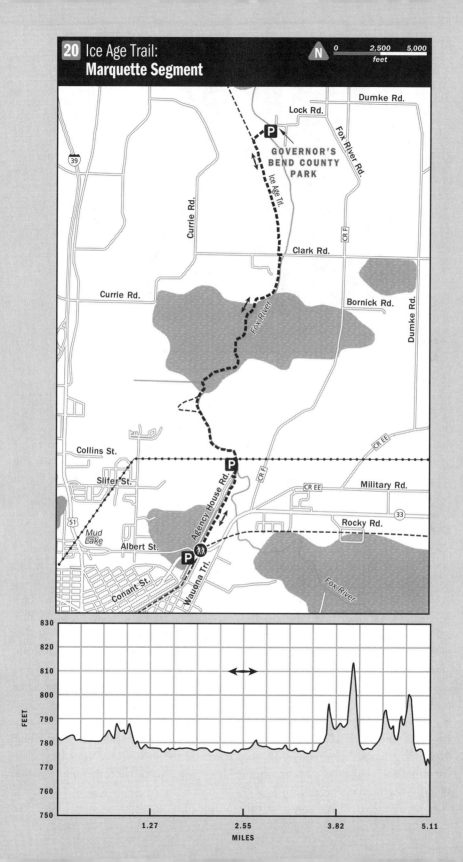

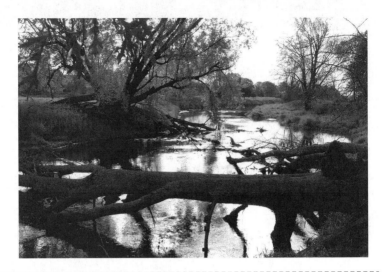

Fox River

as well as a trail kiosk and garbage cans.

The trail heads into trees and follows the water's edge about 15 feet above it on a narrow footpath over undulating earth. At 350 feet it bends left following the curve of the Fox River and comes out into the open for the next 2.8 miles. Following the tall embankment, look out over prairie and farmland on either side of the river. Pass under high-tension wires 0.1 mile from the trees. Across the water is a small evergreen forest. Follow the curve of the river west here. Watch along the trail for raspberries and black caps in June and July.

There are 21 bridges to cross, and you come to your first one 0.3 miles later. Water from the fields to the left drains into the river here and at many other points along your route. Another 100 feet brings you to bridge #20 (counting down until the end). For most of these bridges you have a short steep descent and another quick climb several feet up the other side.

The next three bridges are spaced almost evenly every 200 feet, the third one being a bit longer than the rest and offering handrails. To your left the prairie becomes agricultural fields, primarily corn. The tall embankment keeps them dry, as do the drainage channels. You can see thick forest across the river, which soon gives way to fields so that your view is quite far in all directions.

Bridge #16 is 0.3 miles later, and then the grassy trail becomes lumpy like moguls until you come to a few trailside oak trees hanging over the water at 0.1 mile. The next 0.15 miles crosses three more bridges, the last one over a larger channel. On the other side the river bends right as does the trail, and bridge #12 is at another 0.1 mile with a steep climb on the other side. You enter brush 0.1 mile later and then trees another 0.1 mile after that. There is some minimal shade from the oaks here.

Along the route you can see an abundance of hunting stands, and hiking here during gun deer-hunting season is probably not a good idea. Be sure to wear brightly colored clothing if you decide to go out. There's good reason for all the deer stands; watch for deer paths to the water source in the grass and brush. Past the oaks, you are in the open again and heading north with the river's bend. Look for wildflowers in the spring and summer and milkweed in the fall. Hawks hunt the fields, while kingfishers and herons ply the waters for food.

Another 0.25 miles puts you over three more bridges. The river heads east with oak forest to your left, then rounds another bend to continue north to bridge #8 at 0.3 miles. In the fall you may find salamanders and frogs seeking places to dig in for the winter. Cross three more bridges in 0.2 miles and arrive at an old railroad abutment as the trail heads east again. A 60-foot bridge once spanned the river here. An interpretive sign here tells the history.

Stay alongside the river and avoid farm paths that head left. Pass a tall hunting stand 0.1 mile from the abutment. Then the trail goes north once more continuing 0.15 miles to bridge #4. From there you are 0.2 miles from Clark Road, passing through a few oaks and a patch of sumac just before you climb up to the pavement. Go left along the road 150 feet to an arrow and cross to the right to descend into a band of oak forest that stretches north across the fields. The path here can get soggy as it is a depression in the surrounding terrain. A ridge rises to the left at 0.3 miles, and the trail goes along the east side of it, partly shaded. The trail surface is tricky as decayed railroad ties lay beneath loose soil, grass, and moss. At 0.2 miles pass a cedar and enter a small clump of aspen before crossing bridge #3 over a low point. To the left of the trail is marshy. The trail remains straight, so cross through the open on potentially soggy ground. Cross bridge #2 at another 0.1 mile with open water on either side.

The next 0.5 miles starts out following the edge of the marshy area and gradually closing the gap between the trail and a forested hill to the left. The ground becomes a bit higher and drier, and the trail is mostly shaded. At that 0.5-mile mark, enter a patch of "snake weed," which resembles little bamboo shoots, and then the trail goes east 0.15 miles across a low open field where you cross the final bridge. On the other side, the trail goes right through brush and trees 100 feet on a mowed path before it turns east (left) and crosses onto what is almost an island at Governor's Bend County Park. You'll find picnic tables and grills, and the road crosses a bridge to street parking on the other side of the Fox River, which flows around the bend. This is your turnaround point or a good place for a second car or pick-up to make this hike one way.

NEARBY ACTIVITIES

Visit the 1832 Historic Indian Agency House just before the second trail parking lot on Agency House Road/Rustic Road 69. Call (608) 742-6362 for more information.

21 ROWAN CREEK TRAIL

KEY AT-A-GLANCE INFORMATION

LENGTH: 2.8 miles

CONFIGURATION: Interconnected loops with an out-and-back segment

DIFFICULTY: Easy

SCENERY: Mixed forest, pine forest, wetlands, flowing water

EXPOSURE: Mostly shaded

TRAIL TRAFFIC: Light

TRAIL SURFACE: Packed dirt, some tree roots and boardwalks

HIKING TIME: 1 hour

DRIVING DISTANCE: 22.8 miles

ACCESS: Year-round

MAPS: USGS Poynette; posted at trail junctures

WHEELCHAIR ACCESSIBILITY: None

FACILITIES: None

SPECIAL COMMENTS: Dogs allowed. Do not confuse this park with another Rowan Creek access point closer to Interstate 39. Cross-country skiing is possible in winter, but trails are not groomed.

IN BRIEF

A stroll along one of the finest trout streams in the state also leads to an island of pine surrounded by wetlands.

DESCRIPTION

One hundred feet into the woods from the parking lot is the first trail juncture where you will also find a map board. Go left here as the trail goes downhill heading toward Pine Island. The trail surface may show some erosion and some sandy patches. Another 0.1 mile takes you to another juncture. To your left a 0.7-mile lollipop trail takes you out onto Pine Island. The trail to the right is where you continue deeper into the park when you return.

Go left. One hundred feet later, enter cattail marsh and step onto a floating boardwalk. Cross this to the island where there is a bench alongside the trail to your right. The small island in the middle of the marsh is populated almost entirely by towering pine with a few small oaks scattered along the edges. Just past the bench, cross another smaller boardwalk before you come to the island's loop trail. Go left at the map board.

In the 1930s this area was converted to pine. The trail follows the western edge of the island, loops around and back, and

GPS Trailhead Coordinates

UTM Zone (WGS 84)　16T

Easting　0304396

Northing　4805951

Latitude　N 43° 22' 51.40"

Longitude　W 89° 24' 53.03"

Directions

From where it intersects US 151, take I-39 north 20 miles to Exit 115 for County Road J/CS. The exit loops back, so go left (east) on County Road CS 2.2 miles to find the park on your left. The trailhead is at the parking lot.

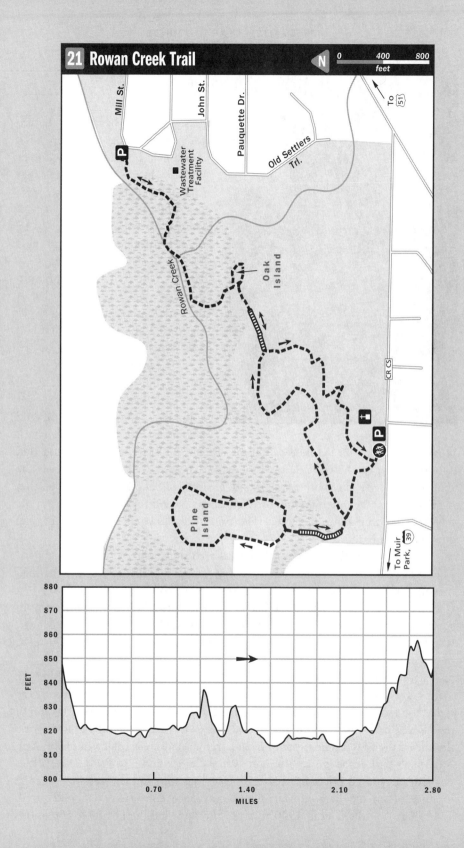

N

0   400   800
feet

Mill St.

John St.

Pauquette Dr.

Old Settlers Trl.

To 51

P

Wastewater Treatment Facility

Rowan Creek

Oak Island

CR CS

P

To Muir Park, 39

Pine Island

880
870
860
850
840
830
820
810
800

FEET

0.70   1.40   2.10   2.80

MILES

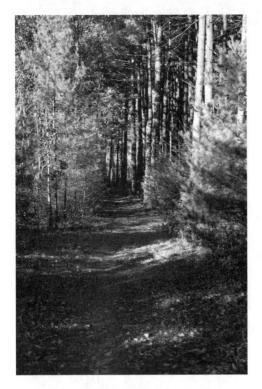

passes another bench just before completing the 0.5-mile loop. Back at the map board, cross back over to the main trail and go left at that first juncture continuing east.

This is mixed forest again, mostly hardwoods, and at 0.15 miles you round a point and head right 200 feet to a trail juncture. The straight trail is a cutoff trail that takes you to the return leg of the park loop and back to the parking lot 0.2 miles away. Go left and find water on both sides of the trail. The area to the right is a stagnant pond. Hike 0.1 mile to a bench where the trail goes up over a hump to another juncture and map board. Straight takes you back to the lot. Go left and cross a cattail marsh on a 200-foot boardwalk. You find another bench on the right on the other side. The first trail on your right is the return path off the diminutive Oak Island. Heading left another 75 feet is another map board and the outgoing trail for Oak Island. Save it for your return from the out-and-back trail along the creek. The trail heads downhill to the left, passing another map board.

As signage for the trail points out, this area shows three distinctive habitats. The upland forest is characterized by dry, sandy soil that plays host to oak, hickory, and red cedar, while the moist lowland forest is primarily ash, box elder, elm, and willow. The difference in trees attracts different residents as well; squirrels, turkeys, and grouse tend toward the upland forest, while barred owls, woodcock, and pileated woodpeckers prefer the lowland trees. The third habitat, of course, is wetlands.

Cross a short wooden bridge and then another bridge, following along the main branch of Rowan Creek. You are in the open here with wet prairie to the right. You have another 0.3 miles and one more bridge to cross before the end of the mowed path where you find the local wastewater treatment plant just beyond the end of the trail. There is parking here on the roadside as well as a picnic area. An asphalt path leads left to a bridge over the creek and into Pauquette Park in Poynette. If you go just a few paces in that direction, you can see the concrete footings of an old dam. Rowan Creek was once converted to a mill pond. The removal of the dam in 1940 restored the flow and the favorable conditions

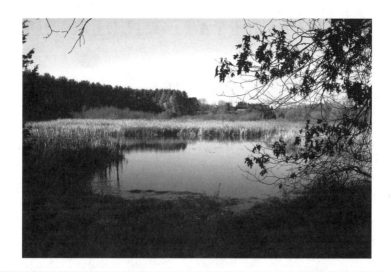

Rowan Creek

for trout.

Head back the way you came along the creek. This is one of the best trout streams in the state. Brown trout spawn in November, and springs upstream keep the water temperature constant in all seasons making it ideal for the trout eggs to hatch in during February. Cross back over the three bridges and come once again to the map board and trail for Oak Island. It is less than 0.1 mile and goes left returning just a bit farther down your return path.

At that point go left and return to the 200-foot boardwalk. On the other side, go left at the trail juncture and map board. You have 0.35 miles left to the parking lot. You will pass the cutoff trail coming in from the right at 0.15 miles. Stay left and follow the trail through upland forest until the next juncture and map board, where you will go left 100 feet out to the parking lot.

NEARBY ACTIVITIES

Stop in at the MacKenzie Environmental Center on the east side of Poynette on County Road CS/Q. The center is run by the Wisconsin Department of Natural Resources and features prairie restoration with hiking trails, a native animal park with a bison herd, and a museum and interpretive center. Call (608) 635-4351 for more information.

22 SWAN LAKE STATE WILDLIFE AREA

KEY AT-A-GLANCE INFORMATION

LENGTH: 3.8 miles

CONFIGURATION: Out-and-back

DIFFICULTY: Moderate

SCENERY: Wetlands, oak savanna, open water

EXPOSURE: Mostly sun, with shaded patches

TRAIL TRAFFIC: Light

TRAIL SURFACE: Crushed rock, unmaintained field paths, an overgrown but sturdy boardwalk

HIKING TIME: 1.5–2 hours

DRIVING DISTANCE: 34.4 miles north of the Interstate 39 and US 151 juncture

ACCESS: 5 a.m.–10 p.m.

MAPS: USGS Portage; www.dnr.state.wi.us

WHEELCHAIR ACCESSIBILITY: None

FACILITIES: None

SPECIAL COMMENTS: Trail is not marked and in many places undeveloped and even unclear. Wear long pants and proper footwear. A short, ankle-deep portage across a 20-foot low point in the trail may be necessary. This is an excellent birding spot.

IN BRIEF

Explore an overgrown trail along a dike through wetlands to an island of oak savanna surrounded by pockets of marsh and open water. Waterfowl and migratory birds abound.

DESCRIPTION

The difficulty here is not one of inclines, but of not always being able to see the trail, and in some cases, blazing it yourself through general boundaries. There are a couple of features that will discourage the casual walker: overgrown trails, some with plants with burrs or spines; a potential walk through ankle-deep water for a few feet during wet seasons; and in some cases, lack of any real trail at all. These challenges, however, are part of the attraction. Even the short boardwalk is often camouflaged by all the grasses and wildflowers growing up between the planks, but this gives the hiker a feeling of walking, not on water, but at least on marshland.

The Swan Lake Wildlife Area is made up of 1,624 acres predominantly of cattail marshes. This trail follows part of a 1.5-mile dike into the thick of it, then a boardwalk to the "mainland," and then a gravel road out to an island in the middle of it all. You can expect to see sandhill cranes, herons, various species

GPS Trailhead Coordinates

UTM Zone (WGS 84) 16T

Easting 0305666

Northing 4821261

Latitude N 43° 31' 8.42"

Longitude W 89° 24' 16.27"

Directions

From its juncture with US 151, take I-39 north 26.5 miles to where it breaks from Interstate 94 and joins WI 78. Continue north on I-39 another 2.4 miles and take WI 33 right into Portage. Go 2 miles to the intersection with US 51 and go right 2.8 miles to County Road P. Go left 0.7 miles. The parking area is on the left. The trailhead is 0.1 mile farther along County Road P on the left.

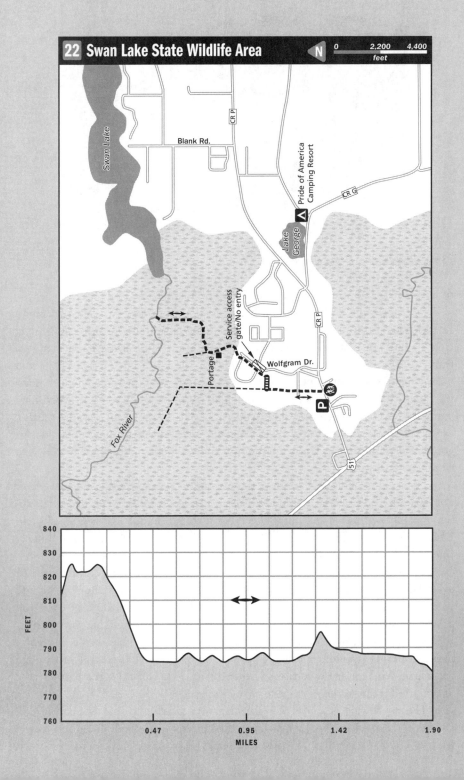

22 Swan Lake State Wildlife Area

N   0   2,200   4,400
feet

Swan Lake

Blank Rd.

CR P

Pride of America Camping Resort

CR G

Lake George

Service access gate/No entry

Portage

Wolfgram Dr.

CR P

Fox River

P

51

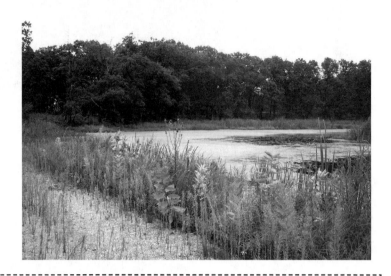

Swan Lake is a haven for waterfowl.

of waterfowl, and other birds, as well as deer, muskrats, and rabbits.

Start from the parking lot and head east 0.1 mile along the edge of County Road P, facing traffic. On your return be sure to pay attention to traffic coming from behind you. Either stay far to the side of the road or cross so that you face traffic for the short distance. The trail begins on the north side of the road behind a large metal gate. Beyond this is a two-tire path through the grassy field following along the line of residences to the right. You will wish you had worn long pants if you come in contact with wild parsley or some of the various thistles, especially when you get to the dike. There are wildflowers through here, a lot of golden rod in particular. Ignore all the spur trails to your right—these merely lead to private backyards.

Locust trees start to take over the terrain as you approach and then enter thick woods and brush at 0.2 miles. The trail is easier to see here, and there are sandy patches. Another 0.2 miles later, pass through the shade of some oaks and then enter the exposed wetlands. To your left is a small pond, and you'll likely find some birds here, perhaps a green heron or some ducks.

The path now follows the dike before you. The trail is not always clear or even there, but the gentle mound of the dike should be apparent. Stay on this and you are fine. You still have a few trees and bushes to your right, but when you pass the last oak tree at about 350 feet along the dike, start watching to your right for the boardwalk, which is only about another 150 feet farther. From that point if you continue straight, the dike continues another 0.75 miles straight through the marsh, where it angles left for another 0.6 miles, coming out at a parking area at Ontario Street on the north side.

The boardwalk is sturdy, but the plant life hides it so that when you look ahead on the path, it always appears as though your path ends about ten feet in front of you. At the end of this 500-foot walkway, you step down into deep grass

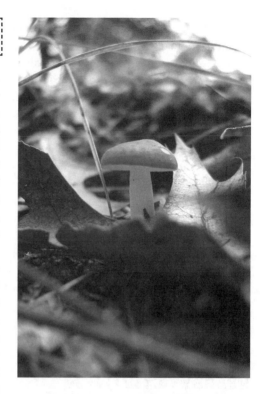

A mushroom appears after a rainy week in August.

and presumably dry, solid earth. Do this carefully because you cannot see where you are stepping. Just a few steps past here is an area of crushed rock and then a gravel road going from right to left. Take a moment to see where you just came out of the grasses and make a mental note. On your return trip, that boardwalk might not be visible from where you'll be standing.

To your right is a service-vehicle access gate and private property. Go left here along the gravel road and enter oak savanna. You may find some spur trails to the right put in illegally by residents off in the neighborhoods east of the area, but stay straight. At 0.4 miles the trail starts to bend left and exits from the woods. A colony of aspen whips line the trail to the left, but to your right, you see right into the marsh with cattails and some open water. As you continue on the gravel road, the aspens taper off, and there, too, you can see all the way west to where the occasional train passes along the edge of the wildlife area just over a mile to your left.

Another 0.1 mile will bring you to a low point in the road where water flows over the gravel to the other side. After heavy rains or in the spring, this might be 20 feet across but no deeper than your ankles. In dry seasons it may take just a running jump to get across. If you don't have waterproof footwear, you might take your shoes off and dry off on the other side.

But this is a nice place to take a break anyway. On the other side is what amounts to an island of woodlands in the midst of the wetlands. Oak savanna meets you here, and to your right is a sort of small bay where waterfowl, such as herons and cranes, might take refuge. Birders will want to find a nice spot among the oaks along the shore to use as a blind.

The path continues on a grassy and perhaps faint vehicle trail into the savanna. Where this trail curves right, you might notice an even fainter trail that continues straight and slightly to the left and takes you out to the edge of the oak savanna along the marsh grasses. This is a nice area to explore as well, offering a view out over the marsh.

The trail herein described follows the path to the right. Some may be content to simply explore the area without continuing to the other side of the "island" 0.7 miles away. The park rules allow you to go anywhere. If you continue on the main trail, you cross a small open field roughly 500 feet from your portage. Stay straight and proceed to the other side, where the corridor through the brush bends left and then right again. It starts to leave the oaks, and a thick impenetrable growth of aspen whips shapes the path. Stay left, following the wall of trees and watching for the corridor in front of you when the clearing widens out a bit. You'll soon come to an open field. Stay left, along those trees and when the aspens taper off, follow the line you are on straight toward another gap in the aspen colony. You will pass a couple of evergreens on your left and walk through a sandy patch. At this point you have no views of the marsh, and it seems less wetlands than an overgrown sandbar. Continuing down the corridor through the aspens, hike through unmowed terrain. Old tire ruts invisible in the tall grass may fill with water or turn an ankle, so be warned.

When you come to a turnaround at the end of the corridor, you see a narrow path through the aspens to the right. Follow it out into the open where there is a trail cut in the grass, most likely made by local critters trying to get close to the water's edge for a drink. This should bring you all the way to the water. This is the Fox River, flowing into Swan Lake to the east, and your turnaround point.

NEARBY ACTIVITIES

Portage hosts a Farmers' Market from 2 p.m. to 6 p.m. on Thursdays in season at Market Square. The 1832 Indian Agency House is on its original site above the Portage Canal, located off WI 33 east of Portage on Agency House Road. It is on the National Register of Historic Places and is open daily for tours from May 15 to October 15 from 10 a.m. to 4 p.m., Sunday from 11 a.m. to 4 p.m. Call (608) 742-6362 for more information.

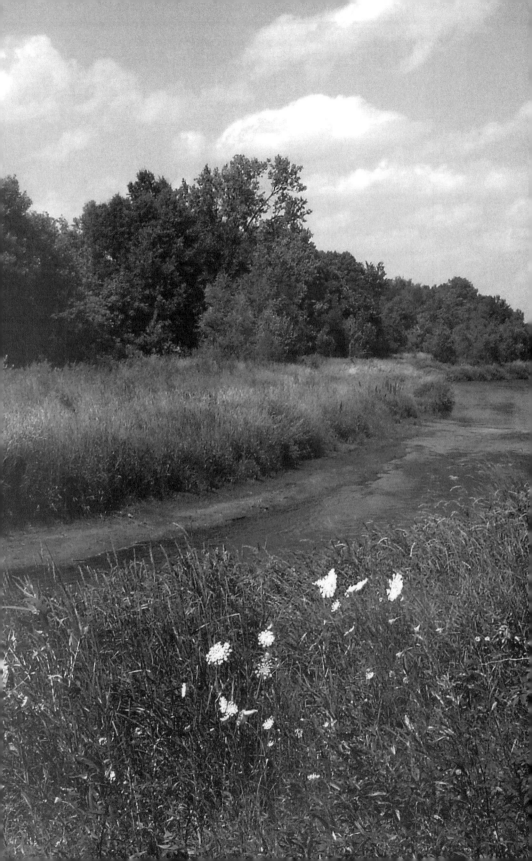

Dane County Trails (23-34)

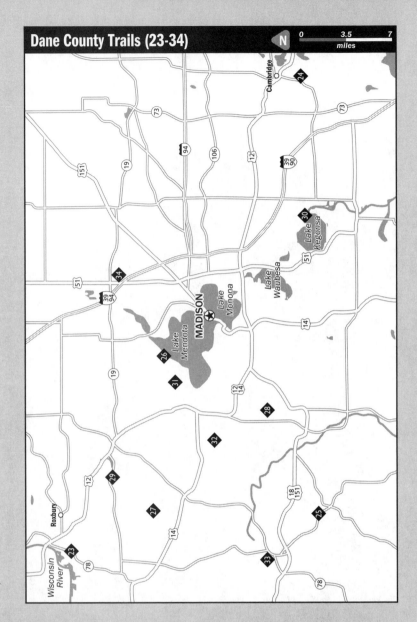

N

0   3.5   7
miles

DANE COUNTY

23 BLACK HAWK UNIT: Lower Wisconsin State Riverway

KEY AT-A-GLANCE INFORMATION

LENGTH: 9.5 miles

CONFIGURATION: Double loop

DIFFICULTY: Easy, moderate, and difficult sections

SCENERY: Mixed forest, prairie, scenic overlooks, effigy mounds

EXPOSURE: Mostly shaded with open prairie sections

TRAIL TRAFFIC: Light

TRAIL SURFACE: Mowed grass, packed dirt, sandy patches, some crushed stone

HIKING TIME: 4 hours

DRIVING DISTANCE: 19.7 miles north from US 14/University Avenue and US 12

ACCESS: 6 a.m.–11 p.m.

MAPS: USGS Black Earth; on map boards at trail junctures and parking lot

WHEELCHAIR ACCESSIBILITY: None

FACILITIES: Portable toilets, shelters, water

SPECIAL COMMENTS: Mosquitoes can be harsh here given the right conditions. Dogs are allowed on leashes except when trails are groomed for skiing.

IN BRIEF

Look out over the Wisconsin River valley from several scenic overlooks as you hike through restored prairies and rich forests with ravines. This is the land where warrior Black Hawk once turned to face the pursuing U.S. Army and militia to buy his people time to escape across the river.

DESCRIPTION

The woods are thick, the prairies full of flowers, and the overlooks show the hilly landscape of the Wisconsin River valley. A spot so beautiful also played witness to a sad bit of history. Black Hawk, a Sauk warrior, led 60 warriors against 700 militia at the Battle of Wisconsin Heights. The bold maneuver—perhaps the only time Black Hawk's band turned around to face the pursuers—was costly to the Native Americans but bought time for nearly 1,000 women, children, and elderly people to cross the Wisconsin River and escape. The success was short-lived, as many were soon slaughtered or drowned at the Battle of Bad Axe, trying to escape across the Mississippi River.

Start up Wachter Road at the special events entryway. The gate is typically closed, and there is a map board next to it. At 0.15 miles go left on a packed-dirt and sand

GPS Trailhead Coordinates

UTM Zone (WGS 84) 16T

Easting   0278390

Northing   4790794

Latitude   N 43° 14' 14.60"

Longitude   W 89° 43' 45.58"

Directions

From its intersection with US 14/University Avenue, take US 12 west 17.5 miles to WI 78. Go left 2.2 miles to find the parking lot on the left where it says WACHTER ROAD. The trailhead is Wachter Road itself from the lot.

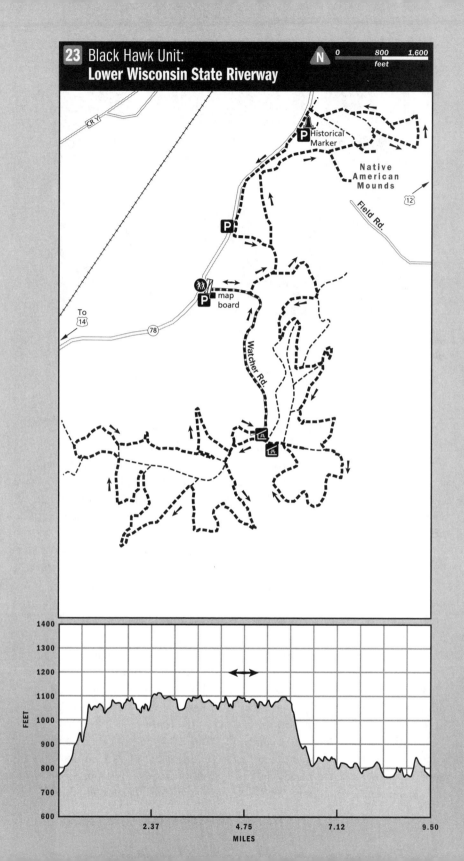

N

0   800   1,600
      feet

CR Y

P Historical
   Marker

Native
American
Mounds

Field Rd.

12

P

To
14

78

map
board

Watcher Rd.

FEET

1400
1300
1200
1100
1000
900
800
700
600

        2.37   4.75   7.12   9.50
                    MILES

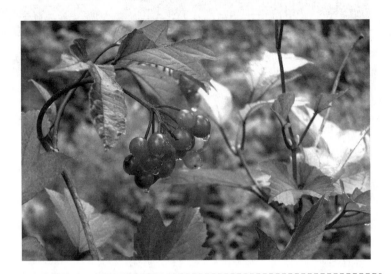

Dew collecting on some berries

footpath into the forest for 0.1 mile, where you will come to a trail juncture. The hike described here divides the park into two halves. Go right for the first giant loop, and then return to this spot to go left for the second loop.

The right path heads 0.3 miles uphill on sandy terrain with pine forest to the left. After the easy pass along the pines, the trail is at its roughest with tree roots, sandy patches, and loose sandstone at a moderate incline. At times the surrounding plants reach into the trail and grab at you as you pass. At 0.3 miles a spur trail goes left into the brush off the official map. It is difficult to see, not maintained, and it follows out along the top of the ridge where it peters out about 0.1 mile into the woods.

Two hundred feet past the spur is an intersection. To the left is private land; go right 0.2 miles, still on dirt and broken rock and a bit steep until you come to a T. Go left on a wide dirt and grass trail. At 0.1 mile the trail rounds a point where a ski trail parts to the right at a map board. Continue straight as the trail curves back around heading south 0.2 miles to another spur trail left. Continue another 300 feet to a clearing. Go straight as a little lollipop trail takes you to what is a scenic overlook when foliage is thin or absent. A sign says as much: TRAIL ENDS AT OVERLOOK. You'll return to this clearing and stay to the leftmost (when returning) path leading out and downhill 0.15 miles to the next juncture with a cutoff trail to the right into the open. There is a map board there as well. Go left and continue down, with nice views to the left.

Another 0.25 miles brings you to the edge of some prairie and a trail that heads to the right over the hill and to the center of the park. Continue straight along the edge of the trees and pass through more woods downhill, round a corner, and come to a small pond with bullfrogs and cattails. From the pond the trail goes left into the woods for a 0.4-mile segment that runs up and down along

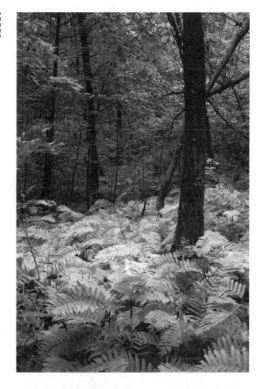

Ferns in the forest

a ravine, briefly passing through open canopy but otherwise shaded. From there head into prairie, passing 0.15 miles through wildflowers to the other end of that prairie cut-off trail you passed earlier at the other end. There's a map here and a straight path that is a ski trail coming down from the hill with the overlook lollipop. Go to the right into the prairie toward a clump of bushes to get the scenic overlook from the top of the hill. Look for the hills of Baraboo and the Wisconsin River valley to the northwest. Double back to the park center and pass a horse pavilion on the left and a boardwalk to the right to another pavilion.

There is a water pump here and portable toilets near a log cabin. Hike past the cabin to the park road. You'll see it heads right and passes a barn off to your right. But go left on mowed paths into prairie. One hundred feet along on your right is your return path to this spot. Go straight another 200 feet to a trail map and juncture of three trails. Go left through prairie surrounded by forest. These paths are easier than the forest trails, with more level surfaces and less of an incline. It's 0.7 miles down this trail to the next juncture. Pass a pond on the left as you come around the back end of the field. There's a nice panorama of the area around you. The path follows the edge of the prairie and heads into trees. At the juncture, go left to follow a 0.8-mile finger loop into the woods. You can also go right here to skip this and the next two similar loops into the forest and head back through prairie to the park center.

When you finish the finger loop, go left at the next juncture to hike the next 0.3-mile loop. A trail to the right allows you to skip it and brings you to that same prairie path that heads east (right) to the park center. At the juncture at the end of this finger loop is a four-way intersection. Right is that prairie path cutoff. Straight continues the larger park loop but cuts off the 0.4-mile loop to the left. Go left on that loop and come to a trail at 0.15 miles that goes left and long out of the park to another park entry. Stay right, and the trail curves right and back, passing a spur trail on the left and continuing to the next juncture, which is the loop's cutoff path on the right. Go left instead, keeping the pines to your right.

There's a scenic overlook on the left at 0.1 mile with two benches on either side of a little clearing. Past here you have 0.6 miles back to the park center bearing left at one trail juncture, which would cut that in half.

Follow the park road past the storage barn 0.7 miles down the hill back to where you first entered the woods near the trailhead (on the right now). Go back into the woods, this time bearing left at the first intersection. This sandy path will take you north 0.1 mile to a juncture. Left goes to another parking lot on WI 78 and is also your return path for this loop. Go straight 0.5 miles on a rolling, grassy trail mostly shaded by thick hardwood forest. Look for some exposed rock above you to the right and wildflowers along the path. You reach a juncture where a trail to the right goes out and back 0.1 mile each way to a collection of Native American effigy mounds.

Returning to this juncture from the mounds, go right (east) another 0.1 mile, pass a trail bearing left, and find a 0.15-mile out-and-back trail on the right steeply climbing to what is an overlook when foliage is down. From the bottom of that spur trail head east (right) another 0.1 mile, crossing a bridge to get to a T juncture. Go right here and take a 0.5-mile turn through brush and then up a ridge to another short spur-trail overlook on the left side of the trail before descending again to the other end of the cutoff trail to your left. The cutoff skips the climb and reduces the distance by 0.4 miles.

From that juncture after your trek over the hill, go to the right, passing a right-bound exit trail to private property and coming 0.1 mile to another juncture. Go right toward the edge of the park along the highway. Another trail goes right to private property; head left along the road 400 feet to a historical marker and wayside. Keep following the trail into the woods running parallel to the highway. Another 0.4 miles takes you to the second parking lot. The trail continues into the woods at the other end 0.15 miles to a juncture you already passed to start this loop. Go right back to Wachter Road, and then go right again down that park road to the original parking lot.

NEARBY ACTIVITIES

Serving deli sandwiches, salads, ice cream, and coffee, and offering a patio overlooking the Wisconsin River, the Blue Spoon Café at 550 Water Street, Prairie du Sac, is a nice place to stop after your hike. Call (608) 643-0837 or go to **www.bluespooncafe.com**.

CAMROCK PARK: Area 2 24

IN BRIEF

A pleasant path through pine and oak forest also takes you on a loop of marvelous prairie restoration and then along the Koshkonong Creek, where it meanders through the wetlands of what was once the Rockdale Millpond.

DESCRIPTION

Many of the hikes in this book expose you to prairie restorations, but this park features a restoration of a different sort. Removal of the Rockdale Dam, which had once held back a large mill pond that flooded much of the area behind the present-day park, allowed the Koshkonong Creek to find its narrow way again. In almost no time at all the resulting mud flats were once again thriving with plant life and abundant wildlife. The removal of the dam has also improved fish migration. One hundred dams have been taken out of Wisconsin waterways since 1967, and in many cases this has meant the restoration of valuable ecosystems.

There are actually three separate parks under the name of CamRock, so be sure you have gone to Area 2. You can view the path on a map board at the trailhead. Enter the woods under a sign across the trail, and at the first fork, go left, following the arrow on a trail sign. The trail follows the direction of the park

---

Directions ———————————➤

From I-39/90/94 follow US 12 14.4 miles east to Cambridge. Halfway through town turn right on CR B and drive 1.9 miles south to the park entrance on the right (west) side. Park in the first parking area on the left side near the entrance. The trailhead is behind you.

KEY AT-A-GLANCE INFORMATION

LENGTH: 2.2 miles

CONFIGURATION: Loop with an embedded loop

DIFFICULTY: Easy

SCENERY: Mixed forest, prairie, wetlands, flowing water

EXPOSURE: Mixed

TRAIL TRAFFIC: Light

TRAIL SURFACE: Packed dirt, mowed grass

HIKING TIME: 1 hour

DRIVING DISTANCE: 16.3 miles east of Interstate 39/90/94 and US 12

ACCESS: 5 a.m.–10 p.m.

MAPS: USGS Rockdale; at trailhead on a map board

WHEELCHAIR ACCESSIBILITY: None

FACILITIES: Shelter, restrooms, water, playground

SPECIAL COMMENTS: Dogs allowed on leashes but with a $3 fee. Biking and cross-country skiing exact trail fees as well. There are three separate sections of park along County Road B, and all of them have trails.

GPS Trailhead Coordinates

UTM Zone (WGS 84) 16T

Easting 0335053

Northing 4760374

Latitude N 42° 58' 41.33"

Longitude W 89° 01' 22.57"

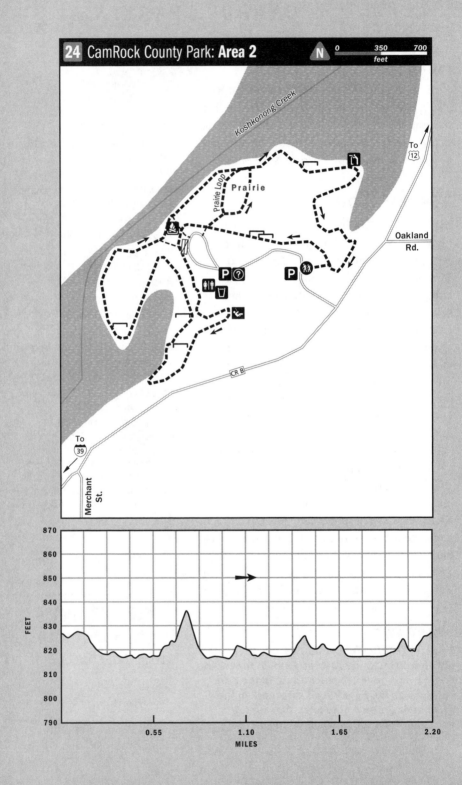

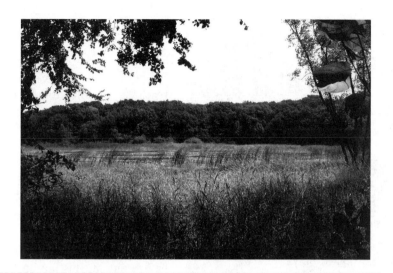

Koshkonong Creek meanders through wetland

road deeper into the park, and within just 400 feet, you pass under a large oak and enter into open prairie with a vast number of restored prairie flowers. Initially the view is blocked by brush and the park road is visible close by on the left. Pass a stand of aspens on your right and a mammoth oak to left, and then the trail becomes grassy as it heads uphill. The field explodes with bergamot, coneflowers, Queen Anne's lace, and black-eyed Susans in the summer months. Crest a small hill and find a couple benches next to a small oak. This is a good vantage point to view the colorful field before you.

Head down the hill on the other side with the prairie to the right. At the next trail intersection, go right as the trail loops 0.2 miles through the prairie and back to this spot. You may find some posted poetry on the trail written by local schoolchildren and inspired by the natural beauty of the park. On the other side of the field, you come to a trail intersection. Go left. This is actually the return trail going right, but take only a few steps until the return of the prairie loop cuts back into the grass and flowers and follows along the edge of the trees. When you come back to the origin of the prairie loop, go right. (The straight path is a stem out to the park road.)

You'll see another trail to the right 200 feet later leading to a clearing around a fire pit. This is also a cutoff trail through to your return trail. To the left is the parking area in the small park-road loop. Just past this trail is a park maintenance road that goes right and also could be a cutoff to the return. A metal gate blocks entry from unauthorized vehicles.

The main trail continues uphill and enters into some Norway pine up to top of hill. A spur trail goes left to the shelter house where you can find restrooms and water. There's also a horseshoe pit and playground in that open mowed area.

Staying on the main trail, pass another cutoff to the right and stay left on a trail carpeted with rust-colored pine needles. Taking the cutoff would shave

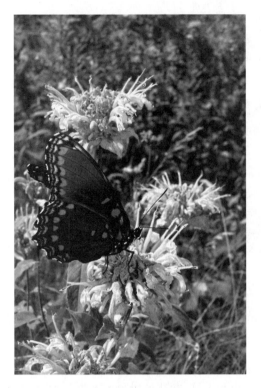

A butterfly in bergamot

0.3 miles off your hike. When you reach an opening to the mowed area, you see a trail marker that points to the right. Follow it; the opening to the left leads out to that playground.

Pine gives way to maple as the trail curves around just inside the park boundary at the county road. There are spur trails out of the park to the left. The path descends easily and at the bottom curves right and switches back. Through the brush to your right, you can see the return trail at a lower level before you reach the curve.

On the return path, look out through the trees to your left to see cattails where once there was a mill pond. Find a bench on the right to enjoy a bit of oak savanna and wetlands beyond, while you can still breathe in the scent of pine trees at your back.

There's a bench at the opposite end of the cutoff trail. Continue past that trail and descend from savanna to the edge of the wetlands. Wildflowers find root here in the shade of the oaks. The path goes down moderately and enters into aspens 200 feet later. The canopy thins here as you come around the bend, but then the trail curls right and heads north into thicker cover. A bench on the right 0.3 miles from the cutoff looks out over cattails and wet prairie. You can see across to the pavilion of CamRock Area 3.

Eight hundred feet beyond this is a mowed area through the brush to the left where you can see out over the muddy banks of the creek. Koshkonong Creek has a bit of current to it, kicking up muddy waters. You can go right to the edge.

At the next trail juncture, you can see straight to the gate at the head of the maintenance road. Go left to stay on the trail. The path follows along the edge of terra firma, while soggier land is just to the left of the narrow line of trees. Pass the cutoff trail on your right that leads back to the fire pit.

You enter prairie once again 0.2 miles from the opening to the creek. Go straight across with the trees and brush to your left, passing the two segments of the prairie loop to your right. Once on the other side of the prairie, the trail goes closer to the edge of the wetlands again, and the brush thins to reveal the marsh beyond. There's a bench facing the marsh, and you can sit with the prairie right up behind you, arguably the better view.

From here the trail is 15 to 20 feet above the level of the wetlands. It enters the woods again, curves right, switches back, and brings you to an observation platform 400 feet down the trail on your left and now at about marsh level. Spend some time here looking for marshland wildlife. The trail turns back toward the county road and follows along the edge of a finger of marsh to your left for another 800 feet. Canadian hawkweed is abundant along here.

The trail turns into the woods once more and follows just shy of the roadway until it brings you back to the first fork you passed near the entry. Go left here to arrive back at the parking lot.

The other two sections of the park offer more trails, although Section 3's paths are aimed more toward mountain bikers.

NEARBY ACTIVITIES

Cambridge is a popular tourist draw with its Victorian storefronts and a surprising collection of shops and galleries. The public beach at Lake Ripley is a good place for a swim after your hike. The town hosts Cambridge Pottery Festival and U.S. Pottery Games the second full weekend in June of each year.

25 DONALD COUNTY PARK

KEY AT-A-GLANCE INFORMATION

LENGTH: 3.4 miles

CONFIGURATION: Lollipop

DIFFICULTY: Easy to moderate

SCENERY: Prairie, flowing water, forest, savanna

EXPOSURE: Half and half

TRAIL TRAFFIC: Light

TRAIL SURFACE: Grass, packed dirt

HIKING TIME: 1.5 hours

DRIVING DISTANCE: 13.3 miles southwest of the Beltline Highway (US 12/18) and Verona Road/ US 18/151

ACCESS: 5 a.m.–10 p.m.

MAPS: USGS Mount Vernon; at trailhead and junctures

WHEELCHAIR ACCESSIBILITY: None

FACILITIES: Pit toilets, shelter, picnic tables

SPECIAL COMMENTS: Dogs require a daily fee ($3; $23 annual) and must be on a leash. There is a self-pay tube in the parking lot.

IN BRIEF

Two good trout streams cross the prairie, and at the edges of the oak-forest hills, you find apple trees and wildflowers.

DESCRIPTION

The Donald/Woodburn family donated the original 105 acres of this park to Dane County. The park has since grown to 480 acres and added a nice picnic area called Pop's Knoll where a shelter and a couple of fire pits rest amid oak savanna. Deer Creek and Frye Feeder, two trout streams, run through the park, crossing prairie and farmland, and the wooded portion of the park climbs a nearby ridge.

From the parking lot go to a service gate in the corner to pick up the trail. To your left is the small hill where the picnic area is. To your right are agricultural fields.

As you walk down the crushed-stone path, you pass pit toilets and a shelter on your left. Then the trail bends right down the hill. You see woods far across the field in front of you and a bit of oak savanna to your left. A stone path leads to the picnic table and fire pit immediately to your right.

Pass under the Pop's Knoll sign after which the trail goes left along the fields and at the bottom of the knoll. Look up to your left

GPS Trailhead Coordinates

UTM Zone (WGS 84) 16T

Easting 0281809

Northing 4759908

Latitude N 42° 57' 38.02"

Longitude W 89° 40' 30.50"

Directions

From the Beltline Highway (US 12/18) go south 7.9 miles on Verona Road/US 8/151 to the exit for County Road G. Go south on CR G 3.5 miles to Messerschmidt Road and go right 1.8 miles to WI 92. Go right just 0.2 miles to the park entrance on the left. At the end of the parking lot to the left is the trailhead at a metal gate.

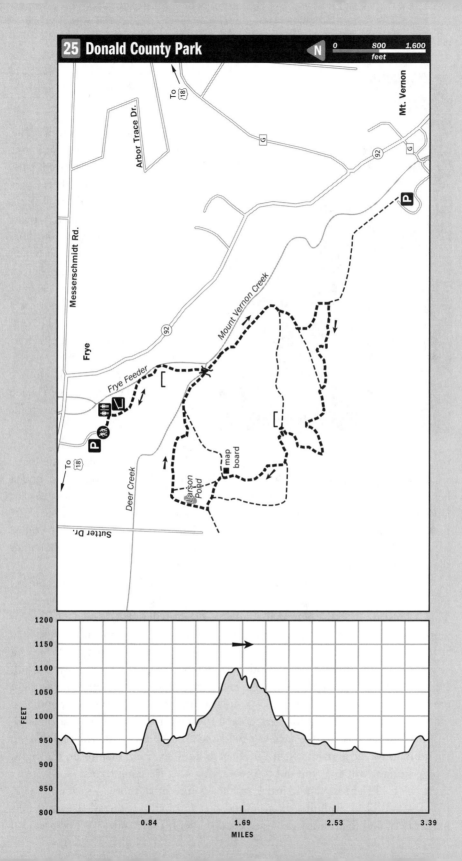

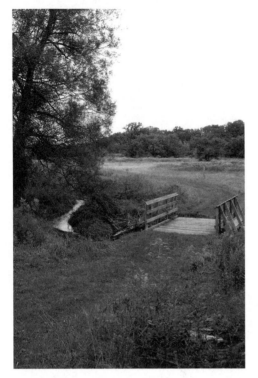

A bridge over Deer Creek

and see some exposed rock. The mowed area ends here, and you begin down a wide mowed path just 0.1 mile from where you started. Just past here the trail starts to follow the small trout stream known as Frye Feeder on your left. Keep following it as the trail bends to the right with its course. Across the stream are a couple of oaks and willows, and the trail bends left again. The stream will take one more big right, and then the trail begins heading toward the woods.

Look for bluebird houses throughout the fields. Frye Feeder will break left, leaving the trail, and just 500 feet later, you cross Deer Creek on a footbridge. The trail slopes up to a trail juncture. This is the beginning and endpoint of the loop. There is a map board across the trail to the left, and to your right you find a bench under an enormous willow. Go left at this intersection, following a two-rut lane closed in by trees but open to the sky. A stand of aspens is to your left. Just past that look for some apple trees that will be pretty in spring and, if you're lucky, might offer a few good munchers in August. The trail is a bit higher than the creek here, and you get a nice view to your left.

The trail curves right 0.3 miles from the map board before a pine plantation, and you come to another juncture as the path curls around the end of the ridge. This is Juncture 2 on the park map, and going right will take you on a cutoff path along the top of the ridge through prairie and eventually into the woods. Stay straight as the trail continues south bending right gently to Juncture 3. Staying straight will cut off some more woods. But for the full trail, go left down the hill. Look for raspberries here in summer, and as you enter into another field, there are some apple trees to the left. Continue through this field, primarily populated with sumac with some wildflowers poking through, to a line of trees at the end. Just beyond them is another farmer's field and a nice view of the rolling hills. Go right along the edge of the field 200 feet to another trail juncture on the right. Going straight will take you out to the parking area for equestrians.

The trail right is at Juncture 4 and heads into mixed forest—primarily oak, hickory, and black walnut—on a packed dirt footpath. The trail rises and falls moderately, and the canopy provides good shade. It is 0.3 miles to Juncture 5 on

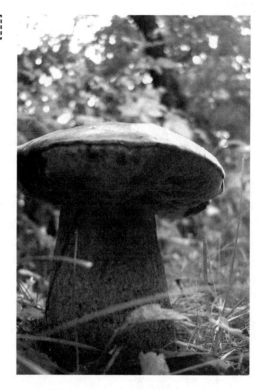

Mushrooms thrive on the damp forest floor.

the park map, and this is where the cutoff from Juncture 3 connects from the right. Stay left. The trail is climbing here and shows some broken rock and tree roots in the surface. Berries may be abundant in midsummer.

The trail winds through thick woods 0.5 miles to Juncture 6, where there's another bench. Go left again, and soon come to a moderate downhill slope with loose rock, sand, and bits of sandstone. It's another 0.1 mile to the next intersection just outside of the woods. Go right, keeping trees to your right and prairie to your left. Another 0.2 miles later, you pass into some tall pines on a trail carpeted with needles over a sandy base. The trail S-curves through and comes back out of woods at Juncture 7, where there's a map board. The trail to the right cuts through prairie and a bit of woods. Go left and pass another spur trail to the right. Stay straight. Soon after there's another trail from the left, which is an alternative trail from where you first exited the woods. This is not on the official park map as of yet. Again stay the course, cross between two low ridges of trees, and come to an arrow directing you to the right. The trail going straight heads out of the park and into private property. Pass some oaks on the right, and just past these is Larson Pond. A short spur trail takes you in closer for a look.

Past the pond at the next trail juncture, go right. Another trail coming in from the right just 200 feet from here is one of the cutoff trails. Stay straight and head back into the woods at 0.1 mile. Find some more pine and then mixed forest with a thick canopy. At 0.2 miles there's a cutoff trail coming in from the right. Stay straight another 0.1 mile as the trail brings you back to the bridge to complete the loop. Cross the bridge again and retrace your steps to Pop's Knoll and the parking lot.

NEARBY ACTIVITIES

Put back any calories you may have burned by stopping in at the world-class Candinas Chocolatier in Verona. To find out more about their decadent delights, call (800) 845-1554 or visit **www.candinas.com**.

26 GOVERNOR NELSON STATE PARK

KEY AT-A-GLANCE INFORMATION

LENGTH: 3.9 miles
CONFIGURATION: Loop
DIFFICULTY: Easy to moderate
SCENERY: Mixed forest, effigy mounds, savanna, prairie, wetlands, stream, lakeshore
EXPOSURE: Mostly sun, parts shaded
TRAIL TRAFFIC: Light
TRAIL SURFACE: Grass
HIKING TIME: 2 hours
DRIVING DISTANCE: 4.8 miles from University Avenue and Allen Boulevard
ACCESS: 6 a.m.–11 p.m. year-round
MAPS: USGS Waunakee; at trailheads and park office
WHEELCHAIR ACCESSIBILITY: Red-Tailed Hawk Trail and a viewing platform and along beach area
FACILITIES: Restrooms, boat landings, fish cleaning station, vending machines, water, pay phones
SPECIAL COMMENTS: There is a designated dog swim area; otherwise your pet must be on a leash. Carryout garbage and recycle bags are available at trailheads. A state park vehicle registration sticker is required. Hiking is not allowed when cross-country skiing is possible. Bikes are not allowed.

IN BRIEF

Explore forest, prairie, savanna, and marshes on the north side of Lake Mendota and take a swim at the beach afterward with a view of the city across the water.

DESCRIPTION

Former Wisconsin Governor and U.S. Senator Gaylord Nelson is perhaps best known as the founder of Earth Day. A passionate environmentalist, he also helped establish the Apostle Islands as a national lakeshore. This 422-acre state park that bears his name sits across the lake from Madison and is easily accessible.

There are several separate trails throughout the park and in total there are 8.4 miles. The selected course starts with the Woodland Trail and takes you through each of the ecological areas. From the northwest corner of the overflow lot, find a map board with nature guides. An access road goes straight past this, but find the trail heading into the woods to your right on a surface of crushed stone.

Boulders are scattered amongst the trees, and flowering bushes and wildflowers are abundant along path. The understory here is thick and offers no views deeper into the woods.

GPS Trailhead Coordinates

UTM Zone (WGS 84)   16T

Easting   0301833

Northing   4778193

Latitude   N 43° 07' 49.96"

Longitude W 89° 26' 10.90"

Directions ⟶

From University Avenue on the far west side of Madison, go north on Allen Boulevard 1 mile to Century Avenue. Go right at the traffic light; after almost 1 mile, this becomes County Road M. Stay on this for 3.8 miles from Allen to arrive at the park entrance on your right. Enter the park and follow the road to the very last parking lot—the overflow lot—on your left. The trailhead is at the right corner of the lot near the entrance.

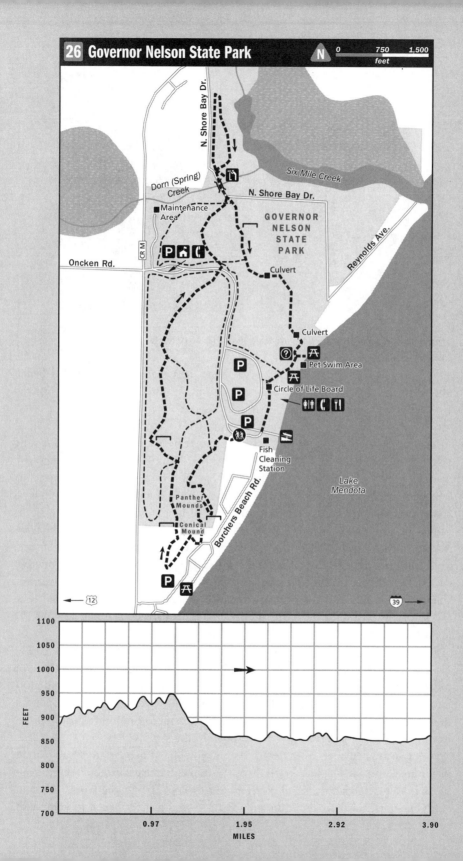

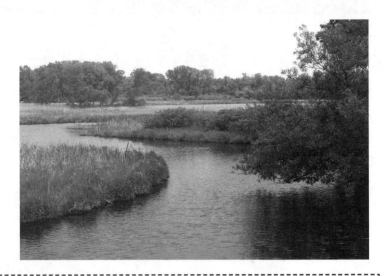

Sometimes known as Spring Creek, Dorn Creek flows to Lake Mendota.

The trail turns to wood chips less than 100 feet in. You'll find a bench 600 feet from the trailhead and also a trail to the right. This is the return for the 1.8-mile Woodland Trail loop. Go straight instead.

The trail is wide and slightly uneven, tilting to the left in some places. After a couple of bends, take the small loop trail left to see a 358-foot long Native American mound shaped like a panther. The 800-foot loop takes you through plenty of wildflowers and yet only about 100 feet from residences just outside the park. Where this trail makes the turn to the right, find a bench with a small overhang. On the left side of the trail beyond a wooden fence is the beginning of the mound, which runs parallel all the way back to the main trail. Ancient effigy mounds were built over long periods of time. Most are conical or linear, but this one is apparently a panther. Mounds may have marked boundaries or events or could have been used to communicate to ancestors. They are still sacred to local tribes and thus protected by law. Stop and read the information board at the end of the trail before continuing left on the main trail.

The trail passes through a row of conical mounds 800 feet from here. The Ho-Chunk Nation occupied this area, which connected major communities via trails linking Mendota, Monona, Dejope, Waubesa, and Kegonsa. You'll find more information and a bench right before the mounds. A wooden fence runs alongside the path and then ends where the trail cuts left from the mounds. Just 300 feet from here is a sandy patch and an area open to the sky.

A spur trail cuts left from here and takes you out of the park to a public road, picnic area, and parking lot. Stay right as the trail curves back around the right and starts heading north to a small clearing and then back into the trees. The trail, sandy in spots, starts to climb the hill, and you find a short bench to your right.

Go to the top of the hill where there are four viewing benches and a memorial rock. The view from here over the trees to the right is quite nice, and a few shade trees make this a perfect place to take a break.

From this clearing there are three trails to the left. The far left trail is part of the Oak Savanna trail and heads south before turning west to run right along the highway. The far right trail is the last section of the Woodland Trail and intersects with Red-Tailed Hawk Trail before returning to the juncture you passed at the beginning of this hike. The central of the three trailheads is yours, and it climbs a steep hill in the sun. This is also Oak Savanna Trail, heading north as it bypasses the last portion of forest. It's listed as the most difficult trail for its rolling hills. Swallows follow you along a wide, mowed path, and some of the birdhouses may be occupied by bluebirds. You can still see and hear the highway from your trail, but it is not so distracting. The name Oak Savanna may be puzzling since you won't see any oaks out here. Current efforts are making headway to remove non-native plants and reclaim the area as savanna.

As you come over the next smaller hill, there's a bench. To the left the road actually disappears behind the hill, and you can see farmland to the north. To the south is the forest you've left. You may see alternative trails that do not follow the map; these are cut by the park for various purposes from time to time and often connect to the trail along the highway.

As you cross the prairie, you come to where Red-Tailed Hawk Trail shares the path, continuing on in the direction of the park office, forward and to the left of the trail line. Stay left and watch for the trail's namesake. Right next to the trail juncture, look up prairie plants on an informational sign or take a rest on a bench. You can find compass plant, prairie smoke, bergamot, blue stems, Indian grass, yellow coneflower, prairie shrub, and many other wildflowers nearby. July shows a profusion of purple, and milkweed grows just behind the bench.

Just before the park road, the trail crosses the path along the road. Exit through the gate and cross the road to pick up the trail again. You are now on Morningside Trail, which goes directly left to the office—where you'll find a phone, restrooms, parking, and an ATM—and then around the edge of the prairie past a maintenance building, or directly back to the parking lots and picnic area. There is sometimes a mowed path straight across the field as well. Take a soft left to follow a branch of Morningside Trail (the right one of the two on the left, which are labeled such).

The trail makes a right-bearing curve across the field a quarter mile through open prairie. Some small trees and shrubs start to appear in the field just past the halfway mark. The next intersection offers a trail going left back along the maintenance area trail. Stay right instead until you come to an exit from the park that goes to the left. There is a small stop sign here. Cross the road, heading toward a bridge; don't take the private drive to the right. Stay on the right side of the road, cross the bridge over Dorn (Spring) Creek, and watch for waterfowl below. This creek feeds into the larger Six Mile Creek farther to your right and then into the lake 0.6 miles from the bridge. On the other side of Dorn Creek, the trail descends to the right from the shoulder of the road.

Go left at the trail juncture if you want to add another 0.5 miles to your hike. The trail follows the road and loops out through the prairie marsh and returns to this spot. The best viewing of waterfowl will be here at the platform to your right as the trail cannot get close to the marshes on that loop. You hear more than you can see at that point as brush rises up on both sides of the trail and a line of trees stands between you and the marsh.

The observation deck is wheelchair accessible and looks out over DornCreek and also Six Mile Creek farther off to the left. An informational sign can help you identify nearby plants such as white turtle head, joe-pye weed, duckweeds, horsetails, cattails, great blue lobelia, and arrow-leaf violets. Backtrack to the park and go left once you cross the private drive entrance and reenter the park.

At a juncture where a trail cuts right back to the trail across the center of the prairie, go straight and enter oak savanna worthy of the name. To the left of the trees, cattails grow out of the marsh. Pass a bench and then come out into the sun again. A trail goes right, but stay the course. Pass a stand of oaks to the left, and then follow the turn as it goes left into scrub brush. Around the bend, look for the skeleton of a dead tree. Cross a metal culvert and plastic posts and beyond that, a patch of willows to the right.

Follow the trail another 0.2 miles as the brush and forest thicken up around you, blocking views in all directions, but granting no shade to the trail. At the end of this segment, the trail passes over another culvert. Eighty feet past this, the trail goes right at a trail post and comes into the shade of some maples.

Here to your left is the pet swim area where there is a small beach and some picnic tables. A map board stands where the trail cuts to the beach.

Continuing past the swim area another 400 feet brings you out of the woods and to the Indianola Beach Playground/Picnic and Concession Area. The path right goes to a parking area and continues as Morningside Trail. There are actually two trails to the left, but one is just a service road and angles back. Stay on the asphalt path to the left. No pets are allowed beyond this point. This area is Indianola Beach, which hosts a concession stand in the summer. Restrooms, a playground, a pay phone, volleyball nets, and a sandy beach round out the offerings. A sign alongside the trail explains the Ho-Chunk circle of life and seasons.

After a dip in Lake Mendota, continue down the asphalt path to get to all the parking lots. If you parked in the overflow lot, you need to follow this to the end, where you also find a boat landing and a fish cleaning station to the left.

NEARBY ACTIVITIES

Just a few miles southwest of Governor Nelson State Park is Mendota Park situated off County Highway M near the intersection of County Highways Q and M near Middleton. The park has 30 campsites and two shelter facilities.

ICE AGE TRAIL: Table Bluff Segment   27

IN BRIEF

Enjoy some rather stunning prairie reclamation where wildflowers abound, then hike over hills and farmland to a scenic overlook.

DESCRIPTION

This segment of the Ice Age Trail opened in fall of 2006, and the prairie segments are awash with color when the wildflowers are in bloom. The trail is marked with posts with arrows or trees with plastic yellow patches, and maintained by volunteers. The parking lot is a grassy area along the south side of the road surrounded by several large rocks. The trailhead is clearly marked.

Start along a mowed path through prairie, which soon gives way to a bit of oak savanna. Far to your right is a red barn and farmhouse. The trail heads down the hill into a small hollow and climbs back up at a moderate grade. You may come across some other mowed paths, but these are merely firebreaks. This next stretch of prairie is the best of the bunch, over-flowing—especially in the summer—with a wide range of native wildflowers: wild berga-mot, black-eyed Susans, gray-headed and pur-ple coneflowers, false sunflowers, Culver's root, and butterfly weed, just to name a few.

On the other side of this 0.2-mile section, the trail heads into the forest predominantly

KEY AT-A-GLANCE INFORMATION

LENGTH: 5 miles

CONFIGURATION: Out-and-back

DIFFICULTY: Moderate to difficult

SCENERY: Prairie, bluffs, mixed forest, farmland and a scenic overlook

EXPOSURE: Half and half

TRAIL TRAFFIC: Light

TRAIL SURFACE: Mowed grass, packed dirt, rugged

HIKING TIME: 2 hours

DRIVING DISTANCE: 8.3 miles west of the intersection of US 14 and 12

ACCESS: Year-round, but the privately owned section is closed during the nine-day gun hunting season in November.

MAPS: USGS Black Earth

WHEELCHAIR ACCESSIBILITY: None

FACILITIES: Pavilion, portable toilet

SPECIAL COMMENTS: Dogs are allowed on leashes. Much of this terrain is private land, and the limited facilities are privately owned, as well, though available for use.

Directions

Go west on US 14 8.3 miles from where it crosses US 12. Just past Cross Plains, take County Road KP north 2.4 miles to Table Bluff Road. Go left 0.3 miles to the small grass parking area and trailhead on the left side of the road.

GPS Trailhead Coordinates

UTM Zone (WGS 84)   16T

Easting   0282847

Northing   4780274

Latitude   N 43° 08' 38.59"

Longitude   W 89° 40' 13.29"

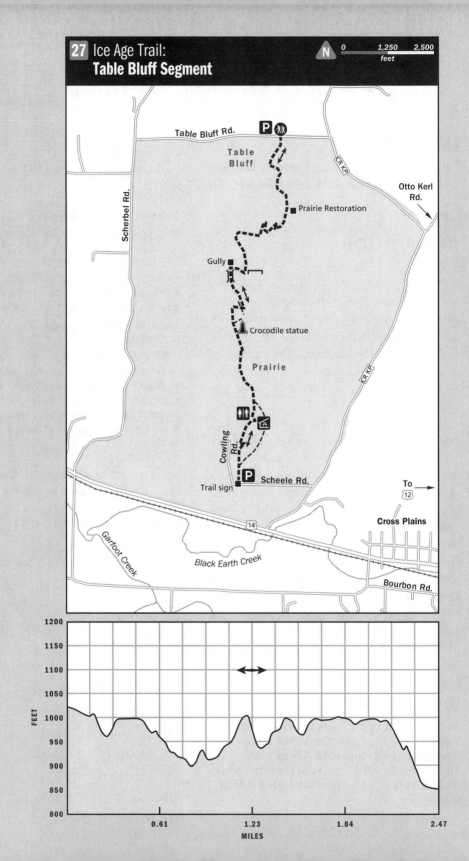

27 Ice Age Trail:
Table Bluff Segment

N 0   1,250   2,500
          feet

Table Bluff Rd.

Table
Bluff

CR KP

Otto Kerl
Rd.

Prairie Restoration

Scherbel Rd.

Gully

Crocodile statue

Prairie

CR KP

Cowling Rd.

Scheele Rd.

Trail sign

P

To
12

Cross Plains

14

Garfoot Creek

Black Earth Creek

Bourbon Rd.

1200
1150
1100
1050
1000
950
900
850
800

FEET

0.61   1.23   1.84   2.47
MILES

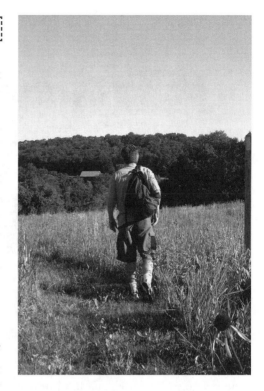

Hiking through prairie flowers

populated with hickory and oak along a rough dirt path. You are skirting a ridge that slopes to the left into thick underbrush. Watch for rocks and tree roots on the trail.

After a switchback the trail surface is not always level and sometimes slopes right with the hill itself. You come to a curve with a fence to your left. The trail goes right out of the woods under a large maple. To the left is private property, so do not take the trail there that may be the most obvious path, depending on recent maintenance or traffic. Stay right, and if the grass is overgrown, look straight ahead for the post with the yellow patch on it that marks the trail. Cross here along the edge of a farmer's field until you reach scattered trees. A trail marker indicates left. At the other side of this small clearing, head back into the woods.

A sign here explains the conditions laid out so that we the public could have access to this segment of the trail. Private owners have granted an easement that does not allow motorized vehicles. You may, however, come across people associated with the property owners who are allowed to use vehicles here. The segment from this point to the southern end of the trail is closed during deer hunting season in November.

The trail climbs over packed dirt with a slope to the left, and in some places rocks have been laid at the edge to maintain the trail and prevent erosion. At the crest of the hill, there is a bench on the left. This area is more open like savanna but then becomes thick woods again for the descent. The trail crosses a gully at the bottom and then bears left along a barbed-wire fence. There is a small rise and another descent that brings you to a small wooden bridge with railings over another gully with a bit of water running through it. From here the trail heads up again.

Listen for the outbursts of crows, maybe the screech of a hawk over the nearby prairies if you're lucky. There are patches of fern here, and since the understory is thick, you may hear more deer than you see. Just past the summit of this next bluff, a private access road crosses the path. Keep straight and watch for the trail post there. Stands of aspen start to appear in the surrounding woods,

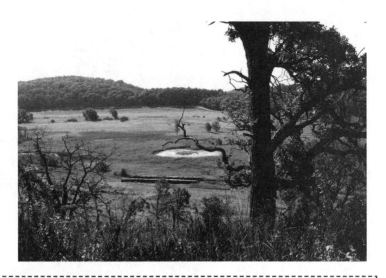

A scenic overlook along the trail

as well as much smaller oaks and hickory than before.

Don't be startled by a small bikini-clad crocodile (or is it an alligator?) lounging to the left side of the path. Just beyond this the trail joins an access road and goes right on a wide, two-tire path through the woods. Come around the bend into a small clearing and head straight across.

It is breezier up here along the top of the bluff, and you enter another patch of prairie full of wildflowers. Pass along its right side and enter into partial shade where in July, you'll find lots of raspberries and black caps.

Oak-hickory savanna holds the top of the hill, and as you pass through the grassy area beneath the trees, you get a bit of sunlight. Emerging around you is the view of the rolling topography of the Driftless Area below and in the distance. Farms poke up from forested areas tucked among hills and swatches of cornfields.

A fork in the trail gives you a crushed-stone private road going left down the hill and its switchback to the clearing at the top. Stay right on this and watch for the trail marker straight ahead just beyond and to the left of a couple of large oaks.

There's often a portable toilet here to the right in this clearing as you come out of the trees, and to the left is a pavilion with picnic tables, which the property owners have kindly allowed hikers to use so long as they do so responsibly. The owners reserve the right to unobstructed use. There are receptacles for trash and recyclables. The view of the surrounding land from the top of this hill is wonderful.

Continue walking heading into tall grass and scattered oaks. To your left and below is some marshland and a couple of ponds. The path is steep through oaks with rocky outcroppings to the left often blocking the view. When you come to a private land sign to the right, bear left and the trail will appear to come to the edge of a cliff. Until you are right upon it, you don't see the path that switches back on dirt and scattered stones, keeping the outcroppings to the left and wildflowers to the right. This is the most charming spot on the trail. Stone steps help you make the next switchback. The trail descends back across the ridge to an arrow that sends you straight down the hill past some smaller oaks. Take the short boardwalk across a marshy spot to the access the road from the southern end of the trail segment. A cable across the road prevents car access. The road up to the left is private.

This access road, with prairie grass to the right and cattails to the left, leads to Scheele Road. Left from there leads to CR KP. You can park here as well as along the east side of the road—maybe you'll have a second car to do the trail one way—but hikers are encouraged to use the designated lot at the trailhead on Table Bluff Road. A map here shows you the way to the northern end.

Eventually this trail connects to the nearby Cross Plains segment of the Ice Age Trail.

NEARBY ACTIVITIES

Arguably the best shoe store in the Madison area and a good source for hiking boots is The Shoe Box in nearby Black Earth on US 14 and Mills Street. Stop by or call (608) 767-3447.

28 ICE AGE TRAIL: Verona Segment

 KEY AT-A-GLANCE INFORMATION

LENGTH: 6.5 miles each way

CONFIGURATION: One way or out-and-back

DIFFICULTY: Easy to moderate

SCENERY: Prairie, woodlands, some suburban overlooks, flowing water, ponds

EXPOSURE: Some shaded portions, a lot of sun

TRAIL TRAFFIC: Light

TRAIL SURFACE: Packed dirt with tree roots, mowed paths

HIKING TIME: 2.5 hours each way

DRIVING DISTANCE: 4.2 miles southwest of Verona Road/ US 18/151 and the Beltline Highway (US 12/14)

ACCESS: Open year-round

MAPS: USGS Verona; *Ice Age Trail Companion Atlas;* sometimes in map box at Military Ridge State Trail parking lot

WHEELCHAIR ACCESSIBILITY: None

FACILITIES: Restrooms and water at Reddan Soccer Fields in Verona and Badger Prairie Park; parking at trailhead, Military Ridge State Trail, and Prairie Moraine County Park

SPECIAL COMMENTS: Be prepared for mosquitoes along Badger Mill Creek, and some of the wooded sections might call for long pants due to scratching foliage.

- -

GPS Trailhead Coordinates

UTM Zone (WGS 84) 16T

Easting 0294620

Northing 4765627

Latitude N 43° 00' 56.08"

Longitude W 89° 31' 13.14"

IN BRIEF

Climb through prairie restoration overlooking Verona, cross through suburbia in the shelter of woods, and follow a creek on this portion of the Ice Age Scenic Trail, which ends in a popular dog park.

DESCRIPTION

From the parking lot there is a wooden sign over the trailhead close to the road. The trail starts out going west along the edge of CR PD for 0.1 mile then breaks left along private property for 200 feet where it goes right across the back of a residence and then heads due south with long-needled pines to the right and prairie to the left for 0.2 miles. Throughout the trail follow the posts and trees marked with yellow patches. You'll find bike trails and spur trails, but the Ice Age Trail is clearly marked.

You come to where the trail bends left, and there is an optional path via the prairie to the left that will skirt around the woods here. The main trail, however, heads into the trees under thick canopy and gently downhill. The packed-dirt footpath is narrow and uneven. At the peak of summer, thorny raspberry bushes may run rampant, and you are going to want to wear pants through here or take the prairie pass around it.

- -

Directions ⟶

Go 1.8 miles southwest on Verona Road/ US 18/151 from where it intersects with the Beltline Highway (US 12/14). Go 2.4 miles west on County Road PD to the parking area on the left. The trailhead is at the northwestern corner of the lot.

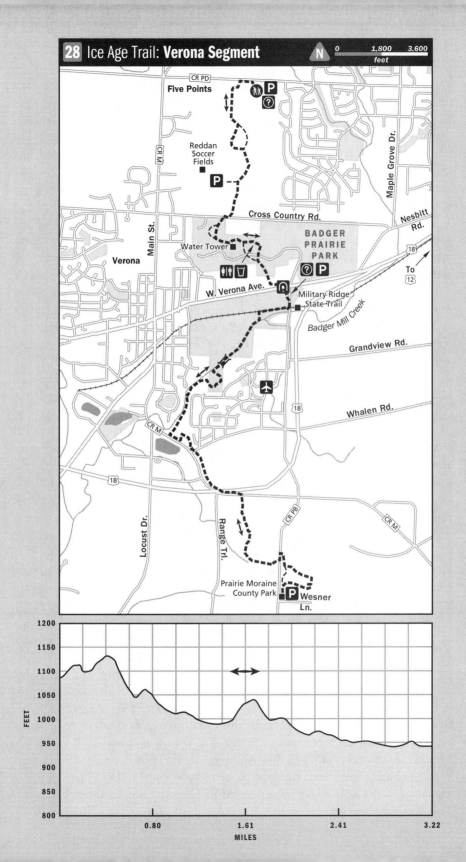

N

0   1,800   3,600
feet

CR PD
Five Points

P

Reddan
Soccer
Fields

P

Maple Grove Dr.

CR M

Cross Country Rd.

Nesbitt
Rd.

18

**BADGER
PRAIRIE
PARK**

Water Tower

Verona

Main St.

P

To
12

W. Verona Ave.

Military Ridge
State Trail

Badger Mill Creek

Grandview Rd.

18

Whalen Rd.

CR M

Locust Dr.

Range Trl.

CR PB

CR M

18

Prairie Moraine
County Park

P Wesner
Ln.

1200
1150
1100
1050
1000
950
900
850
800

FEET

0.80   1.61   2.41   3.22
MILES

At 0.2 miles you come back out of the woods at Reddan Soccer Park. Go left up into prairie where the trail meets the bypass trail coming from the left. Go right here and pass 0.5 miles through prairie rich with native wildflowers and grasses. Pass a spur trail to the right to the trailhead in Reddan Soccer Fields where you find parking, water, and restrooms. Past this, cross a service road, and then come to Cross Country Road. Go right along the wooden fence by the soccer field until you come to an opening marked with a trail sign. Cross the street directly and find a similar gate through the wire fence there.

From here the trail angles slightly to the right. When grasses are short and paths are in need of mowing, you may have to rely on trail posts. The Verona Library is visible far ahead off to the right. At 0.2 miles the trail turns up the hill and starts heading southeast on a line to a water tower on top of the hill.

You pass a bench and come to a juncture. Going straight takes you to the tower. Go left here and the trail soon joins a two-tire path of crushed rock that curves right around the crown of the hill. At the next juncture another trail goes right to the tower and two bike trails head left into the flowers. Stay straight here as the trail leaves the crushed-rock service road and heads into tall grass.

Another 0.1 mile brings you to Badger Prairie Park where there's a playground, parking, and restrooms on your right. The trail bends slightly to the right, goes under the big wooden Ice Age Trail sign, and follows along the parking lot until it crosses the park road. The path continues 0.2 miles more, angling left a bit and crossing a field and an old asphalt road before ducking under some apple trees and arriving at Verona Avenue. There is a storm sewer straight ahead under the road. Go left alongside the road in the grass and look up ahead for a small brick building at the roadside 0.1 mile away. Steps inside will take you down to a tunnel under the highway. The lightbulbs are often broken but there is ambient light at either end, and the tunnel is short.

On the other side go straight to the parking area for the Military Ridge State Trail and Ice Age Trail. There's information about the former Dane County "Poor Farm" that was once nearby. Follow along the asphalt path at the edge of the lot past a map board and picnic tables. There is a map box for this trail to your right.

Continue a short way down the asphalt trail to cross a culvert and go right on the Military Ridge State Trail. Hikers do not need to pay a trail fee, but bikers do. You'll follow the old rail bed 0.2 miles and cross a bridge before the trail goes left through grass and brush and starts south along Badger Mill Creek on the left and unrestored prairie and agricultural fields to the right. This continues for 0.4 miles, and then you'll pass a bat house on the right and enter a stand of pine. Cross the creek on a wooden bridge with metal railings as the trail goes right a short distance to another wooden bridge that crosses another smaller channel. Mosquitoes can get pretty bad through here.

The trail shows some crushed rock in a few low places, but otherwise it can get rather soupy after heavy rains from Military Ridge Trail to County Road M. The next 0.5 miles gives no cover. You see a lot of grass, pine, and aspen to the right, and just brush to the left until you come to a wooden gate. To your right is a covered wooden bridge and residences are on both sides of the trail, but set back from the narrow corridor of woods and the creek, which is still on your right. Go straight across through the next gate and continue another 0.4 miles through shadeless brush until you come to CR M. Go left here without crossing the road and watch for the trail signs as you circumnavigate a landfill. The trail goes left, taking a small loop around the field just past the piles of back fill. The trail comes back to the roadside and looks like it goes through someone's backyard past their wooden fences. It does not, in fact. Stay along the road or in the ditch as you head to the corner of CR M and Whalen Road straight ahead.

Cross Whalen Road to the opposite sidewalk and then go slightly left and up a hill with a water tower. You'll pass a fireplug on the left near the top. Look right and over the view of condos. Facing the road you can see Blue Mound at 1 o'clock in the distance on a clear day.

The trail continues and just descends down the other end of this 0.2-mile ridge. You again pass through a ditch, following trail posts along CR M. The trail uses a wide sidewalk on the overpass to get across US 18/151. At the end of the guardrail at the other side, the trail goes left to the left side of the power lines.

It runs alongside what is still CR M for just over another 0.1 mile before crossing to the right where you can see an electrical box and a trail sign. The trail leaves the roadside and crosses into a low-lying field with a residence and trees to the right. Just 0.1 mile brings you to standing water on your right and a trail that bears left into the woods.

Cross a wooden bridge just inside the trees to another stagnant pond to the left. Another 0.1 mile brings you to a small land bridge through another low area, and then you pass through apple trees to agricultural fields. Go left to the corner of the field and the trail bends right and follows along the edge of the trees. At the corner is a fence to keep you on course. From the turn the trail crosses 0.2 miles through the field to a narrow band of oak-hickory, where it ducks in and ducks back out on the other side and goes left. It follows along another farm field. Deer can be abundant here when corn is planted.

It's only another 250 feet to the woods where the trail heads uphill moderately on a narrow footpath for another 0.2 miles before exiting the trees down a short slope to County Road PB. Go left along the road facing traffic and watch for a Do Not Enter road sign with a small yellow patch on the post. Cross to your right here and pick up the trail on the other side.

Just inside the woods, the trail goes right with scattered rocks and tree roots. CR PB is not far to the right, and a rusty fence keeps you on track from the left. This wooded stretch only lasts another 0.1 mile, and then the trail heads into the open to the left and takes a gentle curve to the right, passing under an enormous oak before heading out through oak savanna and prairie.

From the oak it is 0.2 miles to the crest of the hill, where you will find a trail juncture where the Ice Age Trail will continue in the future. Go right to a trail that goes left to the dog exercise area. On your right is a bench overlooking the prairie. Go right 0.3 miles to the parking area at Prairie Moraine County Park, possibly the most popular dog park in the area. If you are planning on using two vehicles to make this a one-way hike, this is the place to park, where CR PB meets Wesner Lane just 1 mile south of US 18/151.

NEARBY ACTIVITIES

Stop in for a treat at Michael's Frozen Custard at 407 West Verona Avenue in Verona. Call (608) 845-8887 or go online and see their flavor calendar at **www.ilovemichaels.com.**

INDIAN LAKE COUNTY PARK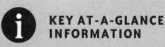

IN BRIEF

Sign in as a visitor in a historic chapel on a bluff overlooking a small lake and then hike parts of the Ice Age Trail and local ski trails over rolling hills.

DESCRIPTION

In the winter of 1856, John Endres and his entire family became infected with diphtheria during an epidemic in southern Wisconsin. The disease was especially dangerous for children, and Endres climbed to the top of the hill above their home and prayed, promising that if his family survived, he would construct a chapel there. Indeed everyone survived, and Mr. Endres made good on his promise and in 1857, constructed the tiny St. Mary of the Oaks, containing an altar with a praying Virgin Mary, a picture of Jesus, and various other religious objects. Hikers can—and often do—sign the guest book there.

It is arguably the main attraction at this 453-acre county park where a portion of the Ice Age Trail skirts a small lake left by retreating glaciers. In fact, a segment of the Ice Age Trail is also located in this park, and the path I mapped out contains a portion of that in addition to some of the great trails deeper in the woods.

KEY AT-A-GLANCE INFORMATION

LENGTH: 4.7 miles

CONFIGURATION: Loop

DIFFICULTY: Easy to moderate

SCENERY: Hilly woods, a historic chapel, prairie, and a small lake

EXPOSURE: Half shaded, half exposed

TRAIL TRAFFIC: Light

TRAIL SURFACE: Grass, packed dirt

HIKING TIME: 2–2.5 hours

DRIVING DISTANCE: 2.2 miles west on WI 19 from US12

ACCESS: 7 a.m.–10 p.m.

MAPS: USGS Black Earth and Springfield Corners; map board at trailhead

WHEELCHAIR ACCESSIBILITY: Grassy paths around the lake

FACILITIES: Restrooms, pavilion, picnic tables

SPECIAL COMMENTS: Dogs can be unleashed in the designated area, but owners must pay a fee at self-pay station in the parking lot to the west just off the highway. Portions of this park are part of the Ice Age Trail, and the cross-country skiing trails are excellent and challenging.

Directions

Take US 12 north from Madison to WI 19. Go west 2.2 miles to the park entrance on the left. Follow the park road 0.4 miles to the parking lot. The trailhead to the Ice Age Trail is straight at the end of the lot near a map board. This hike, however, starts to the east of the lot at the bottom of steps that disappear into the woods.

GPS Trailhead Coordinates

UTM Zone (WGS 84) 16T

Easting 0287065

Northing 4785192

Latitude N 43° 11' 22.18"

Longitude W 89° 37' 13.57"

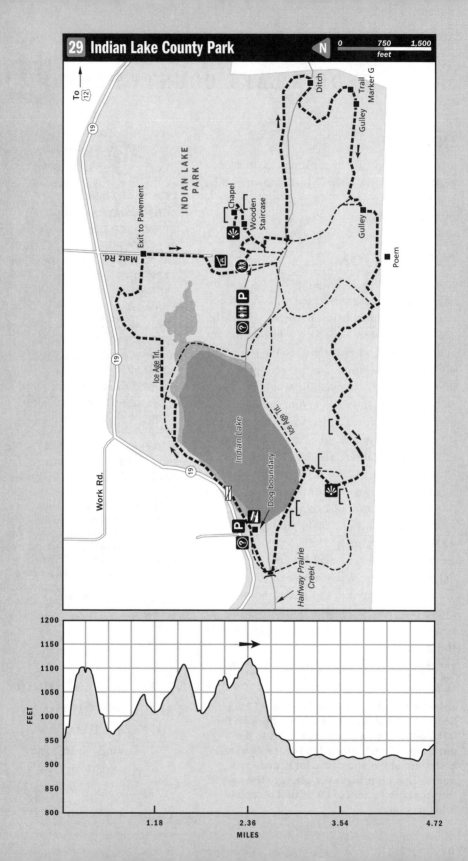

29 Indian Lake County Park

N

0   750   1,500
feet

To 12

19

INDIAN LAKE PARK

Exit to Pavement

Matz Rd.

Chapel

Wooden Staircase

P

Ice Age Trl.

Ice Age Trl.

Indian Lake

Dog boundary

P

Work Rd.

19

19

Halfway Prairie Creek

Ditch

Trail Marker G

Gulley

Gulley

Poem

FEET

1200
1150
1100
1050
1000
950
900
850
800

1.18   2.36   3.54   4.72

MILES

St. Mary of the Oaks Chapel

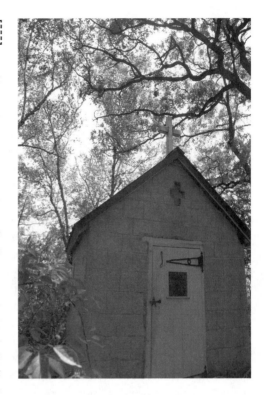

In the parking lot there are pit toilets, and nearby is a pavilion with a few picnic tables. At the south end of the parking lot, find a map board, which marks the head of the Ice Age Trail segment. But don't start here; rather follow the edge of the parking lot left from here and walk to the edge of the woods to the trailhead. A boardwalk and steps start up the hill for the first 100 feet toward the chapel, and then the trail becomes crushed rock.

Cross an access road that runs left to right and continue up the hill. Expect a bit of huffing and puffing. Another 500 feet up, the slope through oak-hickory forest brings you to an intersection where a trail goes to the right over an unshaded swell. Stay left for now, though you will be returning for this other branch after your visit to the top of the hill. Just past here are a few more steps and then a boardwalk. Toward the top of the hill, the trail becomes packed dirt through an area rather good for raspberries in July. The trail does a turn, back to the left, and brings you to the chapel. Many visitors find a bit of peace up here in the woods, although the Catholic affiliations draw protests from those who don't feel a religious site should be maintained within a public county park.

The trail continues past the chapel and out onto a cliff where there's a nice lookout over the lake below. Sit on the bench here amid wildflowers and take in the view of lake and rolling farmland and forest.

Go back down the hill to the intersection at the end of the boardwalk and go left along the top of a ridge with slopes to either side. Go left off the top of the ridge just before a large oak, where the path takes you down a steep and narrow footpath and to open prairie. If you went right at the large oak up top, you would descend to the access road you crossed earlier. But the path you are on also rejoins the access road and a mowed area 500 feet from the top of that ridge. Straight ahead are a couple of picnic tables and a log cabin shelter used as a warming house in winter. Part of the Ice Age Trail is straight ahead and slightly to the left going to the left of some trees that separate it from the shelter area. To the right is part of that access road. Instead go left at this juncture and follow the long trail around the back of the park with plenty of woods and a hilly terrain before coming out on the other side in prairie and overlooking the lake.

Your trail has a wooden post marker that reads #1. Cross the field until you reach the trees at 600 feet. This is a nice stretch for prairie flowers in the spring and summer, especially bird's-foot violets in spring. The trail passes into a clump of trees for 300 feet before returning to the open prairie. Another 800 feet later, a line of trees begins to the right. Beyond this as the trail begins to curve right with the edge of the forest, find a bench on your left. The trail curves all the way back the other direction and enters a forest with a very high and thick canopy. Cross a culvert there and from here the hiking is typically moderate or a bit more. The trail starts to slope up and follows around a bend through a sharp dip in the terrain and then more climbing. The understory is thin through here, and you really get a sense of the undulating lay of the land beneath the towering trees.

Follow the trail's curve to the right and pass a wooden trail marker not long before you look down to your left into a deep gulley in the woods. From here the path goes uphill once more. Trees creak in the wind like old rockers or perhaps a ship. At the top of the hill, the terrain slopes down to your right. The trail also descends to a cutoff trail with a marker labeled 2/3, indicating two of the three numbered skiing/hiking trails in the park.

Don't go right, which is the initial part of the Ice Age Trail, but go left. You soon after encounter a wrong-way sign. Don't worry, this is for cross-country skiers to avoid head-on collisions.

Just 200 feet past here is another 2/3 trail marker with a path heading back to the right. Take the soft left following the #2 trail. Again ignore the wrong-way indicator (except during ski season) and pretend you are a rebel. Pass another gulley, this one to the right.

The trail heads to the right and along here to your left through a ridge; beyond that is farmland just 100 feet through the trees. Watch for a posted poem 700 feet along a rather straight stretch until you come to a bend to the left where the trail starts a slow climb and comes to another fork. Stay left again. The trail climbs to your highest point on this hike 0.3 miles later. From here is the steepest descent. Imagine that this is *up*hill for cross-country skiers going the "correct" way. The trail descends about 200 feet in altitude more than 0.3 miles. Halfway down you pass a bench.

From the forest, head into the open with aspens to your left. Seven hundred feet later the trail comes to a scenic overlook and bench where there's an intersection with the Ice Age Trail heading left. Read the amusing sign about crows here to the right and take in the view of the lake and prairie. Descend an open field toward the lake, stopping for a break if you need one at another bench halfway down.

At the bottom of the hill, the trail goes right back to the parking lot, but continue left to go around the lake. This area of the park has gone to the dogs—literally. Pet owners delight in one of the few areas where they are allowed to unleash the hounds. Benches look out over the lake to the right at a couple of spots along here. Some willows line the water. Trails are cut each year through the field to the left. Stay on the main trail along the lake until it breaks left and crosses the field 700 feet to a bridge where the Ice Age Trail rejoins and crosses Halfway Prairie Creek. Cross and go right until you reach a parking lot on your left. This is most convenient with hikers with pets. Here you can check another map board and self-pay the dog fee. To your right is a boat landing. Go straight across between the lot and dock and pick up the trail on the other side. A short way down the trail, pass through a gate. This area offers partial shade under the taller trees that run between the highway to your left and the lake on your right.

You arrive at a farmer's field most often planted with corn or alfalfa on your left. On your right watch for a small point that leans out into the lake. This is a nice spot to have a look for waterfowl. Past this point the grassy trail moves away from the water's edge and becomes marshy. Cattails and willows dominate the surrounding terrain, eventually giving way to cottonwoods before the trail opens up again to the open sky.

This is the lowest segment of the trail and on some older maps it may even look like you are hiking in the lake. In wet seasons this path will get soggy. At the corner of the farmer's field, go left with willows at your right. The trail follows a gentle S around the field's edge and then leads you to the pavement of the park entry road. Follow this back to the parking lot to complete the loop.

NEARBY ACTIVITIES

The Tree Farm is located just a couple of miles west of Indian Lake at 8454 Highway 19, Cross Plains, WI 53528. They sell Christmas trees for the holiday season, but are also an excellent pick-your-own vegetable, herb, and flower farm. Call (608) 798-2286 or go online to find out what's ripe for the picking: www.thetreefarm.net.

30 LAKE KEGONSA STATE PARK

KEY AT-A-GLANCE INFORMATION

LENGTH: 5.3 miles

CONFIGURATION: Multiple loops

DIFFICULTY: Easy

SCENERY: Prairie, marsh, forest, lakeshore

EXPOSURE: Mostly sun

TRAIL TRAFFIC: Light

TRAIL SURFACE: Mostly cut grass or packed limestone, some dirt, asphalt

HIKING TIME: 2.5–3 hours

DRIVING DISTANCE: 8.5 miles south from the intersection of US 12/18 and Interstate 39

ACCESS: 6 a.m.–11 p.m. year-round

MAPS: USGS Stoughton; on the DNR Web site and at park office

WHEELCHAIR ACCESSIBILITY: Yes, on Lakeshore Trail, Prairie Trail, and the boardwalk

FACILITIES: Restrooms, picnic areas with grills, campground, changing rooms, vending machines, pay phones, water

SPECIAL COMMENTS: Dogs are allowed on leashes, and there is a pet swim area. Much of the property is wheelchair accessible, from picnic tables and restrooms to a railing for lake entry at the beach.

GPS Trailhead Coordinates

UTM Zone (WGS 84) 16T

Easting 0318142

Northing 4760227

Latitude N 42° 58' 22.39"

Longitude W 89° 13' 49.18"

IN BRIEF

This lakeside park offers several short hikes or one long one that takes in varying landscape that includes restored prairie, a pine plantation, oak forest, and a marsh. Afterward go for a swim.

DESCRIPTION

This park was once part of a great river valley that was here more than a million years ago. The last of the glaciers passed over this area, and where they stopped, they left a line of glacial deposit called a terminal moraine located today just a few miles south of Lake Kegonsa. The meltwater flowing from the shrinking glaciers filled some of the former river valley with sand, gravel, and large boulders, forming dams in some places and raising the base significantly. The result is the chain of four lakes in the Madison area.

The park has several trails that can be combined, as they are here, to make a long hike through a variety of terrain. If you just want to take White Oak Nature Trail and Prairie Trail, you should take the first right after the park office for trail parking. For the complete hike, go to the beach parking area

Directions

From its intersection with US 12/18, drive south 5.2 miles on Interstate 39 to the County Road N exit. Turn right (south) and at 0.6 miles turn right on Koshkonong Road, taking it 1.7 miles to its end at Door Creek Road. Go left 1 mile to the park entrance on your right. After checking in at the main office, follow the park road as it curves back around under an overpass and then take the second right to beach parking. The trail begins at the sidewalk near the beach.

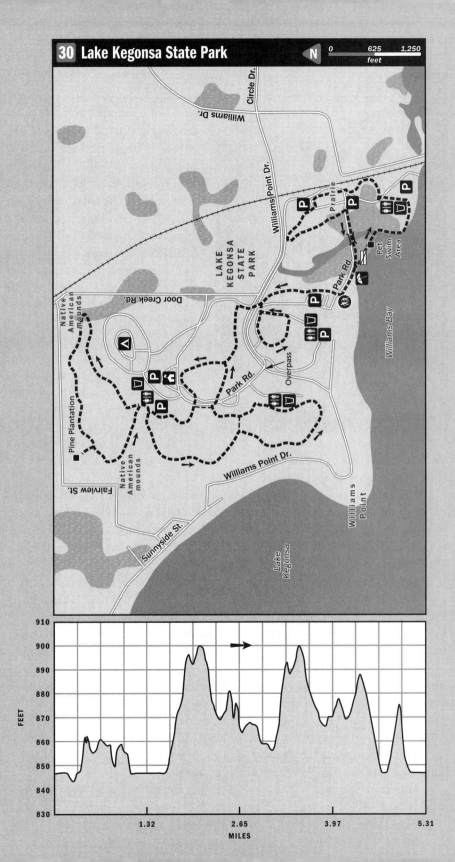

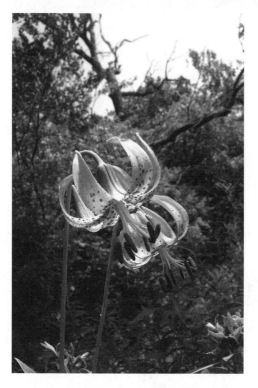

and find the paved walkway at the corner of the lot near the changing rooms.

Pass the small beach area on your right. The trail takes you through a pleasant picnic area along the lakeshore. Four hundred feet down the path, you'll pass a gate in a wooden fence and then the pet swim area on your right. The trail crosses a culvert that connects the marshy area to your left to the lake on your right, and then goes under tall cottonwoods as it loops through the mowed area past benches and a small dock before arriving at another parking area. Stay left here and walk past the pit toilets and through the parking lot to the park road. Just out of the parking lot, look for a yellow sign on the right side of the road that marks the trail.

This little half loop ventures through mixed forest for 750 feet before rejoining the road. At the end of this segment is the Williams Knoll picnic area where you can still see the old foundation of the carriage house of John Williams, who once owned much of the park land when he came to Wisconsin in the 19th century.

Follow the park road now to the right. Just past the parking lot on the left is a trail entrance to the Oak Knoll Trail, which begins with prairie. The trail left heads straight back to the pet swim area. Go right here along the park road through a nicely restored prairie full of native species of wildflowers. At the next small parking lot, go left following the lot's edge and follow the trail around to where it connects to a left-to-right trail along the edge of the trees. Left takes you back in a small prairie loop; go right along the edge of an oak-hickory forest with the prairie now to your right.

The trail cuts through the woods across a mowed circle and reemerges amid coneflowers, bergamot, black-eyed Susans, and Queen Anne's lace. Here is another junction with a trail leading right to the road. Go left with the prairie on your right and look for Turk's cap lilies through here.

After only 400 feet, you are back into woods with aspen and black walnut until another 400 feet later you find that trail back to the pet exercise area.

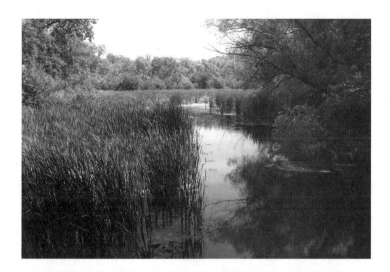

Wetlands near Williams Bay

It's 800 feet back to the wooden fence by the beach, and halfway there you cross a bridge that offers a very nice view of the marsh on both sides. Return to the parking area and take a stroll down the short boardwalk to the right to look for waterfowl in the marsh.

Continuing from the end of the boardwalk, walk along the right side of the lot heading north. To your right the marsh is visible in early spring or after the leaves are gone in fall. You'll come to a second parking lot, and at the end of the grassy median in that lot, look for a trail sign.

Walk 700 feet through more prairie to a trail juncture. The path on the left crosses the road to Bluebird Trail; save this for the end if you'd like. Go right and cross the park road. On the other side is a metal gate. Go around the gate and again cross a road, Williams Point Drive. Cross at an angle to a sign that reads TRAIL TO CAMPGROUND. Walk through a short corridor of foliage and then into open prairie. The trail forks here. To the right are the campgrounds. Go left on an exposed path with prairie on your right and shrubs to the left.

At 900 feet go right at the trail juncture, crossing the prairie and then bearing left at the opposite side. This is the closest point to the park office, and you'll pass a small spur trail that would let you out there. Continue until the next place to cross the park road. On the other side, the trail goes left or right. Stay right following the curve of crushed limestone. This is the Prairie Trail and is wheelchair accessible. Look for compass flowers in the field. At the next juncture, go right into woods. Here there is a sign for identifying wildflowers. Lead plant, spiderwort, purple prairie clover, butterfly milkweed, and various grasses are residents here, and this sign helps you find them.

It's only 100 feet to the head of the White Oak Nature Trail and its 14 numbered stations that correspond to the self-guided nature tour booklet.

There should be some at the trailhead if you didn't pick one up at the park office. A playground and flush toilets are here next to the parking lot.

White Oak Nature Trail is a 1.2-mile loop with packed-dirt surface and a lot of tree roots. The rise and fall of the land make this more strenuous than the prairie segments but nothing more than moderate. Tall oaks and various other trees provide plenty of shade. Look for black raspberries here in late June. Going right you encounter Native American ceremonial mounds at 0.3 miles where the trail curves left within the park boundaries. Another 0.4 miles brings you to the entrance of the Pine Plantation. Go right here and have a look at the red needle carpet and the most fragrant part of the forest. Back on the main trail, pass more mounds to the right. Then the trail climbs back up to the trailhead once again, where there's a bench if you need a break.

From White Oak Nature Trail, go right and take a crushed-limestone trail to your right that passes through a fire pit area and out into the prairie again. Go right at the trail junction as the path takes you 0.3 miles south across the edge of the prairie to the next juncture. To the left is a cutoff for the Prairie Trail. Instead go right on the group camping trail, a 0.6-mile loop around more prairie. As the trail curves and heads back, it passes through a shaded corridor of locust trees before coming back into the open at a baseball diamond to the left of the trail.

The trail rejoins the Prairie Trail as you continue with it to the right until you come once again to a crossing of the park road. On the other side, pick up a trail that goes left along the road or right into the prairie. Take that right path and follow it straight across the prairie 0.3 miles to where it comes once again to where you started into the fields. Go right here through the brush and cross the two park roads to arrive at a sign that reads TRAIL TO BEACH. Here you have the option of going right across the parking lot entry road to hike along a small hill covered with wildflowers on a 0.3-mile loop that is Bluebird Trail. On this trail you immediately come to a fork. Going left up the hill, you come to another juncture. Go right. The trail left leads to a picnic area on top of the hill where there are pit toilets and water. As the loop comes back around, you see an exit to the road on your left as the trail continues right through a stand of aspens. Soon you are back where you started, and you can cross the road to the Trail to Beach and head right back to the parking area.

Note: A self-guided hike through the forest includes a booklet available at the office or White Oak trailhead. All vehicles require a park sticker ($7 daily, $25 annual for vehicles with Wisconsin plates). The park participates in the Junior Ranger/Wisconsin Explorer program (see Preface, page xv).

NEARBY ACTIVITIES

Cinema Café at 124 West Main Street in nearby Stoughton combines big-screen movies with homemade pizza served while you enjoy the show. Call (608) 873-7484 to find out what's playing.

PHEASANT BRANCH CONSERVANCY
(with Pheasant Branch Creek Trail)

IN BRIEF

An outstanding conservancy project that features a little bit of everything: a stunning view of Madison and the Capitol, restored prairie and wetlands, a big spring, and a mixed-forest hike along a creek that crosses back and forth over the trail in six places.

DESCRIPTION

The village of Pheasant Branch was a stagecoach stop back in 1847 near what is now Century Avenue. The Stamm House, where travelers might spend the night or get a bite to eat, is still there and serving. Much of what is here today, preserved in the conservancy, was once converted to farmland. As Middleton grew and developed land, the run-off water also increased. The little Pheasant Branch Creek became overwhelmed and started putting too much sediment into Lake Mendota. The municipality rerouted the creek a bit in 1970, through the marshes you see today, so that much of that sediment and the pollutants in the runoff can be filtered before the creek empties into the lake.

From the Orchid Heights Park trailhead, start south on asphalt through a pleasant

KEY AT-A-GLANCE INFORMATION

LENGTH: 7.6 miles

CONFIGURATION: Loop and an out-and-back

DIFFICULTY: Easy with one moderate climb

SCENERY: Prairie, oak savanna, wetlands, mixed forest, running water, springs

EXPOSURE: Shade and sun

TRAIL TRAFFIC: Moderate

TRAIL SURFACE: Crushed rock, boardwalk, packed dirt, stepping stones

HIKING TIME: 3 hours

DRIVING DISTANCE: 1 mile from the intersection of County Roads M and Q in Middleton

ACCESS: 7 a.m.–10 p.m.

MAPS: USGS Middleton and Madison West; posted map boards

WHEELCHAIR ACCESSIBILITY: Yes

FACILITIES: Restrooms, water, vending machine

SPECIAL COMMENTS: Dogs allowed on a leash. The Pheasant Branch Trail requires you to use stepping stones to cross five concrete "bridges" submerged in the ankle-deep creek.

Directions

From the intersection of CR M and CR Q in Middleton, go north 0.4 miles on CR Q to Rolling Hill Drive and turn left. Take the first right 300 feet later on Larkspur Road. Follow this to its end less than 0.2 miles and turn right on Valley Ridge Road. Go 500 feet and take the first left on Sedge Meadow Road. Cross two speed bumps and take the first left, which is the entrance to the parking lot at Orchid Heights Park. The trailhead is at the map board near the restrooms.

GPS Trailhead Coordinates

UTM Zone (WGS 84)   16T

Easting   0298461

Northing   4776977

Latitude   N 43° 07' 7.37"

Longitude   W 89° 28' 38.42"

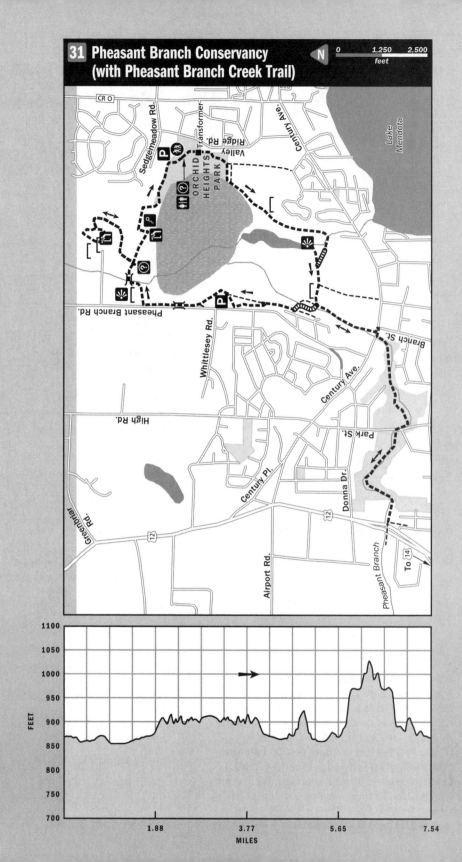

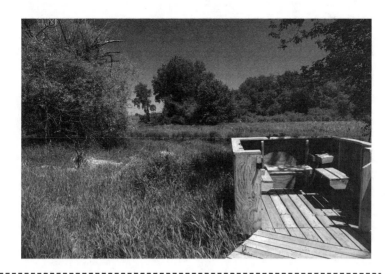

A viewing platform overlooking open water

recreational park. To your right you can see ponds and marshland popular for migrating birds in the spring and fall. The path is shared with bicyclists, and there is no shade through here. At 500 feet pass a transformer station. Beyond this the field is not mowed. You see oaks to the left and prairie to the right. Watch for hawks and field birds.

Stay on the trail to the right at the first intersection and find a crushed-rock trail. You reach a line of trees and another trail juncture. A trail goes straight, up a hill toward a water tower, and out of the park 0.3 miles to the south on Highland Way. Go right with trees to your right, prairie to your left, and follow the edge of the field as it bends south and enters mixed woods at 500 feet.

The path is shaded and the understory is waist-high, allowing you to see deep into the woods to the left. Pass a bench on your left, and 0.3 miles from where you entered the shade, come out again with houses up on the ridge to the left. Shade is limited to a few box elders and cottonwoods along the path. You reach a bridge over Pheasant Branch Creek at another 0.3 miles. From here it breaks from the residential zone and 200 feet later joins a boardwalk wide enough for bikes, pedestrians, and two-way traffic. A spur trail cuts right through a wooden fence 500 feet farther along and leads to a platform overlooking the marsh where you may see wood ducks, mallards, herons, and sandhill cranes.

The boardwalk ends just 300 feet from this spur trail, and another trail 200 feet after that bears left out to Century Avenue. Neither spur trail allows bikes or dogs. You come to a trail intersection with a bench to your right. Now you have a choice. The trail straight across the bridge before you and the one to the left are essentially the same and connect on the other side of the creek. (The one to the right allows bikes.) Choose these to skip the creek trail. The trail to the left leads out to Century Avenue, where there is a trail kiosk with history and

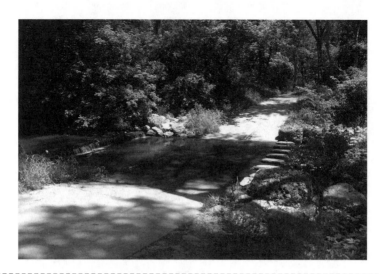

Stepping stones where the creek crosses over the trail

other information, a couple of restaurants, and a gas station for refreshments and restrooms. This is also the connection to the Pheasant Branch Creek Trail, which makes a 3-mile out-and-back segment of this 7.6-mile hike.

Go left 0.3 miles to the park entrance on Century Avenue. Cross at the traffic lights at Branch Street and Century Avenue to your left. Go right (west), cross the bridge over the creek, and enter Pheasant Branch Nature Preserve. Bikes and dogs are permitted here as well. There's a map board on the right and water on the left. Cross the creek five times on concrete stepping stones. Bicycles ride through several inches of water that flow over each concrete "bridge."

The trail is partly shaded by black walnuts and oaks, and you can see the creek flowing toward you, tumbling over rocks. The trail curves right and opens up in a hollow with houses tucked back in woods on either side. The trail comes to a dip and your first crossing at 0.2 miles with a dozen steps across a 20-foot concrete creek bed. Five hundred feet later, the trail crosses the creek again. On the other side of the creek, a small meadow opens under the trees. The trail bends gently to the right and 0.2 miles from this crossing is the next. The trail climbs the last 100 feet to street level. A sign marks the entrance near a service gate, and there's a map of the trail. Cross Park Street; the trail continues on the other side, where you'll see two giant storm sewers to the right. Left is a marshy area, and a bench is to your right.

Just 0.4 miles from Park Street is the next creek crossing, and the final crossing is another 500 feet after that.

Just on the other side of the creek, wood-beam-and-dirt steps lead up to the back of Middleton Alternative High School. Continuing past the steps, the path becomes asphalt and takes you either left up to Parmenter Street or straight under the overpass of the Old Beltline Highway to more groomed trails at

Confluence Pond, Deming Way, Northern Fork Trail, and even out past Middleton Airport. This is the turnaround for this hike, and you must retrace your steps back across Century Avenue into the conservancy once again to the trail intersection with the bridge over the creek.

Back at that juncture, the bridge to your left (west) is foot traffic only and follows a narrow boardwalk; bikes follow the trail north along the creek and cross a bigger bridge before rejoining the other trail. Cross the bridge and follow the boardwalk as it takes a right-angle right turn and then meets the main trail again. Go left here and see condos up the slope before you. The crushed-stone path is wider and exposed. At the next T-intersection, go right. The trail left leads out of the park to the condos.

From here the path runs straight, and at 0.2 miles there is a trail left and up the hill to the parking lot where there is a nice overlook of the park and a bench to enjoy it from. Go straight if you don't want to take the hill.

From the parking lot, a paved bike trail follows the road north, but go right on the footpath through savanna. The trail descends sharply and connects again to the main trail. Go left to find the end of the asphalt trail from the lot and a gate in front of you. Go right along Pheasant Branch Road for 0.3 miles, crossing a small footbridge over a swampy area at 500 feet.

Then the trail cuts right at 90 degrees from the road, and continues through prairie, crossing a bridge and taking you 0.2 miles to a trail juncture. To the right is an informational kiosk. Straight ahead takes you 0.6 miles back to the parking lot, and a soft right leads down a short slope to a lower level of prairie and marsh.

Go left up the moderately steep mowed-grass path that takes you 1 mile on a path that goes up along the slope of the hill around the back to the top. From that point the trail does a loop through oak trees around the crown of the hill. Starting left on the loop, come to a wonderful scenic overlook and a bench. From here you can see all the way to the Capitol in downtown Madison. When you return to the kiosk area, look for that sloping trail down another level. Take that path, rather than the main trail, 800 feet to an observation platform where you can see springwater bubbling up through the sandy soil in a small pool.

From the platform go right up the hill to rejoin the main trail. Pass another information kiosk immediately on your right, and it's just another 0.4 miles along the crushed-rock path back to the parking lot.

NEARBY ACTIVITIES

Capital Brewery in Middleton offers tours and hosts a beer garden on summer evenings. Check them out at **www.capital-brewery.com** or call (608) 836-7100.

32 POPE FARM PARK

 KEY AT-A-GLANCE INFORMATION

LENGTH: 2.9 miles

CONFIGURATION: Loop

DIFFICULTY: Easy, some moderate

SCENERY: Prairie, farmland, a ravine, scenic views of the Capitol

EXPOSURE: Mostly sun

TRAIL TRAFFIC: Light

TRAIL SURFACE: Mowed grass, some dirt, and cedar chip

HIKING TIME: 1–1.5 hours

DRIVING DISTANCE: 2.2 miles west of the Beltline Highway (US 12/14) and Old Sauk Road exit

ACCESS: 7 a.m.–half an hour after sunset

MAPS: USGS Middleton; on signs at trailheads and several trail junctures

WHEELCHAIR ACCESSIBILITY: Around scenic parking area and possibly some grassy trails

FACILITIES: Portable toilets, water, picnic tables

SPECIAL COMMENTS: No dogs allowed. The park is a work in progress, and trails will adapt to the needs of the park and crops, so the map may vary from time to time.

IN BRIEF

Learn about the glaciers as well as Native American and pioneer agriculture as you climb a couple of recessional moraines of prairie and farmland offering views all the way to Madison's Capitol dome.

DESCRIPTION

With urban development seemingly racing west from Madison, how fortunate it is that the Pope family of the Town of Middleton has set aside this 105-acre park that is partly a working farm. The view of the Madison Capitol in the distance alone makes this park worth a visit, but as you walk the top of two moraines, you take in prairie and farmland with some great educational signage along the way. Rhyolite present in the stone fence that climbs the hill is evidence of the tremendous earth-moving of the glaciers of the Ice Age. The closest regional deposit of this stone is in the Lake Superior basin.

The trail starts up the hill along the edge of a stone fence on your left. You pass prairie restoration on your way up. At 750 feet you reach parking for the scenic overlook where there are a couple of portable toilets. Just past this are two simple amphitheaters to the right fashioned with sitting stones and several

---

GPS Trailhead Coordinates

UTM Zone (WGS 84) 16T

Easting   0291088

Northing   4772367

Latitude   N 43° 04' 30.88"

Longitude   W 89° 33' 58.12"

Directions

Exit the Beltline Highway (US 12/14) at Old Sauk Road and go 2.2 miles west. The park entrance is on the right. Park in the first parking lot on your left. The trailhead is at the northwest corner of the lot.

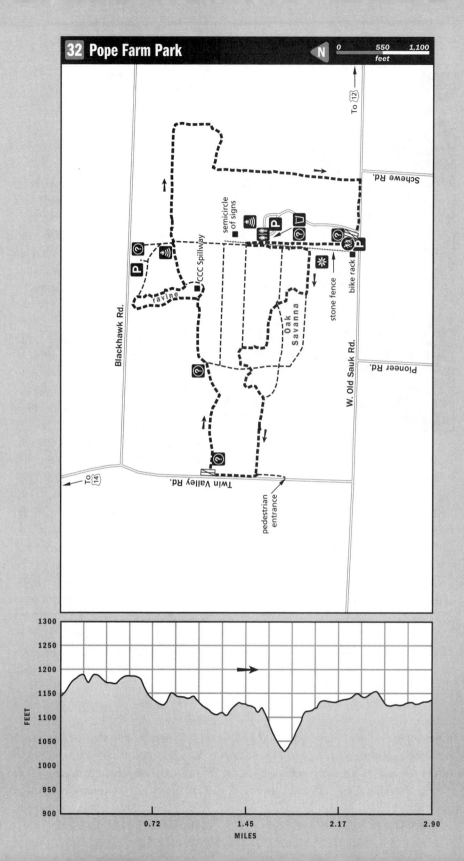

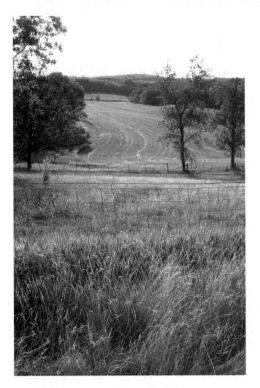

educational signs. The view east is all the way to the dome just over 9 miles away.

Recessional moraines are rock and soil deposits left where the glacier paused as it receded, and there are two of them here. You are standing on the first; signage challenges you to find the second.

To your left is an opening in the stone fence. Cross here to the other side to find the wide mowed trails arranged in geometric order over the fields. You have options to go back and forth across the field between the various plantations. Go left back along the stone wall with a field of sunflowers to your right as the trail takes you downhill to two small gardens. The plants here exemplify the crops of the Native Americans and the early pioneers. Just before them the trail goes right with the sunflowers on your right and a farm fence to your left. Only 500 feet later, the path goes to the right up the hill. (Future development may open up this trail to go straight here with the ridge to the right and continuing west to the agricultural fields of the western side of the park.) At the crest of the hill, find oak savanna at the left. A trail goes right back toward the stone fence or follows left along the top of the hill, keeping the savanna on your left. There is a gate just past here on your left. This trail goes down through the oak savanna and follows the lower edge of the hill, heading west with oaks above you to the right. This area is sometimes closed.

If you skip the gate and go along the top of the ridge, you come to a circle of stones. The trail bends right then brings you to another juncture. Right leads you back to the fence again. Go left alongside grain crops and down the hill with that oak savanna still off to the left.

At the bottom of the hill, go left. Right is a cutoff trail skipping the western fields of the park. As you head left, take your first right as the trail goes along the north edge of an oak-covered hill. (Going straight brings you to that trail through the savanna beyond the gate you passed.) The trail ascends to a flattened top and offers a nice view of the neighboring farm. You can also see the oak savanna trail where it rejoins the fields and follows up the hill along the southern limit of the park and parallel to the path you are on. A path from your perch on this hill doubles back to it.

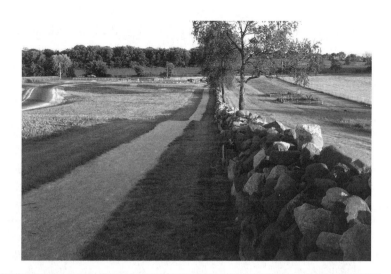

A stone wall alongside the trail

Head west following the trail toward Twin Valley Road. To the left is a little country church and more crops just outside the park. You can expect deer here in the early morning or toward dusk especially. Across the field to the right is mixed forest along the return trail, and you have a bit of altitude on the field to see it all.

Walk the 0.2 miles to the end of the field at the edge of the road. To the left a trail takes you to a pedestrian entrance from Twin Valley Road. Go right along the road to the opposite side where there's another map board. Go right again with the woods, at your left, populated by young black walnuts and long-needled pines and occasional oaks.

Keep along the edge of the woods as the trail goes left with the property line where another juncture also offers you a path to the right that would take you back to where you've been. There's a map board here. You are now coming back into the middle section of the park, and from the map board it is another 750 feet to the next trail to the left. Keep along the edge of the woods until there.

The path left goes into the woods along a deep gully heading north with cedar-chip trail on either side of it. The cut in the earth is a nice dramatic contrast to the rolling hills, but before you head into the shade, continue forward on the trail less than 200 feet to see a bit of regional history.

On your left will be a spillway constructed by the Civilian Conservation Corps and used to capture the force of runoff. The rainwater enters the spillway and gathers in a basin before being released into the gorge, reducing its speed and preventing excessive erosion.

Backtrack to the trail into the woods. This footpath descends through predominantly locust, cottonwood, and oak. Along the right is a deep gully. Be careful of the trail edge, especially when cedar chips are fresh and give a false sense of stability. It's only 800 feet to the road where you cross the bottom of the gully and climb back up to the other side to follow the trail back through the woods toward the spillway.

When you come out of the trees, go left, which is due east. If you haven't guessed already, this is the second moraine. You'll reach another small stone amphitheater that overlooks the Black Earth Creek Valley and a ski jump in the distance.

Continuing east here you have choices. Left takes you to the parking area along Blackhawk Road; right goes back to the stone fence and ultimately to where you started. Going straight is part of the Country Road Trail and takes you through more crops along the edge of the eastern section of the park, which really does have the feel of a country road minus the traffic and perhaps the dust. You are 0.4 miles from the parking lot if you go right. The trail before you will loop around 0.9 miles to the lot.

Go straight where the prairie is loaded with wildflowers: coneflowers, bergamot, black-eyed Susans, sunflowers, and many others. You can find a mulberry tree along this route as well as a couple of apple trees where the trail comes all the way around to Old Sauk Road before it turns west again along the roadside to the parking lot.

NEARBY ACTIVITIES

For a great local Friday fish fry (or homestyle cooking any other day), check out The Village Green at 7508 Hubbard Avenue in Middleton. Call (608) 831-9962.

STEWART COUNTY PARK

IN BRIEF

Multiple loops take you through a ravine and thick woods and over a hill of restored prairie for a fantastic view of the countryside. A spring-fed creek feeds the diminutive Stewart Lake.

DESCRIPTION

Stewart Park was the first park in the Dane County park system. Central to the property is Stewart Lake, which was created by a dam on a spring-fed creek. Located just north of Mount Horeb, it is nestled in at the edge of some of the residential neighborhoods but offers good wilderness and a hilltop view of the surrounding countryside.

Restrooms are located right at the parking lot. The trail begins at the end of the parking lot and follows an asphalt path from the lot right along forest. Water runs down this channel after heavy rains. There's a pavilion to the left and a playground in this mowed area.

Walk toward Stewart Lake and enter the trees at 0.1 mile where the asphalt ends and

KEY AT-A-GLANCE INFORMATION

LENGTH: 3.6 miles

CONFIGURATION: Four interconnected loops with cutoffs

DIFFICULTY: Moderate

SCENERY: Mixed forest, prairie, flowing water, lake, dam, ravine, wildflowers

EXPOSURE: Half and half

TRAIL TRAFFIC: Light

TRAIL SURFACE: Packed dirt, mowed grass, short stretch of asphalt

HIKING TIME: 1.5 hours

DRIVING DISTANCE: 19.6 miles west of the Beltline Highway (US 12/18) and Verona Road juncture

ACCESS: 5 a.m.–10 p.m.

MAPS: USGS Cross Plains; on a map board deep in the trail system

WHEELCHAIR ACCESSIBILITY: None

FACILITIES: Toilets, shelter, playground

SPECIAL COMMENTS: Dogs require a daily fee ($3; $23 annual) and must be on a leash. Cross-country skiing also exacts a daily fee ($5; $20 annual).

Directions

From the Beltline Highway (US 12/18), go southwest on Verona Road/US 18/151. Drive 15.6 miles and take Exit 69 to Mount Horeb and US Business Route 18/151. Merge with County Road ID, follow it 1.4 miles to a roundabout, and take the second exit to continue on CR ID/Business Route 18/151. Continue 0.6 miles to County Road JG (North Washington Street) and go right for 0.1 mile, turn left on Wilson Street (still CR JG) for one block, then turn right onto Lake Street (also still CR JG) and follow it 0.7 miles to the park entrance on the right. The trailhead is at the far end of the parking lot on the right.

GPS Trailhead Coordinates

UTM Zone (WGS 84)   16T
Easting   0276356
Northing   4766496
Latitude   N 43° 01' 5.65"
Longitude   W 89° 44' 40.42"

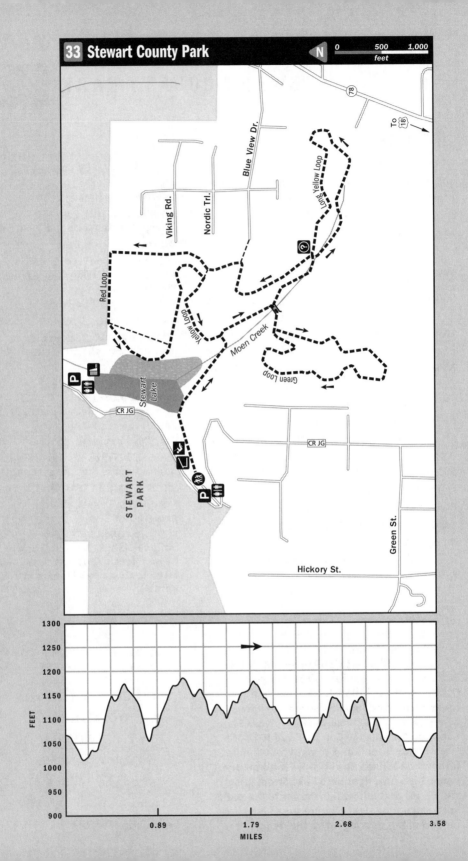

N

0   500   1,000
feet

78

To
18

Blue View Dr.

Viking Rd.

Nordic Trl.

Yellow Loop

Red Loop

Yellow Loop

Moen Creek

Green Loop

Stewart Lake

P

CR JG

P

STEWART PARK

CR JG

Green St.

Hickory St.

1300
1250
1200
1150
1100
1050
1000
950
900

FEET

0.89   1.79   2.68   3.58

MILES

> The trail enters a ravine.

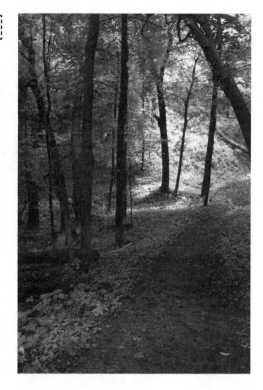

crushed stone begins. It is mostly shaded here by the trees going up the hill to your left. Pass first some stone blocks and then some timbers holding up the earth on that side of the trail. Cattails, brush, and a few trees separate you from the lake on your left. The path curves to the right, and you can look for some blackberries through here in August as well as several varieties of wildflowers.

Just 0.2 miles into the woods, pass a brick pump house and see a trail sign at the head of a mowed path just beyond it. Moen Creek is to your left. The trail crosses a culvert and then bends left at a fire plug to the right of the trail.

You then come to a fork in the trail. The trail to the left is your return path. Go right through oak, hickory, and black walnut. Look for Indian pipe through here, a white tubelike flower that has no chlorophyll but lives off of nutrients from fungi and decaying trees. At the next fork 0.1 mile later, go right and cross a footbridge over the creek. This is the beginning of the 0.8-mile Green Loop with a couple of steep climbs. To shorten your hike, continue straight rather than crossing the bridge.

Right after the bridge is a culvert, and then the trail goes right. The trail heads into the bottom end of a small ravine. In the ridge to your left, you can see exposed sandstone. Pass a bench on the left and come to another fork. Go left up the hill following the direction of the ski trails. This is steep, and if you go right instead, it is just slightly more gradual in its climb to the top of the opposite ridge.

At the top the path levels out in a small mowed area where skiers can rest after that 0.1-mile climb.

The trail curves right just inside the park and continues, slightly uphill. You pass through a scattering of wildflowers and the canopy opens a bit to the sky. As you come into a small piece of prairie nearly overrun by sumac, pass along the backyards of a few houses. Straight across the field is a bench. From here the trail starts down moderately through young black walnuts and a scattering of flowers and grasses. As you come down around the curve and into another clearing, you see the terrain slope into the groove of that ravine.

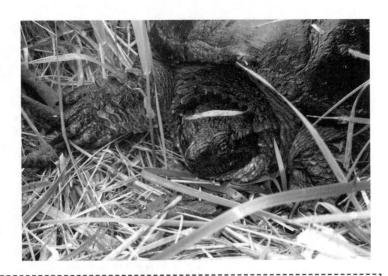

A snapping turtle near Stewart Lake

At the bottom the path curves right and then back again to cross the ravine on a land bridge. To your right it slips down deeply. The trail bends right and follows along the other ridge into forest again with the land sloping to your right. You'll come to an arrow that points down and reads STEEP SLOPE, but it is actually not as steep as your ascent on the other side. You are in a wide open space beneath the canopy, and this is a nice view of the shape of the ravine. The trail bears left at the bottom and leads you back to the bridge and the main trail.

Go right and a short trail brings you up to the main trail and continues right 0.1 mile to a four-way trail juncture where you find a map board. If you stay on your course through this clearing, taking the trail to the right, you follow the Long Yellow Loop, which is 0.5-mile loop returning to this spot. To skip this, look for a trail to your left that goes back in the direction you came from.

The Long Yellow Loop goes uphill and crosses prairie with a nice variety of wildflowers, including coneflowers, black-eyed Susans, false sunflowers, and cup plant. It passes through a stand of pines and then brings you to some oak savanna on the right. A blue trail arrow attached to a bluebird house points the way left. Leave the woods for prairie over hilly terrain with trees to your right. The trail heads downhill to the clearing and map board to complete this loop.

Now stay right as you pass the map board and take the trail there. It continues up through black walnuts and soon levels off into prairie 0.2 miles from the map board. The trail curves along the boundary of the park passing a spur trail out to Blue View Drive. From there it is another 300 feet to a cutoff trail to the left, which would take the 0.8-mile Red Loop off your hike. Going right, continue over the hill and up the next through prairie passing a bench on your right and then a spur trail to the right to Viking Road. You reach the top of the hill just 700 feet along the Red Loop. Looking around along the horizon, it is obvious you are in the

Driftless Area of Wisconsin with its rolling unglaciated terrain. You see farms and hills in the distance and the Mount Horeb water tower to the south. Continue to the end of the field where the trail rounds a corner to the left and heads downhill with trees and brush on either side.

At Birdhouse #12 a cutoff trail goes left along the prairie, but stay straight into the forest through tall pine. The surface is packed dirt with scatterings of hickory nuts. As the trail curves left, you lose the cover of the canopy, and as you round the bend, you meet up with the prairie alternative trail from Birdhouse #12. As you continue, the hump of the hill rises to your left, obscuring the horizon with a bulging prairie. The trail bends right along the edge of the forest and brings you to the end of the Red Loop, where there is a map board and that cutoff trail joining from the left. Go right and downhill on packed dirt at a moderate grade 0.2 miles to the beginning of the Long Yellow Loop. Look for exposed rock on the left as you descend. At the trail juncture you see the fireplug down the trail to the right. This is the return path that leads you back out past the pump house to the parking lot.

You can walk across the dam at the north end of the lake. There is a parking lot as well as toilets. From the first parking lot, go right, continuing down CR JG. Odds are you'll see deer in the park, and if you're lucky, you will see one of the lake's resident snapping turtles.

NEARBY ACTIVITIES

Stop in at the Mustard Museum at 100 West Main Street in Mount Horeb to see a collection of more than 4,600 mustards. It's not just for looking—you can take some home as well. Go to **www.mustardmuseum.com** or call (800) 438-6878 to find out more.

34 TOKEN CREEK

KEY AT-A-GLANCE INFORMATION

LENGTH: 3.7 miles
CONFIGURATION: Loop
DIFFICULTY: Easy
SCENERY: Prairie, marsh, flowing water, and some mixed woods
EXPOSURE: Only partly shaded
TRAIL TRAFFIC: Light
TRAIL SURFACE: Mowed paths, some packed dirt, and a boardwalk
HIKING TIME: 1.5 hours
DRIVING DISTANCE: 0.5 miles north on US 51 from the Interstate 39 juncture
ACCESS: Year-round, 5 a.m.–10 p.m. except for campers
MAPS: USGS De Forest; available at trailhead or from campsite manager
WHEELCHAIR ACCESSIBILITY: Yes, on boardwalk and most grassy trails
FACILITIES: Restrooms, campsites, playgrounds, disc-golf course, vending machine, bridle areas, and shelters
SPECIAL COMMENTS: Dogs are allowed on leashes or unleashed in fee-controlled dog areas. The fee is $3 daily and $22 annually. A smaller fenced area is reserved for small dogs. Horses share some trails with hikers and since the animals can be spooked, they have the right-of-way. Disc golfers pay a $5 daily fee for using the course.

IN BRIEF

Follow a trail and boardwalk along a clear country creek, explore sedge meadow and prairie, and finish the day with a round of disc golf.

DESCRIPTION

At the end of the last Ice Age, drainage of this area was blocked and the soggy land supported plant life that, as it died and decayed, became the alkaline peat deposits now beneath the marsh. In the 1930s dredging lowered the water level, allowing prairie to invade. Sedges lost out to lavender asters, sunflowers, and goldenrods, which bloom in late summer. Token Creek and some wetlands remain, but prairie closes in around them as the creek makes its meager way to the Yahara River via the northern reaches of Cherokee Marsh to the west.

From the park gate, continue to Shelter #2 just past the campgrounds. Find a map board at the trailhead across from the shelter. A map box to the left should have trail maps, or you can go to one of the campsite hosts and ask for one.

Starting from the trail board, follow along the road to the tall grass. A cross-country ski trail starts here and follows the

GPS Trailhead Coordinates

UTM Zone (WGS 84) 16T

Easting 0311511

Northing 4783695

Latitude N 43° 10' 57.05"

Longitude W 89° 19' 9.64"

Directions

Take US 51 north out of Madison until you pass under the I-39 interchange. Almost a half mile north of here, find Token Creek Lane, just past a truck stop on the right. Turn here and follow the lane to the park entrance gate. From the gate follow the park road 0.25 miles and park on the right side near the trail board.

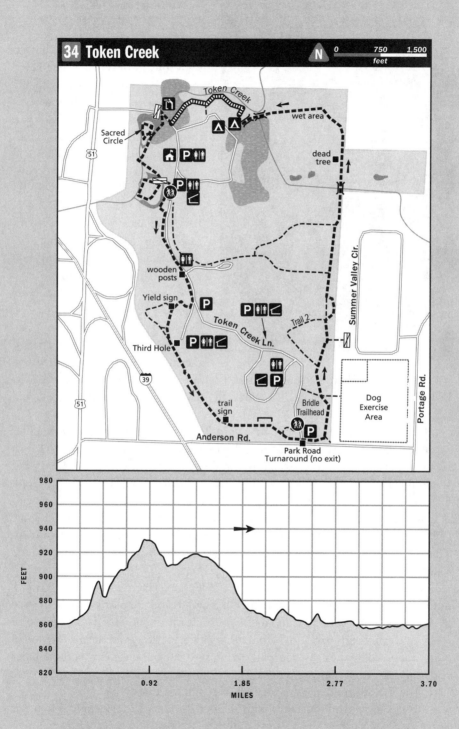

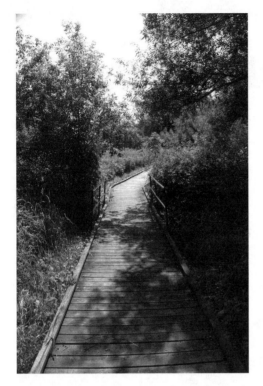

A boardwalk follows Token Creek

road deeper into the park, but go right toward the creek edge to pick up another trail. Go left with the creek on your right following a mowed path. This takes you through tall grasses and some willows before the trail turns left and connects to that original cross-country trail. Go right and find a trail marker for Trails 1, 2, and 3. Follow along the edge of the park road. You can see the highway intersection from this clearing, and through this first portion of the park, you will have traffic noise and the occasional plane passing overhead from the nearby Dane County airport. The trail is open to the sun for 900 feet, and then you pass into woods. There's a spur trail to the left to the road. After this juncture the hiking trail joins the horse trail. It is mostly shaded by a mix of maple, oak, and black walnut.

Come back out to the road and a gate. The trail is really the grassy shoulder of the road. Stay right alongside it and pass between two wooden posts. Pass a roadside parking area, after which the trail goes right back into oak forest and slopes down. Follow it as it curves right gently down the hill through oaks. Look for a few young shagbark hickories through here. The forest is bustling with chipmunks, squirrels, and stirrings in the undergrowth as the trail dips at some cedar chips. At a yield sign at a trail juncture, go left and reemerge into the sun. This is the closest to the highway that you will be, and highway noise can be quite loud here.

Pass behind the third hole of the disc golf course and find the end of Trail 1 at this juncture. Continue straight on Trail 2 and 3. You are partly shaded by pine as you walk along with the fairway to your left on the other side of the line of trees. The trail bends to the right and back with a gentle S, and the air is redolent with long-needle pines. As you pass a clump of sumac, the pines become taller and you pass a trail sign as the trail turns left just inside the boundaries of the park. You can see residences to the right through the trees.

To the left is grassy meadow with a few trees starting to take hold. From this point traffic noise fades significantly, and there is a bench in the shade to the right where you can sit and watch birds active in the prairie. Just past this find another trail marker as the trail bends right through a short corridor of sumac before crossing the field to the end of the park road and a turnaround there. Trails to the left just before this are part of the bridle trails and an exercise circle for the horses.

Cross the turnaround and enter the woods again on the other side. There's an entry trail to the park from the right 400 feet from here, where the main trail goes left along the western boundary of the dog exercise area. There is parking along Anderson Road just outside the gate. Continue to the left on the mostly shaded trail of cedar chips that soon give way to grass and packed dirt. The trail bends left and brings you to another trail marker at the entrance to the pet exercise area to your right. Pass the entrance and follow the cut path with trail marker 2 and 3.

Stay on straight Trail 3. The left path is Trail 2, which eventually loops out and back through the meadow to your left through the disc golf fairways to rejoin this trail again. Pass a spur trail on the right to a private gate, and then as you reach the other side of the open field, the return trail for Trail 2 is on your left. Soon after you come to another fork in road. Go right here for a short loop with no horse access that curves out and back a bit farther up the trail. Go right at the trail marker when you return to the main. Just past here is a cutoff trail that leads back to the parking lot. Stay to the right instead and head out into open meadow again. At the other side, come to the Trail 2 juncture that goes left toward the parking lots. Go straight on Trail 3. Look for an old red barn with a rooster weathervane through the trees outside the park to the right. On the other side of the field, another trail heads left to a bench. Go straight and check out the enormous aspens with massive trunks to your left. To your right just outside the park, see another park with playgrounds. A couple of unofficial trails cross 30 feet of tall grass to get there.

You are now walking along a ditch with some standing water to your left. Cross a creek with wooden railings. Prairie awaits you at the end of the brushline; look for a tall dead tree next to a low area with standing water and algae on your left. Watch for some sandpipers and perhaps cranes or herons. Swallows skim the tops of the grasses. Duck back into thick woods on a packed-earth trail often showing tracks of deer and other animals. The shade lasts another 600 feet, and you have to cross a low muddy area about 6 feet across with a culvert in the middle before crossing another meadow.

At the other side a bridge, the trail crosses a tiny creek and the path returns to shade. Now you can see Token Creek to the right before crossing another bridge. Look for lilies along the water's edge. The trail ventures left into a campsite. Go around the site unless it is unoccupied; the trail picks up on the other side where a strip of old asphalt heads back into the tall grass. Pass under some trees to find the beginning of the boardwalk. It goes left at a right angle and passes through a swampy area with an abundance of willows as it follows Token Creek curving right. This is the nicest part of the trail, easy to walk, secluded, and putting you right along the waterway through brush and sedge meadow. A boardwalk spur goes left to the wheelchair-accessible campsite. Stay straight and cross a bridge over another small creek feeding into the bigger Token Creek. Willows provide some shade up to the end of the boardwalk at the park road. Educational signage here gives information about the 0.5-mile boardwalk segment of the trail and touts the springtime sky dance of woodcocks, which can be seen in open areas of the meadow.

You have the option of following the park road back to the parking lot. Otherwise go right to the park entrance gate, where there is an observation platform across the road overlooking a wide area of the creek. This segment of the trail is also a dog exercise area. The trail continues to follow the creek, and cedar trees start to appear. Come to a gate on your left and a trail to the right over a culvert (which may suffer from erosion and washouts) onto a small island in the stream. It's a short loop around and back, and you can find a "sacred circle" built by friends of the park where cedars surround a small boulder. Blackbirds pay close attention to you in late spring when they nest around here. On the opposite side of the island take the fork to the left; the right trail is a short dead end, but you can climb out onto the rocks in the stream from there.

Go right back on the main trail and pass a small spur that merely goes through the grass to the water's edge. Just past here find a volleyball court to the left but keep right, continuing along the creek visible now through the weeds to the right. The next intersection is another island loop. Go right over a concrete bridge with a culvert that allows this narrow branch of the creek to pass. Cross onto a second larger island. The trail follows the perimeter, offering some looks into the water and a couple of maple-shaded spots in an otherwise sunny meadow.

Returning to the concrete bridge, cross back to the main trail, go right, and then take the branch to the left to get to your car, which should already be visible from here.

Winter is nice for hikes along the boardwalk and nearby portions of the trails, where you can easily find animal tracks—and the woodcocks' sky dance is not something you see just anywhere.

NEARBY ACTIVITIES

Pine Cone Restaurant right outside the park is a truck-stop and greasy spoon with cheap eats and coffee—nothing fancy, just hearty highway fare. Call (608) 249-8778 for more information.

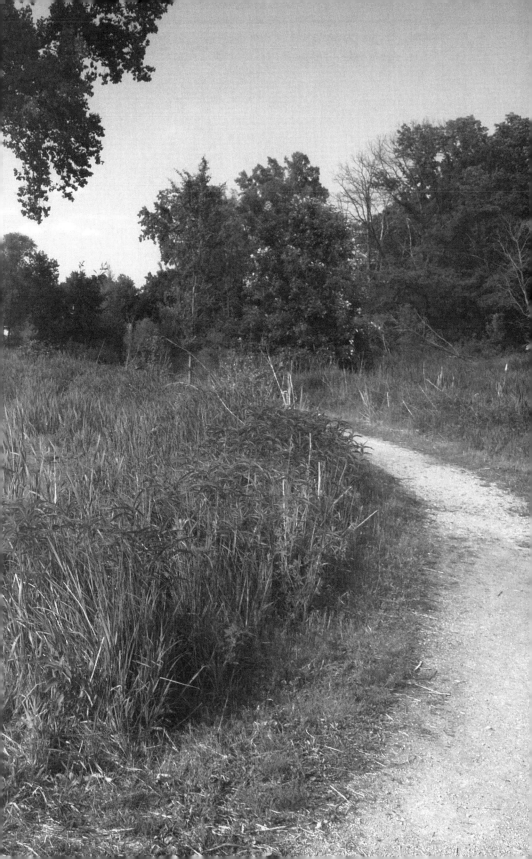

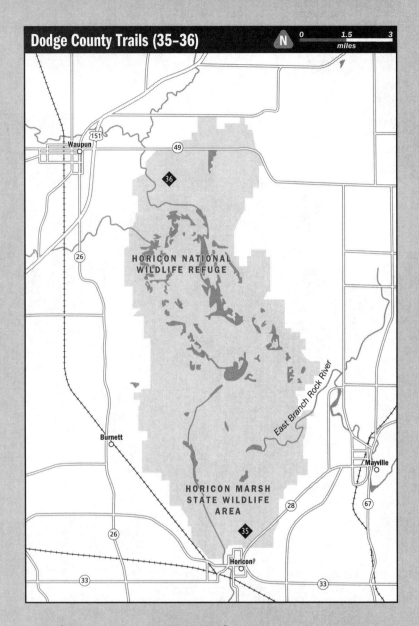

Dodge County Trails (35–36)

N

0   1.5   3
miles

Waupun
151
49
36
26
HORICON NATIONAL
WILDLIFE REFUGE

Burnett

East Branch Rock River

Mayville

HORICON MARSH
STATE WILDLIFE
AREA
28
67
26
35
33
Horicon
33

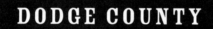

DODGE COUNTY

35 HORICON MARSH STATE WILDLIFE AREA

KEY AT-A-GLANCE INFORMATION

LENGTH: 4.7 miles

CONFIGURATION: Three connected loops

DIFFICULTY: Easy

SCENERY: Vast marshlands, waterfowl, some forest

EXPOSURE: Mostly sun, some shade in forests

TRAIL TRAFFIC: Light

TRAIL SURFACE: Crushed rock, grass, and dirt

HIKING TIME: 1.5–2 hours

DRIVING DISTANCE: 45.2 miles from US 151 and Interstate 39

ACCESS: 5 a.m.–10 p.m. year-round

MAPS: USGS Mayville South; available in park office

WHEELCHAIR ACCESSIBILITY: Observation deck only

FACILITIES: Two park offices offer restrooms and water. Observation decks

SPECIAL COMMENTS: This is an ebird.org birding hot spot. There are special extended office hours during the migration periods. Don't forget your binoculars.

IN BRIEF

Walk along the dikes in one of the state's most significant bird migration points.

DESCRIPTION

Horicon is the largest freshwater cattail marsh in the United States. In spring and fall, the waters teem with migrating waterfowl. To call this a quiet hike would be a lie as geese, herons, grebes, teals, and even pelicans come in droves and create quite a bit of chatter. More than 250 species of birds pass through here each spring. Within the marsh, Fourmile Island and Cotton Island are rookeries hosting the largest nesting colonies of blue herons and egrets in Wisconsin. There are so many birds nesting there, in fact, that the overpopulation is having harmful effects on the soil and trees.

Before your hike, stop in at the park office to get a birding checklist and a Junior Birder pamphlet for the kids. You should also go to the observation deck next door for an overlook of where you are about to explore.

The trailhead is at the parking lot just 0.15 miles before the office on the left. There is a map board here. Follow cedar chips 0.15 miles through mixed forest and emerge at the edge of the marshland. Interpretive signs lie throughout the trail. Outside the woods

GPS Trailhead Coordinates

UTM Zone (WGS 84) 16T

Easting 0368668

Northing 4813629

Latitude N 43° 27' 50.58"

Longitude W 88° 37' 24.71"

Directions

From its intersection with I-39, take US 151 north 34.3 miles to WI 33. Turn right and go 10 miles east to Horicon. Turn left on Palmatory Street and go north 0.9 miles to the parking lot on the left. The trailhead is on the north side of the lot.

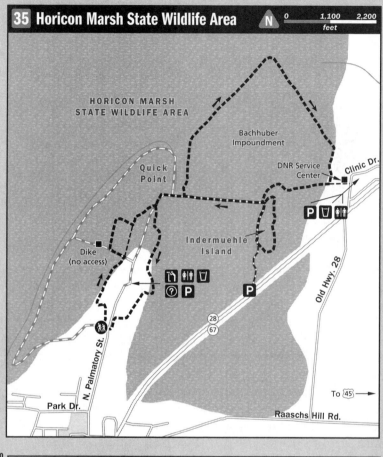

35 Horicon Marsh State Wildlife Area

HORICON MARSH
STATE WILDLIFE AREA

Bachhuber
Impoundment

DNR Service
Center

Clinic Dr.

Quick
Point

Dike
(no access)

Indermuehle
Island

Old Hwy. 28

N. Palmatory St.

28
67

Park Dr.

Raaschs Hill Rd.

To 45 →

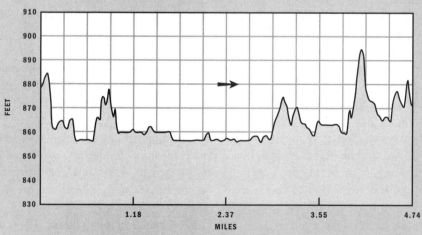

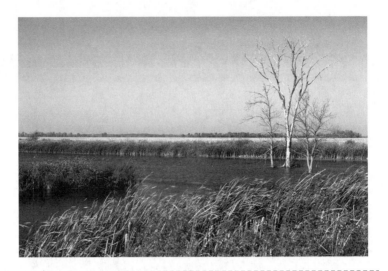

Bachhuber Impoundment shelters abundant waterfowl.

a service road goes left to right; stay right as a mowed path cuts through prairie at the bottom of a sloping hill to your right. The park office is above as is an observation platform overlooking the wide expanses of cattails and open water. Brush will obscure the view from the trail for the first 0.15 miles, and then another 0.1 mile brings you to a trail juncture. The service road goes straight and up to the right. Go left here out into the marsh along the back of a dike. This 0.3-mile squared loop will return to the service road 0.15 miles farther north. As you venture out into the marsh, you come to a right turn at 0.1 mile; public access on the straight path beyond this point is prohibited. Marsh lies on either side of the trail. In addition to birds, be on the lookout for a lot of turtles sunning themselves.

At the end of the loop, you come back to the service road where you go left into hardwood forest. The trail comes to a juncture at 0.15 miles. To the right is a wide service road trail, and just up that trail is the return loop around the hill to the parking lot. But save it for later; you're going left here. Another 0.1 mile takes you out of the trees and to a pump house on the left. Another much larger loop than before follows the dike around a large portion of marsh known as Bachhuber Impoundment, which has a lot of open water pockets sheltering hordes of waterfowl. Watch for tiny snakes and frogs on the path as well. The dike trail begins around behind the pump house. The trail runs 1.5 miles out and around before returning along the bottom of another ridge where a Department of Natural Resources service center overlooks the marsh. A trail heads up the hill there to the parking lot and center.

Go right on the return road, heading back toward the pump house. The trail curves 0.4 miles around the edge of a forested "island," leaving you at another juncture. Go left here as the trail goes onto Indermuehle Island for a 0.6-mile loop on a grassy trail through the woods. Two thirds of the way around (if you start left), is a trail out to another parking lot on WI 28.

As you come back off the island, walk 0.4 miles to the pump house and then continue back into the woods on the trail you took to arrive. This time at the trail juncture go left, and then make another quick left after that. The trail descends closer to the marsh with partial shade before you head out into the open again through prairie just a bit higher than the cattails.

From the juncture to the parking lot is another 0.7 miles. First you will pass a trail on the right that cuts out to the park office and observation deck. Go left here instead as the trail curves down around woods to the right and then runs parallel to the ridge. It ends with a turn around the end of the ridge where it brings you to a gate at the roadside. Directly across the road are the parking lot and the trailhead.

NEARBY ACTIVITIES

Dodge County Ledge Park at N7403 Park Road, Horicon, offers overnight camping, hiking trails, and a nice overlook of the Horicon Marsh. Call (920) 387-5450 to find out more. You could also check out the Horicon Aquatic Center, a recreation center on North Cedar in Discher Park in Horicon. Call (920) 485-3522 for more information.

36 HORICON NATIONAL WILDLIFE REFUGE

KEY AT-A-GLANCE INFORMATION

LENGTH: 4.3 miles

CONFIGURATION: Three connected loops

DIFFICULTY: Easy

SCENERY: Prairie and marsh

EXPOSURE: Mostly sun

TRAIL TRAFFIC: Light but moderate on the Egret Trail and boardwalk

TRAIL SURFACE: Mowed grass, crushed limestone, boardwalk

HIKING TIME: 1.5–2 hours

DRIVING DISTANCE: 52.2 miles from US 151 and Interstate 39

ACCESS: During daylight hours year-round

MAPS: USGS Waupun North and South; posted in parking lots and at trailheads

WHEELCHAIR ACCESSIBILITY: Only the boardwalk

FACILITIES: Pit toilets at two parking areas

SPECIAL COMMENTS: Dogs must be leashed and on trails. This is an ebird.org birding hot spot, and the best time to go is in the spring or fall during migration season. There is a park visitor center farther east of this section of the refuge with more information about the flora and fauna.

IN BRIEF

Low-lying hills offer great views of prairie and wetlands, and a floating boardwalk allows access to the marsh and its bounty of wildlife.

DESCRIPTION

This is the federally run portion of the marsh, so there is no state park fee. It is the largest freshwater cattail marsh in the country and birders treat this as a mecca during the migration periods when more than 250 species pass through. The scenic park road is a 3-mile loop. If you are looking for a short visit to the marsh, just skip to the Egret Trail and floating boardwalk right near the trailhead. Otherwise start from the Red Fox Hiking Trail trailhead across the road from the lot entrance. There is a map posted here. Just 200 feet into the prairie, the trail forks after a short boardwalk over a low area. Go left through open prairie showing an abundance of wildflowers.

The trail loops 0.35-miles over the hill, passing close to some trees and then finally into the woods. The shade only lasts 0.1 mile, and then you head back into prairie. Just outside the woods, you come to the top of a hill where there's a bench to sit and take in the nice view of prairie and marsh beyond.

GPS Trailhead Coordinates

UTM Zone (WGS 84)   16T

Easting   0365184

Northing   4830849

Latitude   N 43° 37' 6.31"

Longitude   W 88° 40' 15.11"

Directions

From its intersection with I-39, take US 151 north 48.1 miles to WI 49 near Waupun. Go 2.1 miles east on WI 49 to the park entrance on the right. Enter the park and drive 1.7 miles to the parking lot for the Egret Trail on the right. The trailhead is across the road from the lot entrance and marked with a sign that reads RED FOX HIKING TRAIL.

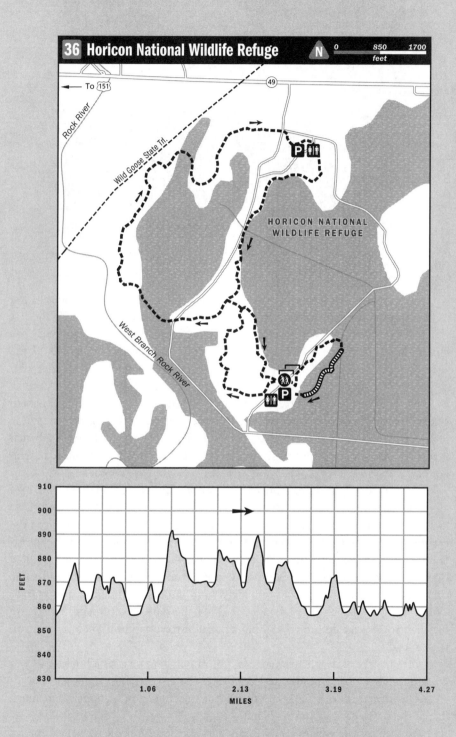

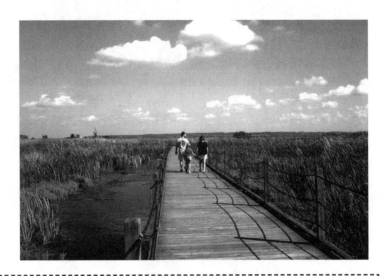

The floating boardwalk on Egret Nature Trail

Just down the hill another 300 feet, you come to a juncture. Going to the right returns you to the parking lot and completes the Red Fox loop. To the left is a 300-foot connection to the Redhead Hiking Trail. At this next juncture, go left through open prairie 0.2 miles to the park road. On the other side of the road, the trail continues through a row of trees before it comes into an area with cattails to the right.

The trail heads toward trees and brush, and at 0.2 miles, you find a bench. The path bends right and downhill through open forest. At the bottom you come to a nice little clearing that sits at the edge of some open water. There is a bench here that makes a good spot to sit and take it all in. This is a likely place to find a heron.

Another 0.1 mile leads you over another boardwalk, and then you hike along the edge of a ridge with trees to your right but no canopy. As the trail starts to climb from here, you find a bench with another good view 0.2 miles from the boardwalk. The trail passes over the top of a hill, curves right toward the forest, and then continues back down the hill to another boardwalk at 0.2 miles. Follow the path back through open prairie once more, climb another low hill, and come to a bench overlooking open water. Bring your binoculars; the birds are not that close. From the bench it's 0.4 miles back to the park road passing two more benches, some large cottonwoods, and a patch of trees and brush before rising up to the road.

On the other side, the trail makes a short climb and passes a boulder as you cross one more hill of prairie and 0.15 miles before arriving at the parking lot closest to the park entrance (not yours). You can find pit toilets here but much like at the other parking lot, no water.

Go right at the edge of the lot to a service road from the corner of the lot and a small park office/kiosk which is open only intermittently. At the corner of the lot, go left midway down the side of the parking lot to find the head of the next trail segment. Continue on crushed limestone as the trail takes you through prairie 0.75 miles to the end of the Redhead Trail loop, passing close to the edge of the park road and through some brush near the end. A short pass through the woods also brings you through a gap in an old rock wall. Back when this was farmland, the farmers had to do the painstaking work of removing stones—which, thanks to the glaciers, there is an abundance of—from the fields. From the rock wall, it's prairie until that connecting trail. Go left at the trail juncture, taking the connecting trail back to the Red Fox Hiking Trail and going left. Another 0.35 miles takes you back to the trail fork where you go left across the boardwalk and out to the park road.

At the road go straight across and up a short trail on a small knoll. To the right is the parking lot and ahead there are three benches. Go left on a boardwalk a few feet as it takes you at an angle to the roadside where the crushed-rock trail and park road cross a marshy area with a low concrete curb to the right overlooking open water. There is a bench halfway across the 200-foot gap. On the other side, the trail breaks right and heads into the shade of hardwood forest. This 0.6-mile loop briefly passes through the trees and then comes out on a floating boardwalk through the cattails. Just past the trees is a trail to the left out to the road. Go right as it takes you to the boardwalk that zigzags through the marsh. Find an observation deck to the left at the first juncture. It has benches and a roof over it for shade. There is a second platform, much lower to the water and unshaded, 0.1 mile past the first one. From the end of the boardwalk, take a short asphalt path back to the parking lot.

NEARBY ACTIVITIES

Across the highway from the park entrance is the privately owned and volunteer-operated Marsh Haven Nature Center. There is a short trail and a 30-foot observation tower here, and the center itself offers a variety of information and houses a small museum. Admission to the museum is $1. Call (920) 324-5818 for more information.

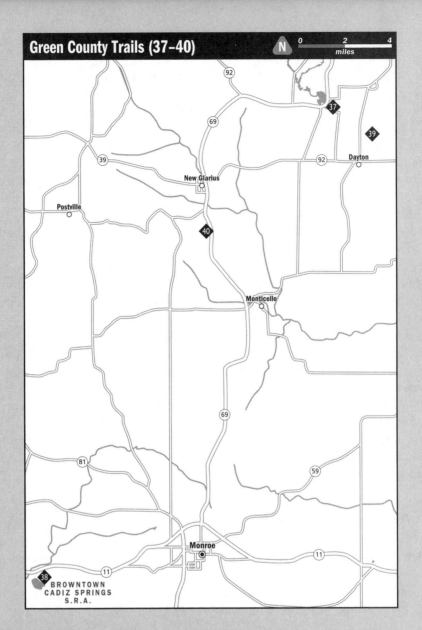

Green County Trails (37–40)

N

0   2   4
miles

92

69

37

39

39

92   Dayton

New Glarus

Postville

40

Monticello

69

81

59

Monroe

11

38
BROWNTOWN
CADIZ SPRINGS
S.R.A.

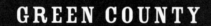

GREEN COUNTY

37 BADGER STATE TRAIL

KEY AT-A-GLANCE INFORMATION

LENGTH: 9 miles (each way)

CONFIGURATION: Out-and-back/ one way

DIFFICULTY: Easy

SCENERY: Farmland, mixed forest, an old train tunnel, a river

EXPOSURE: Mostly shady

TRAIL TRAFFIC: Light to moderate

TRAIL SURFACE: Crushed limestone

HIKING TIME: 3.5–4 hours (one way)

DRIVING DISTANCE: 9 miles south from the exit for WI 69 from US 18/151 near Verona

ACCESS: Open year-round

MAPS: USGS Belleville and Monticello; www.badger-trail.com; dnr.wi.gov/org/land/parks/ specific/badger

WHEELCHAIR ACCESSIBILITY: Yes

FACILITIES: Restrooms at trailheads only; no facilities on the trail

SPECIAL COMMENTS: State trails do not charge fees for foot traffic. Bring a flashlight for the tunnel and perhaps a light jacket if you are susceptible to cold. If you plan to hike the entire length, be sure to bring enough water. Though there is ample shade along the segment, sunscreen is always a good idea.

IN BRIEF

Hike the highlights of southern Wisconsin's latest and arguably greatest rails-to-trails effort as it passes along the line between glaciated and unglaciated terrain, plunges into the dark of a long tunnel, and crosses the Sugar River.

DESCRIPTION

Badgers are burrowing creatures, and when European immigrant miners came to southwestern Wisconsin—then a territory—for the lead-mining boom in the early 1800s, the seeds were laid for the state's nickname, the Badger State. This hike might make a badger out of you as well as it passes through a 1,200-foot tunnel through an unglaciated hill. The Badger State Trail was inaugurated in July 2007 and is a fantastic conversion of rail bed that connects Madison to the Illinois state border and that state's trail system. If you like the hike, come back with your bike and take it from where it begins on Purcell Road north of Paoli. Future paving will finish the connection to the end of Madison's Southwest Path and Capital City Trail to the north.

In Belleville, right across Pearl Street from the parking lot and trailhead is Library Park with picnic tables and a gazebo. If you go west on Main Street (WI 92), you can find several

GPS Trailhead Coordinates

UTM Zone (WGS 84) 16T

Easting 0293096

Northing 4748224

Latitude N 42° 51' 30.94"

Longitude W 89° 31' 56.61"

Directions

From US 18/151 in Verona, take WI 69 south 9 miles to Belleville. Turn left on East Main Street and take the immediate first right. One block later at Pearl Street, turn right. The parking lot and trailhead is on your left behind the public library and post office.

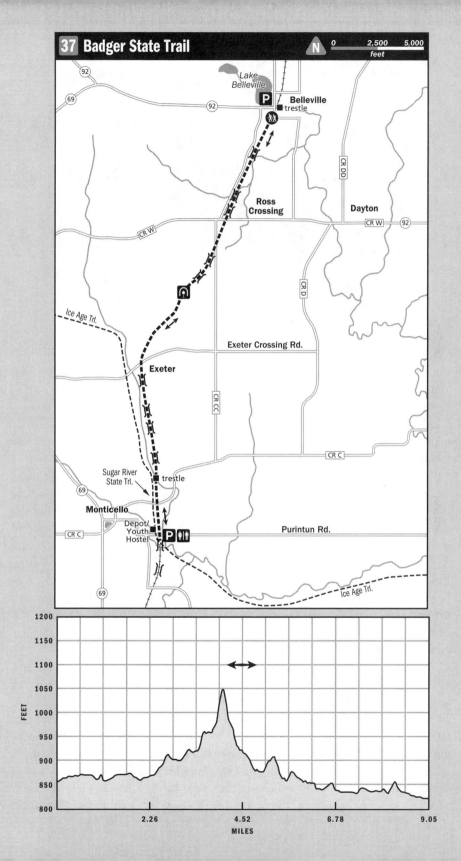

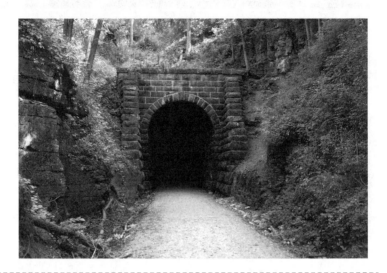

1,200-foot Stewart Tunnel

restaurants and bars. The building in the middle of the park is a community center, and though it has restrooms, it is not always open. The public library has restrooms, or you can seek them out at restaurants on Main Street. There is a place to lock up bikes and a self-pay tube for the trail pass if you choose to ride the trail instead of hiking it. For a good look at the Sugar River, head north on the trail 700 feet (about two blocks from the library) to an old steel railroad bridge.

From the parking lot behind the library at 135 South Vine Street, start south along the trail. Cross Vine Street at an angle and then School Street. From here the trail is unshaded for 0.7 miles until the first bridge on this segment. On the entire Badger State Trail there are more than 40 bridges and trestles, in fact, and you cross several of them.

Wetlands ease up around the trail through here, and 0.4 miles later you cross Fahey Road. Another bridge lies 0.6 miles from here and yet another 0.3 miles beyond that. From there it is only 0.2 miles to County Road W which heads west 4.5 miles to New Glarus, a small town with a strong Swiss heritage. Before or after your hike, stop in to find Swiss culture, great eats, and the popular New Glarus Brewery.

Past County Road CC at 0.4 miles, the rail bed was cut into the earth, and the trail becomes a narrow corridor of trees crossing another bridge 0.6 miles later. On the other side of Tunnel Road, find a nice patch of wildflowers before crossing a bridge and entering the channel up to the tunnel. Enjoy rough-cut rock covered with moss walls in either side of the trail as you approach the dark opening of the Stewart Tunnel, named for the engineer behind the construction of the entire line. The 1,200-foot passageway will be a little chilly even in the heat of summer, and throughout it you can expect to be hit by a few drips in the dark. You can't see the other end of the tunnel due to a bend in its course, so a flashlight is recommended. Part of the tunnel's arch is built of brick; other portions are cut stone, and there is a corrugated metal section as well. About halfway through, you will hear a noise that may disturb you. It is almost as if there is a beating heart there in the earth, a pulsing noise. Fear not, this is merely the cooing of pigeons perched somewhere in the dark. The reverberations of the tunnel have some interesting effects on the sounds. Exit the southern end of the tunnel between stone-block walls.

What lies before you is equally amazing when you think about it. You begin crossing what is essentially a land bridge. You can see that the surrounding terrain slopes down perhaps 100 feet on either side of the path, and treetops rising up from below are at eye level. This rail bed is not the earth and stone removed from the tunnel. In fact, this material had to be hauled in before the equipment to build the tunnel could reach the hill behind you. This must have been some serious manual labor.

At 1.2 miles you cross Tunnel Road again. You reach Exeter Crossing Road at 0.3 miles and Marshall Bluff Road another 0.7 miles after that. From here you might call it "the segment of bridges." To the right is more marshland. You cross a bridge in the sun at 0.4 miles, another bridge at 0.8 miles, and *another* bridge 0.4 miles later, until you finally reach the scenic Little Sugar River after 0.3 miles. You might not be surprised, but here there is a bridge.

Look into the woods at eye level to the right of the bridge and forward. The Sugar River Trail passes through the trees there, and you may see other hikers or bikers. Another 800 feet past the bridge, a trestle crosses the trail high above. It is a road to nowhere these days. It also crosses the Sugar River Trail. Two different railroad companies operated the former rails that ran these two trails, and you can see where one side of the trestle is different from the other. Each company built and paid for its half and then the two portions were connected to make the crossing.

Just past here a spur trail spans the 30 feet of woods between you and the other trail. From the trestle it is another 0.3 miles to County Road C. At the road the Sugar River Trail is 100 feet to your right, making the same crossing. Now you cross more wetlands. Weeping willows are common here.

You are 0.6 miles from the end of this hike. Halfway there, a spur trail breaks right and takes you into Monticello. Main Street has a few places to eat. The Dining Room is a recommended dinner stop (after 5 p.m. Wednesday–Sunday; [608] 938-2200). Stock up for the trail at Gempler's Market, where you can get good sandwiches at the deli.

You can see that the trail continues past your stopping point at County Road EE. The Sugar River Trail intersects just 800 feet farther on. The next 12-mile stretch of the Badger State Trail has no facilities until you reach Monroe. The parking lot shared by both trails is to the right (west) on CR EE, where you will find restrooms, water, and an old depot. This depot doubles as a youth hostel.

Look for wild turkeys and deer along the trail as well as hawks and songbirds. Black caps (black raspberries) can be found in many partly shaded places in early July.

Monticello is the best place to start if you want to get on the trail just for the tunnel or combine the Badger and Sugar River trails for an outing. You also have some options for making this hike shorter. There are 3.9 miles between Belleville and the tunnel, but the distance is 4.9 miles if you approach from Monticello. Dropping off a second vehicle at one of the two parking lots is another possibility: remember it is 9 miles *one way*. Crossing roads offer unofficial roadside parking, and the closest cutoffs to the tunnel are the two trail intersections with Tunnel Road. From the south it's 1.2 miles to the mouth of the tunnel; from the north it's only 0.3 miles.

Tunnel Road can be reached by driving west from New Glarus 4.4 miles on County Road W to where County Road CC goes south. The northern end of Tunnel Road is 1 mile south on your right. Continuing south on CR CC another 1.5 miles, go right on Exeter Crossing Road to find the southern end of Tunnel Road 1.4 miles on the right.

NEARBY ACTIVITIES

In Belleville, Community Park is a short walk from the library. Check out Lake Belle View where the main and west branches of the Sugar River come together. In Monticello, you can fish or go kayaking or canoeing in Lake Montesian, which features a wheelchair-accessible pier and a bridge to an island. Nearby community gardens are a nice place to walk as well.

BROWNTOWN-CADIZ SPRINGS RECREATION AREA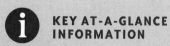

IN BRIEF

The dikes through these two lakes are great for birders, and the trails continue beyond, following a spring creek through woodlands and then crossing prairie and farmland.

DESCRIPTION

The trail begins on an asphalt path along the back of a dike between two dam-made lakes—Beckman Lake to the west and the smaller Zander Lake to the east. Early in the morning you can expect a lot of birds and a few anglers along the dike. Swallows sweep over the grasses and open water, while great blue and green herons hunt along the shoreline. The trail bends left (east), and by 0.25 miles grasses, cattails, and brush close in on the right side. Two hundred feet later, the dike enters brush completely. The trail is then mowed grass.

At 0.5 miles find a trail to the right. Just 75 feet past here is a return trail going left, which would take you back around the diminutive Zander Lake via some woods for a very short hike. Take the trail to the right and cross a wooden bridge over the spring creek that feeds the lakes. Be aware this footbridge can be quite slippery even with a bit of dew. The trail enters thick woods and 400 feet later comes to a juncture.

KEY AT-A-GLANCE INFORMATION

LENGTH: 4.2 miles
CONFIGURATION: Figure eight
DIFFICULTY: Easy
SCENERY: Lake, wetlands, mixed forest, prairie
EXPOSURE: Half and half
TRAIL TRAFFIC: Light
TRAIL SURFACE: Packed dirt, mowed grass
HIKING TIME: 2 hours
DRIVING DISTANCE: 47.7 miles southwest from the Beltline Highway (US 12/18) and Verona Road (US 18/151)
ACCESS: 6 a.m.–11 p.m.
MAPS: USGS Browntown; at thevpark office
WHEELCHAIR ACCESSIBILITY: Along parts of the dike. A toilet and fishing pier/boat launch are accessible as well.
FACILITIES: Pit toilets, water, playground, boat launch, shelter
SPECIAL COMMENTS: In the past the park map has been horrifically inaccurate; confirm that it has been updated since 2007. Changes in mowing patterns may also make this book's map slightly inaccurate in some places. Dogs are allowed on leashes. All vehicles require a state park sticker ($7 daily, $25 annual for vehicles with Wisconsin plates).

Directions

From the Beltline Highway (US 12/14/18), go left 7.3 miles on Verona Road/US 18/151 to WI 69. Follow WI 69 south for 33.2 miles to Monroe. Go west on WI 11 for 6.1 miles. Turn left on Allen Road, go 0.8 miles to Cadiz Springs Road, and turn right, continuing 0.3 miles to the park entrance on your left. Park in the first lot near the end of the dike, where you will find the trailhead.

GPS Trailhead Coordinates

UTM Zone (WGS 84)   16T
Easting   0272765
Northing   4718307
Latitude   N 42° 35' 1.42"
Longitude   W 89° 46' 8.99"

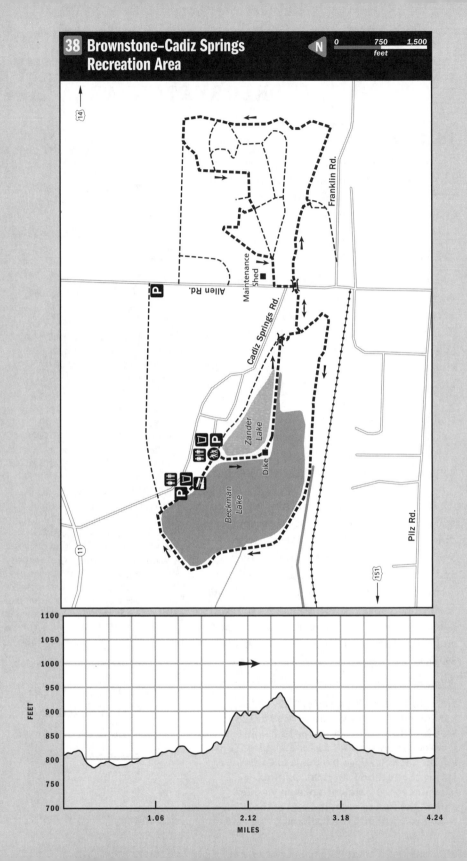

38 **Brownstone–Cadiz Springs Recreation Area**

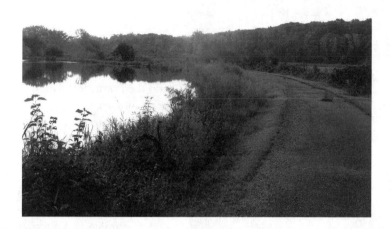

The dike between the two lakes

Go left here. The right path is the second loop of the figure eight that heads around Beckman Lake.

Another 0.1 mile takes you out to Allen Road. Down the road to your left is a bridge over the creek, but the trail resumes directly across the street. Enter open woods thick to your left and pass along the edge of a field on your right, which was supposed to be restored to prairie; funding has been delayed.

It's 0.25 miles to the next trail juncture, and halfway there you catch glimpses of the creek through the brush on the left. At the juncture a trail goes right out to Franklin Road. Stay left and pass through a row of trees and brush to a field on the other side. Another 0.25 miles takes you through the open to the next juncture. Go left. The trail to the right heads out of the park (as probably would any other mowed paths to the right along this section).

Enter the woods, cross over the tiny creek, and then follow the path slightly to the right up into some more trees. Another 0.2 miles takes you into a clearing, and 0.15 miles across that clearing, an alternative trail heads off left and into the woods opposite. Stay straight back into the forest passing another trail on the left and continuing 0.15 miles back into the open and the northeastern corner of the park. Go left with power lines and agricultural fields running parallel to the right of the path. Going straight would take you out to Allen Road to bypass the wooded portions of the trail.

Rather, go left at the next juncture as the trail angles away from the park boundary curving until it is heading due south. Stay straight on this, passing a connecting trail on the left and then following along the edge of the woods to the left as well. The trail turns right and follows between sumacs and a farm field on your right and the woods on the left. Follow it into the woods 0.3 miles from where you left the power lines. Two hundred feet in is the next juncture, and you follow it

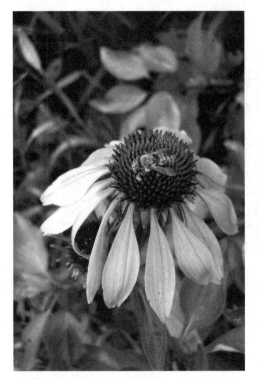

A bee probes a coneflower

first to the right and then left as it skirts the woods once more. The trail curves north along the trees and then turns left where you see a path into the woods. Follow this 0.3 miles through mixed forest to bring you to a clearing and trail juncture with the park maintenance shed on the right. Go right, straight out to Allen Road. Go left on Allen Road, cross Cadiz Springs Road and the bridge to find your return trail on the right—the same trail you emerged from for this half of the park.

Backtrack 0.15 miles to the trail juncture and now head left. The path goes 0.4 miles through woods with open canopy and then emerges next to Beckman Lake, taking you another 1 mile around the edge of the water, passing several benches along the way. At the west end of the lake, the land slopes down to your left and you have a view out over pasture to the farmland and hills beyond. On the north side of the lake, you pass a service road that can take you out to Cadiz Springs Road and across to an optional out-and-back trail into oak forest. Stay along the lake and pass parking, pit toilets, and a playground as well as a boat launch before you reach your starting point 0.15 miles later.

NEARBY ACTIVITIES

Whether you are a train enthusiast or not, this little roadside attraction shouldn't be missed: The Toy Train Barn at W9141 Highway 81 in Argyle showcases a real-life engineer's collection of vintage trains running amid several cleverly designed and animated settings. Admission is $5 per adult and $2.50 per child, and it is open year-round 10 a.m. to 5 p.m. Call (608) 966-1464 or visit **www.whrc-wi.org/trainbarn**.

ICE AGE TRAIL: Brooklyn Segment 39

IN BRIEF

Get some up-close views of sandstone formations in the forest and take in vistas over the prairies on this rugged segment of the national trail.

DESCRIPTION

Many of the glacial formations in the area are said to have been left when the last of the most recent glaciers retreated north 10,000 to 20,000 years ago. The moraines on this segment of the trail are believed to be from glaciers of an earlier advance more than 60,000 years ago.

The trailhead is in the gravel parking lot at the southern end of the segment. A map is posted there. The path heads north 0.2 miles across open prairie and follows various trees along the way marked with yellow painted squares, which are useful in winter. The trail is maintained, but often the grass gets a little long. It is exposed here. Entering the woods, the trail begins sloping gently downhill and becomes packed dirt with a covering of dead leaves.

Just 0.4 miles later, you enter a clearing. Fire lanes go off to either side but are overgrown though still possible for further exploration. There is a plethora of wildflowers through here.

KEY AT-A-GLANCE INFORMATION

LENGTH: 9 miles

CONFIGURATION: Out-and-back

DIFFICULTY: Moderate to difficult

SCENERY: Prairie, mixed forest, glacial moraines

EXPOSURE: Some shade, a lot of sun

TRAIL TRAFFIC: Light

TRAIL SURFACE: Narrow packed dirt footpaths with roots and rocks; grassy paths

HIKING TIME: 3.5–4 hours

DRIVING DISTANCE: 10.4 miles west from US 14 and WI 92 south of Madison

ACCESS: Open year-round

MAPS: USGS Attica and Oregon; posted maps at trailheads

WHEELCHAIR ACCESSIBILITY: None

FACILITIES: A single water pump on the trail

SPECIAL COMMENTS: Some portions of the wooded areas are overgrown a bit with snagging plants such as raspberries and similar thorny tendrils. Long pants are advised.

Directions

From Madison head south on US 14 (Park Street) and continue 13.7 miles from where it passes under the Beltline Highway (US 12/18). Turn right (west) on WI 92 and follow it 9.2 miles west to Hughes Road. Go north (right) 1.2 miles, following the road as it turns left. The parking lot is on your right. The trailhead is at the parking lot.

GPS Trailhead Coordinates

UTM Zone (WGS 84) 16T

Easting 0295772

Northing 4746424

Latitude N 42° 50' 35.24"

Longitude W 89° 29' 57.12"

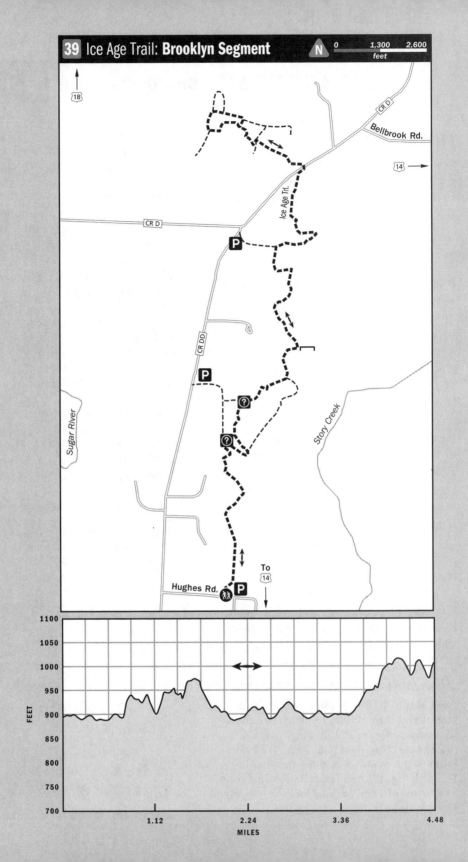

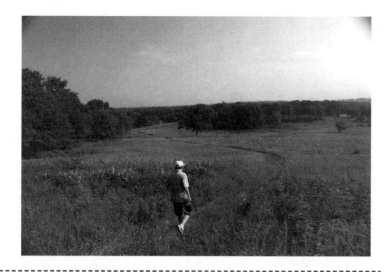

Descending into prairie from a forested ridge

The trail starts uphill soon after and passes through some small oaks coming to the crest of the hill before it sloping down, partially shaded by the canopy.

The trail veers left, but go straight according to the yellow patch on a tree. There are sandy patches here along the trail. As you come over the crest 150 feet later, you have a few steps of tree roots and earth.

There are plenty of tree roots under the dead leaves, so mind your footing. You'll go over another hilltop 400 feet later and then follow the trail down a slope along pine trees that have carpeted the surface with needles.

At the bottom of the slope, the path might be difficult to see if no one's been through in a while, but bear straight ahead as it heads back into woods. The trail curves and comes up to a small pine grove with a trail marker and map showing where you are. Follow the yellow arrow to the right. The path to the left takes you out to an alternate parking lot.

Continuing along the trail, look left and see some of the exposed sandstone from the glaciers' cutting work. The trail is downhill and mostly sand with scattered rocks and tree roots for about 700 feet. Above your head on both sides is exposed rock.

Head into a small clearing. One trail goes left and another goes straight. The official trail is left and takes you higher up to a water pump just before the path heads into the woods. The trail to the right sidesteps the woods and can be an alternate return through the prairie on your way back to the trailhead.

The next 0.6 miles is through forest. At the highest points, the trail looks down the rocks to the left and the slope to the right. You can see quite far down the hill through the forest and gain an appreciation for the rise and fall of the land if the trail hasn't already made that pretty clear. From here you will descend almost 100 feet in 2,100 feet. To the left the land slips into a groove between two hills. The trail dips into this and crosses, and when you climb to the opposite side, you find a trail map. To the left is the trail to the parking lot at County Road DD. Go right and enter a clearing. In summer you can find raspberries and their thorny shoots. The thorns, combined with the mosquitoes and ticks, make long pants a good idea in most weather.

Head to the bottom of the next gully and bear right. Follow along the bottom of the gully with a ridge rising up on either side of you. Foliage blocks views of exposed rock except in early spring or late fall. Look to the right almost 1,000 feet from the map board and there is a Department of Natural Resources (DNR) trail. Go left up the hill, staying with the yellow arrows as the trail passes through more wild berries before it widens and becomes grassy as it comes into a clearing. At the next intersection, go left. The trail to the right returns through the prairie. Stop for a nice view of the valley below this point known as Crane Overlook.

From here the trail descends to the left through a grassy meadow. Land rolls away with clumps of forest dotting the landscape. Pass a trail post, and the land drops even farther. As the trail levels off a bit, stay straight along the top of the ridge, keeping the view on either side. To the left see a traditional red barn. Lichen-covered rocks peek through the prairie grass as you come to a bench 30 feet left of the trail. Pass a row of oak and pine to see across the prairie to the woods beyond. Find another trail marker just before the trail descends through grass and wildflowers. Tire ruts from park vehicles may lurk below the grass on the trail, so be careful.

You come to the woods. This next 0.6 miles is on a narrow trail and can be the worst of the snagging plant life, so be prepared. Raspberries are a midsummer reward. When you exit the trees, you come to a trail marker that leads you right where you'll find a map board. The trail left heads out to a parking lot.

Now the trail is open with tall grass and trees not far off to either side. As you pass another trail marker, the prairie opens up and your view stretches for a couple miles. A double tire lane heads into the field and takes you 0.2 miles to a rocky platform with sandy patches overlooking a berry patch and the prairie beyond.

The trail might be hard to follow over this surface, but as you come over the rise, just keep straight, and you should see the trail marker at the edge of the forest. Go left here 500 feet along the edge of the forest, but don't expect any shade. The trail heads right into a mix of forest and grassy patches for another 0.2 miles before you see signs of civilization again. Pass a trail marker on your right and head across an open meadow with raspberries on both sides. Head for the clump of woods on the other side and pass along the left side of them. The trail enters shade there and curves with the edge of the trees until it crosses the road. Be careful of traffic rounding the bend to the left of you.

Cross CR D to find a giant oak with a no trespassing sign. This lollipop portion of the trail is 1.5 miles long. Go left along the uncut field to a mowed path along this field's edge. There's a trail map and a yellow sign that says

FOOT TRAFFIC ONLY. A house with a wooden deck will be before you. To remain on the easement, follow the edge of the cut grass that goes slightly to the left. At an enormous oak see a yellow arrow on a trail post sending you right into the forest. Private land is very clearly marked.

The trail is exposed, crossing a mix of grasses, wildflowers, and brush. Long-needle pines appear, and the trail slopes up at a yellow-marked black walnut tree where you'll find fire lanes going either left or right. Go straight up the hill, and at the top, find a prairie restoration. The official trail goes straight along edge of forest but then breaks right bearing through the center of the prairie. The gentle curve goes back to the edge of the trees to the left. You may see bluebirds here, and the wildflowers are abundant. The park does a controlled burn in the spring.

State trails are in the process of being developed, so you may find some alternative paths outside the perimeter of the prairie. The official trail follows around the field and crosses the open field to the north, which attaches to this central prairie as a transept does to a cathedral. You can follow the DNR trail around its edge if you want to extend the hike or just continue around the central prairie until you come to where you originally entered from the trail up the hill.

Retrace your steps and follow the trail all the way back to your car. The alternate parking lots give you options for a one-way hike as well. There is no official parking near the 1.5-mile lollipop segment north of CR D.

NEARBY ACTIVITIES

Lake Belle View in Community Park in nearby Belleville to the west is a pleasant spot for a post-hike picnic.

40 NEW GLARUS WOODS STATE PARK

KEY AT-A-GLANCE INFORMATION

LENGTH: 3.8 miles
CONFIGURATION: Loop
DIFFICULTY: Moderate
SCENERY: Prairie, mixed forest, scenic overlook
EXPOSURE: Mostly shaded but exposed in prairie sections
TRAIL TRAFFIC: Light
TRAIL SURFACE: Packed dirt, mowed grass, some tree roots and rocks
HIKING TIME: 1.5 hours
DRIVING DISTANCE: 17.5 miles from US 18/151 and WI 69 near Verona
ACCESS: 6 a.m.–11 p.m. year-round
MAPS: USGS New Glarus; brochure
WHEELCHAIR ACCESSIBILITY: Restrooms and an accessible wildlife blind on the Walnut Trail
FACILITIES: Toilets, water, picnic tables, playground, campsites
SPECIAL COMMENTS: The park produces a trail guide that corresponds to numbered stations throughout the Havenridge Nature Trail. There are also shorter, easier trails plus a paved connecting trail to the Sugar River State Trail. All vehicles require a park sticker ($7 daily, $25 annual for vehicles with Wisconsin plates). The park participates in the Junior Ranger/Wisconsin Explorer program (see Preface, page xv).

IN BRIEF

Explore the woods south of New Glarus, teeming with wildlife. Trails run through rolling restored prairie and hardwood forest offering nice vistas, and the park's nature guide and interpretive trail make it an educational experience.

DESCRIPTION

The farmland around here undulates with the rolling terrain of the unglaciated corner of southwestern Wisconsin. When European settlers arrived, they interrupted the burns—natural or by Native Americans—that kept the prairie and oak savanna healthy. Because of this woods went unchecked and brush filled in beneath the tree cover. Today, some prairie sections have been restored through burns and reseeding with native species. Some of the native plant life, however, rose naturally out from beneath the ashes of prescribed burns after lying dormant there for many years.

Chipmunks and ground squirrels create quite a chatter as you hike the New Glarus Woods, and you'd have to be rather unlucky not to scare up at least a deer or two. The prairie sections are vibrant with color and savanna is beginning to come back in some places. The hardwoods attract some interesting

GPS Trailhead Coordinates

UTM Zone (WGS 84)   16T

Easting   0284809

Northing   4740521

Latitude   N 42° 47' 13.18"

Longitude   W 89° 37' 51.68"

Directions

From US 18/151 near Verona, go south 3.8 miles on WI 69. Go right on County Road PB for 5.1 miles, then turn right on WI 69/92 and follow it 8.4 miles through New Glarus to County Road NN. Go right here 400 feet to find the park office. Parking is just off the county road another 400 feet past the office. The trailhead is on the left side opposite the parking area.

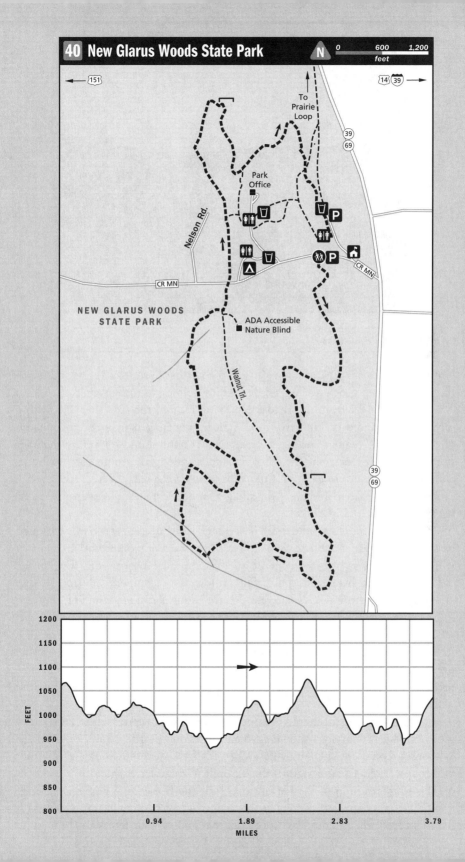

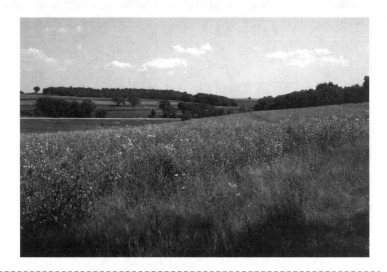

A field of native prairie flowers

bird species such as the scarlet tanager and the northern oriole. The rise and fall of the trail will keep your pulse up a little, but it's nothing too exhausting.

Cross CR NN from the roadside parking lot and the trail descends with a surface of dirt and occasional tree roots. The park managers maintain the breadth of the trail with regular cutting, but the path is natural and uneven, sometimes sloping to the left or right. Numbered signposts along the route correspond to entries in the *Havenridge Trail Companion Booklet* available free at the park office. It's informative and great for all ages, and it includes quotes from famous naturalists.

The first stretch of the trail is a long, slow descent primarily through basswoods, maples, and black walnut. Wildflowers are abundant. At 0.2 miles you will have come down to the edge of a fantastic prairie restoration. You can see WI 69 from here over rolling hills full of flowers in summer. The trail follows along the edge of the woods, sloping down this hill and then climbing the next into open hardwood forest another 0.2 miles farther.

The shade is short-lived, and 900 feet later, you are back into the prairie following the perimeter. Coneflowers are abundant. Look left out across the prairie and see a quarry in the distance. Continue down the hill and up once more and you are back into the trees. The growth here is closer together and with smaller trunks.

When you come back into the open after 500 feet, there's a bench up ahead with an educational sign showing you the various prairie plants of southern Wisconsin, complete with drawings. Then it's back into the woods for another 900-foot stretch. To your right is the 0.5-mile Walnut Trail which cuts 1.1 miles off this southern loop of the Havenridge Trail and bypasses any further prairie.

The trial is open to the sky at this point. When you reach trail marker 13, 0.3 miles from the Walnut Trail trailhead, the land to your left is the beginnings of oak savanna. Look carefully to see some patches of wetland where a creek runs through it.

Hike another 0.3 miles to where the trees start to thin, exposing prairie. When you finally enter the field, you are at the farthest point from the highway, and even the occasional hum of truck tires fades over the hill behind you. At 400 feet from the edge of the woods, cross a culvert that channels a small creek, almost invisible in the deep grass, and the trail starts to turn right. You can see where this water runs as a long band of trees and brush sprouts out of the middle of the prairie.

Six hundred feet later, cross the creek again and go uphill to the trees. The trail follows along their edge to the left and then passes just inside the woods with a barbed-wire fence to your left marking the end of the park property. Agricultural fields lie beyond it. This is the "quietist" part of the forest, though the chipmunks might have a different idea about that.

This section of the trail goes gradually uphill 0.8 miles to the end point of the Walnut Trail and then another 350 feet to CR NN. This is a possible cutoff point, and you could walk the highway 0.3 miles to the parking lot to your right.

Go directly across the road where the trail drops off the edge of the asphalt just like at the beginning, going downhill through forest dominated by basswood for the first 0.4 miles. Halfway down this segment, there is a cutoff trail to the right that leads to the park office, toilets, and water.

Where the trail starts to go uphill, it also starts into a curve to the right. Four hundred feet past here is a bench on the right and a mowed area through the brush to the left that allows you to step to the edge of the prairie beyond. The view from this hilltop is out over the valley of New Glarus. The trail heads south again another 0.2 miles to where it follows along the ridge with a deep gully to your left. You'll cross that gully where it comes up almost to the trail level. A cutoff trail here leads to the park office to the south (right). Go north (left) along the opposite ridge as it does a half loop around until 0.3 miles later, you are heading south again. Here you arrive at a trail juncture. To the left a trail leads you out to the asphalt connection to the Sugar River State Trail just inside New Glarus and also a recent 1.1-mile prairie put in at the northern end of New Glarus Woods.

Stay right just a few steps more to another fork. You have a choice; either trail takes you back to the playground area near the parking lot. Along both you will find educational signage. Since the entire loop is only 0.4 miles—you're standing at its turnaround point—you might want to do one, come back down the other, and retrace your steps out. This Basswood Nature Trail is also a nice little loop by itself with an educational twist if you are short on time or energy. In spring, look for jack-in-the-pulpit and wild geraniums.

Go left at this fork, and at 0.1 mile, pass a spur trail out to a parking lot. There's a drinking fountain here and the trailhead of that Sugar River Trail connection is to the left at the end of the lot.

You'll exit the woods 0.1 mile later near some toilets, and a playground is off to the right. CR NN is straight ahead, and you should see your car from here.

The other end of the Basswood Trail is just past the playground equipment to your right.

Hikers with kids can get a Junior Explorers discovery backpack (each is themed: birds of prey, insects, etc.) available at state parks and local libraries. The packs contain guidebooks with activities for kids to work on with parents. They can turn them in to earn a free patch. Look at the park brochure for information about weekly guided nature activities.

NEARBY ACTIVITIES

The town of New Glarus has a strong Swiss heritage and is worth a visit. Stop by Maple Leaf Cheese and Chocolate Haus for ice cream, more than 80 locally made cheeses, and incredible homemade fudge. Call (888) 624-1234 or go to **www .mapleleafcheeseandchocolatehaus.com** for more information. The award-winning New Glarus Brewery just across WI 69 offers self-guided tours and sampling. Check them out online at **newglarusbrewing.com** or call (608) 527-5850.

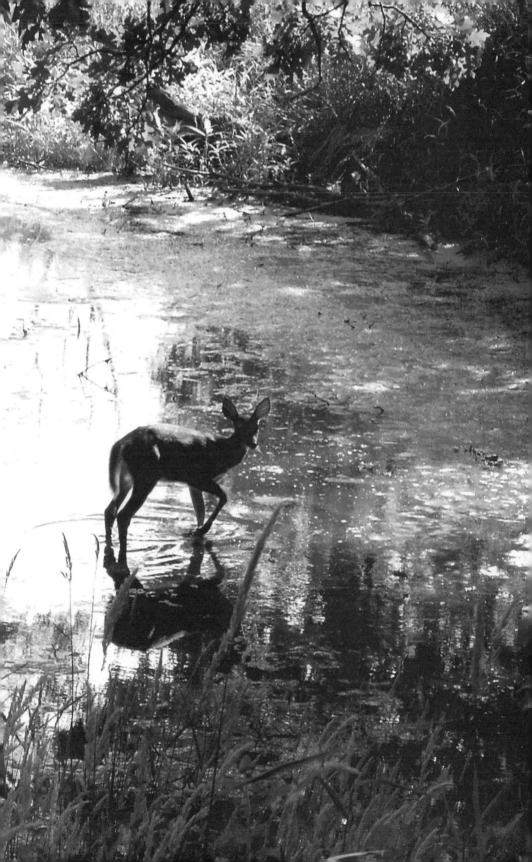

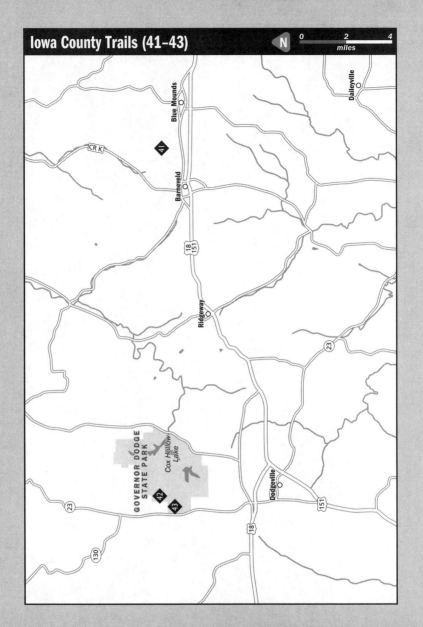

Iowa County Trails (41–43)

N

0 ——— 2 ——— 4
miles

Blue Mounds

Dalleyville

CR K

41

Barneveld

18
151

Ridgeway

23

GOVERNOR DODGE
STATE PARK

Cox Hollow
Lake

42

43

Dodgeville

151

18

23

130

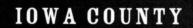

IOWA COUNTY

41 BLUE MOUND STATE PARK

 KEY AT-A-GLANCE INFORMATION

LENGTH: 5.6 miles
CONFIGURATION: Loop with many shorter alternatives
DIFFICULTY: Moderate to difficult, but easy with cutoffs
SCENERY: Mixed woods, some prairie, scattered boulders and tiny streams, two scenic overlooks
EXPOSURE: Mostly shaded with some exposed prairie portions
TRAIL TRAFFIC: Light
TRAIL SURFACE: Crushed rock, packed dirt, loose rock, tree roots
HIKING TIME: 2.5–3 hours
DRIVING DISTANCE: 24.8 miles west from the Beltline Highway (US 12/18) and Verona Road/US 18/151
ACCESS: 6 a.m.–11 p.m. year-round
MAPS: USGS Blue Mounds; at visitor center and major trail junctures
WHEELCHAIR ACCESSIBILITY: None
FACILITIES: Restrooms, water, camping, swimming pool, playground, observation towers, showers, pay phones
SPECIAL COMMENTS: All vehicles require a park sticker ($7 daily, $25 annual for vehicles with Wisconsin plates). Only the mountain-biking trails are open to hiking when the other trails are groomed for skiing. In winter, call the park at (608) 437-5711 to be sure.

- -

GPS Trailhead Coordinates

UTM Zone (WGS 84)   16T

Easting   0267278

Northing   4767726

Latitude   N 43° 01' 35.68"

Longitude   W 89° 51' 22.84"

IN BRIEF

This is the highest point in southern Wisconsin and a brilliant collection of trails ranging from easy woodland portions to more demanding but scenic detours into uneven terrain along a woodland spring creek. The geology of the park and the views to the faraway horizon are competing stars here.

DESCRIPTION

Check out the observation tower first for an amazing view of sometimes more than 50 miles.

The hike begins to the left of the tower, as you approach it, on Flint Rock Trail. A crushed-rock path with wood-beam steps descends through scattered rocks and boulders and zigzags through mixed forest. Warm shallow seas that covered this area millions of years ago left evidence in fossils in some of the rocks. A trail sign invites you to look for them. Good luck.

At 0.1 mile a trail goes left to the campgrounds, but keep going straight. Find some interactive interpretive signage through here, which is great for kids. Many shallow

- -

Directions ⟶

From the Beltline Highway (US 12/14/18), go left 22.7 miles on Verona Road/US 18/151 to County Road F. Go right 0.2 miles and then left on County Road ID 0.5 miles. Turn right on Mounds Road for 0.5 miles to where it turns left and becomes Mounds Park Road. Follow this 0.3 miles straight to the park entrance. Follow the park road 0.6 miles past the visitor center all the way to the picnic area. Follow the one-way road to the right 0.3 miles to the parking area for the West Observation Tower. The trailhead is to the left of the tower.

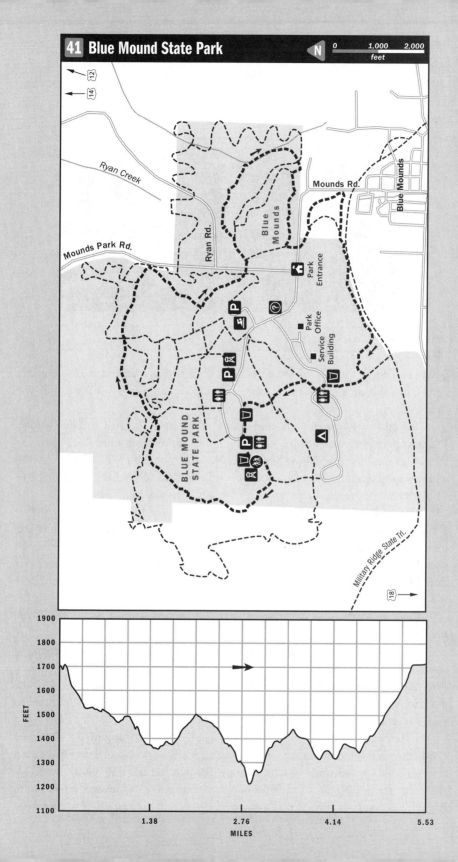

N

0   1,000   2,000
feet

12
14

Ryan Creek

Mounds Rd.

Blue Mounds

Blue Mounds

Ryan Rd.

Mounds Park Rd.

Park Entrance

Park Office

Service Office Building

BLUE MOUND STATE PARK

Military Ridge State Trl.

18

FEET

1900
1800
1700
1600
1500
1400
1300
1200
1100

1.38   2.76   4.14   5.53
MILES

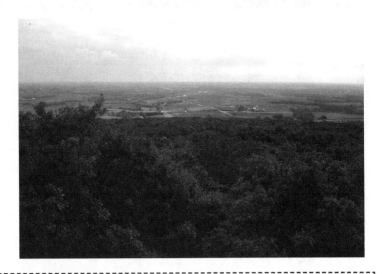

The view from the observation tower

gullies run down the hill from the right and continue down the slope to your left. After rains this area seems more like a rain forest. Another 0.5 miles brings you to a spur trail and a bench out of the shade.

You cross a lot of culverts, and finally at 0.4 miles, a small wooden bridge. Just past here is an intersection. Go straight and continue on Flint Rock Trail and the return path for the Willow Springs Trail. Go left here on Willow Springs Trail where you find a map board and just beyond that the Holy Schist Trail going left. This packed-earth trail is narrow and generally for mountain bikers.

The trail continues another 0.4 miles to a wooden bridge and just past that a big trail intersection. To the left is a narrow dirt path, which is the Chert Dip bike path. To your right find a similar path, also for mountain bikes, the Basalt and Pepper Trail. A soft right is the turn of Willow Spring Trail and John Minix Trail. But you go straight and remain on the John Minix Trail heading east. There is a map board to the left.

Erosion on the trail is common, and after big rainstorms parts of the trail might be washed out.

Cross two footbridges and a large culvert runoff channel before arriving at the next trail intersection 0.2 miles away where the Chert Dip Trail crosses. Another 0.1 mile takes you to a map board and a spur trail to the left out of the park to Mounds Park Road crossing the Chert Dip Trail, which runs parallel to the road at this point.

Continue straight and enter prairie 0.1 mile later. Crossing it you find more crushed rock on the trail as it passes through a forest with minimal understory but a lot of fallen wood under a tight canopy. It's another 0.1 mile partly in woods then out into wildflowers and willows before you arrive at the next intersection. Right takes you back toward the center of the park and the east observation tower.

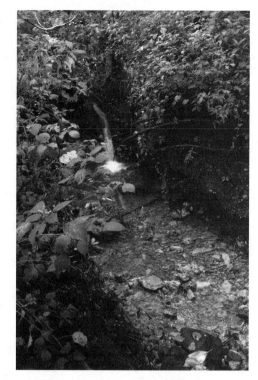

A spring in the forest

Go left here back into woods with brush along the trail. The next 0.2 miles take you over two bridges and two culverts. After the second bridge, the Gneiss and Smooth Bike Trail crosses your path, and you come to Mounds Park Road. On the other side, the trail continues as the Pleasure Valley Trail. Find a map board and trails going left and right. Go left on the grassy trail; to the right is a cutoff to skip the Pleasure Valley Hiking Trail, which is challenging, but for me the most beautiful part of the park and a nice place to linger.

The grassy trail heads down through evergreens, exposed. You come to a trail juncture. Going straight is the grassy Pleasure Valley Bike Trail, and just past this juncture on the left, the mountain bike Overlode Trail goes left. The Pleasure Valley Hiking Trail, however, goes left into the woods passing a bench on the left and apple trees to the right.

As you head into the cover of the canopy, you come across a creek to the left. Look for a tree with an elbow bend to it near the base. This appears to be a Native American marker tree or a pretty good coincidence. The spring-fed creek bubbles over rock as it descends, and you get a closer look as the trail goes down a short distance and then switches back left and brings you right to the water. You cross on the rocks, so watch your footing. On the other side, the trail can be hard to see, but it generally follows the creek downhill with the water no farther than 20 to 30 feet to your right. The path goes down over rocks and is very uneven. You come to a very large maple, and the trail goes around it to the left, where you see wood logs to the right side of the trail.

The path turns right toward the creek and a sign with a trail arrow. Cross over a 10-foot, 15-inch-wide wood beam over the creek. Straight ahead is a hill. Cross another creek on another wood beam. This stream joins the other off to your left. The trail continues alongside the creek and brings you to six wooden steps. The path goes over some rock behind a large boulder and crosses a short bridge. Go up another short series of steps where the trail resumes, still following the creek.

The trail curls around that hill to your right, comes back to the creek edge, and faces the hill. You see water coming out of the cracks of the wall of rock in front of you. The trail sign says GO LEFT. The stream is to the right now, and the trail is low enough to where in wet seasons the water might come up over it. Pass over a two-plank boardwalk to the other side of the creek. You must hop some rocks to get across the creek at the next crossing soon after. A crushed-rock path awaits on the opposite bank; follow it away from the creek. But the trail brings you to another creek; cross on a wide wooden bridge with railings and a nice little cascade to the right.

The path goes uphill with creeks to either side as you climb out of a ravine 0.3 miles to the top on a moderate to steep grade crossing over a giant culvert with wooden railings just before the mountain bike trail crosses. There is a metal gate at the top. At the juncture right after this, go right. Left takes you out of the park to an access road.

Another 200 feet takes you to another juncture. Go left to take the Pleasant Valley Bike Trail, an easy path through open fields with intermittent tree coverage and wildflowers. This will take you 0.3 miles to another juncture and trail map. Go left and cross Mounds Park Road.

On the other side, the trail goes left into the woods. Go left at the next map board and juncture on Walnut Hollow Trail, which takes you on a 0.4-mile half loop through a bit of prairie and then a forest of black walnuts. You come to the other end of the cutoff trail and continue straight. You can see the Military Ridge State Trail to your left, and the trail goes uphill moderately, crossing two bridges and several smaller gullies as it winds its way 0.7 miles to the asphalt connecting trail between Military Ridge and the park. Go right here 0.1 mile to the camping area turnaround. Follow the road straight up to the main park road where a sign points right to the office. You go left along the right side of the park road. Pass another road to the left to pit toilets and a pay phone. Take the crushed-rock trail here to your right that reads TRAIL TO PICNIC AREA. Cross a wooden bridge and come to a map board. Go left up to the picnic area, passing a storage shed on the left and then crossing a mountain bike trail. From the park road to where you emerge in the picnic area is 0.4 miles. From there go left, following along the edge of the road until you arrive back at the parking lot and west observation tower. There's water here along the road.

Note: The park participates in the Junior Ranger/Wisconsin Explorer program (see Preface, page xv).

NEARBY ACTIVITIES

The Cave of the Mounds National Natural Landmark, more than 1 million years old, is the most impressive cavern in the Midwest, and full of impressive formations. It is open year-round and only minutes from Blue Mound State Park. Call (608) 437-3038 or go to **caveofthemounds.org**.

GOVERNOR DODGE STATE PARK: Lost Canyon Trail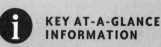

IN BRIEF

Visit a waterfall in a canyon and a cave in the bluffs, and cross hill and vale along Twin Valley Lake before returning through a canyon full of trees and a creek.

DESCRIPTION

The first segment of the path is the only wheelchair-accessible part, but it is recommended for all park visitors. Most everyone stops to walk the asphalt path to see the spring-fed Stephens Falls, which tumbles down into a canyon hidden in the trees.

Just 0.1 mile takes you along a narrow spring creek on the left side of the trail to a juncture. Go straight to see the falls; there is an overlook and also a path of rock steps switching back down to the bottom of the canyon. Return to the trail juncture and begin the Lost Canyon Trail, crossing the bridge and passing the Spring House where the waters emerge from the earth. Go uphill on grass, pass through a stand of tall pine, and enter into prairie. Just outside the woods, this prairie portion of the trail hits a T. Go left. The right trail is the return of 2.5-mile Gold Mine Trail.

Pass through prairie, crossing the park

KEY AT-A-GLANCE INFORMATION

LENGTH: 8.8 miles

CONFIGURATION: Loop

DIFFICULTY: Moderate

SCENERY: Flowing water, a waterfall, a cave, hardwood forest, rock formations, a lake

EXPOSURE: Half and half

TRAIL TRAFFIC: Light

TRAIL SURFACE: Packed dirt, mowed grass, crushed rock with a short asphalt segment

HIKING TIME: 3 hours

DRIVING DISTANCE: 44 miles from the West Beltline Highway (US 12/ 18) and Verona Road/US 18/151

ACCESS: 6 a.m.–11 p.m. year-round

MAPS: USGS Pleasant Ridge; at the park office

WHEELCHAIR ACCESSIBILITY: 0.25-mile asphalt trail to Stephens Falls overlook

FACILITIES: Restrooms, water, picnic tables, boat landing, concessions, campgrounds

SPECIAL COMMENTS: Portions of the trail are shared equestrian trails. All vehicles require a park sticker ($7 daily, $25 annual for vehicles with Wisconsin plates). Pets must be leashed except in designated pet swim areas.

Directions

From the West Beltline Highway (US 12/14) go southwest 37.4 miles on Verona Road/ US 18/151. At Exit 47 for Dodgeville, take US 18 west for 1.9 miles and then turn right on Bequette Street/WI 23 for 3.3 miles to the park entrance on the right. Take the park road 0.25 miles past the office and go straight at the first intersection following the road 0.8 miles to the roadside parking lot at the trailhead to Stephens Falls.

GPS Trailhead Coordinates

UTM Zone (WGS 84) 15T

Easting 0733721

Northing 4767817

Latitude N 43° 01' 37.53"

Longitude W 90° 07' 52.95"

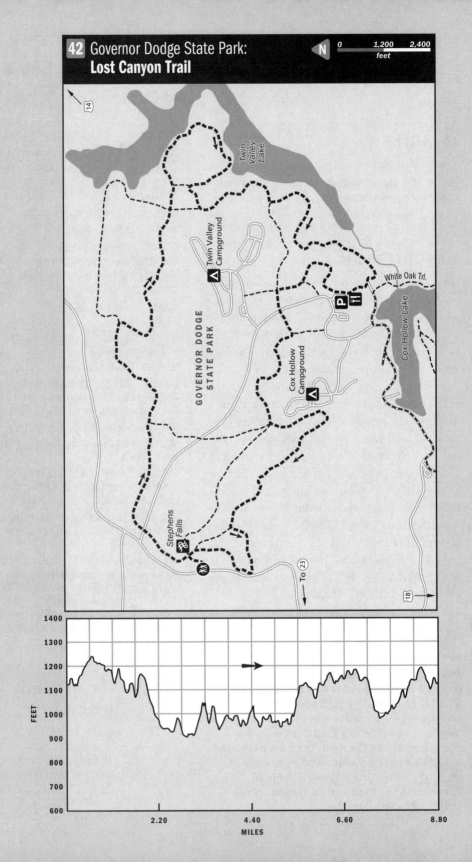

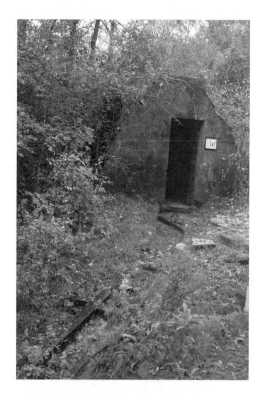

The spring house

road at 0.3 miles and arriving at a juncture 0.1 mile later. A trail to the left connects to the equestrian trail. Go right on a two-tire path with scant shade through oak, walnut, basswood, and hickory. At 0.4 miles you pass the Gold Mine Trail on the right for an optional return to the area of the falls. Stay straight and another 0.6 miles takes you to a spur on the right out to the equestrian trails. The Lost Canyon Trail goes right, passing through sumac. To your right is a fine view of the prairie as you head downhill. Pass a bench as the trail curves left around the edge of forest and into trees at 0.15 miles. The trail becomes mostly shaded through the woods as you continue 0.65 miles to the next horse trail juncture, passing a small creek at 0.35 miles.

Across the wide grassy horse path, stay straight, heading uphill into a loop that rounds the large bluff before you. At 0.1 mile an optional cutoff trail to the right skips the loop. Go straight another 0.5 miles, passing close to the shoreline of Twin Valley Lake before arriving at a spur trail to the right. This heads up the ridge 0.1 mile to the crown where you can find a cave. Follow the signs, and the trail climbs to the top; go right and back down to the right a bit in front of the rocky bluff face to find it.

Back on the main trail, descend to the right, pass cattails along the shore, and reach the cutoff trail at 0.4 miles. Go left heading into woods to another trail juncture. This is the horse trail coming in from the right, so stay left, and 0.1 mile later enter into prairie. The lake is to the left; follow a grassy trail amid wildflowers. Go left at 0.1 mile at the next juncture and continue through prairie with your best view of the lake. You can see the bluffs you just visited across water.

The trail goes back into woods for 0.2 miles, following the edge of a gully, with exposed rocks to your right and sand on the trail. The trail crosses left over a culvert and then heads back into the open for another 0.4 miles of prairie and brush. Cross a culvert into the woods and continue with shade for 0.3 miles. You start to hear Mill Creek flowing off to your left in the open. Another 0.2 miles brings you to the concessions and a parking lot. There are toilets and water here. A trail to your left will connect to the Military Ridge State Trail. Go right along the edge of the parking lot to the next corner. The trail heads up into the woods and bends right as it climbs. A line of rocks separates the trail from another trail to the amphitheater area.

From the lot it is 0.1 mile to the amphitheater entrance. Continue past on asphalt, passing a wheelchair-accessible parking spot. An arrow looks like it leads you to the right into the woods, but it is only to indicate that you should not follow the curve of the asphalt but stay straight on the grassy trail that leads you through prairie and an aspen colony 0.3 miles to the woods again.

Just inside the trees, come to a poorly marked intersection. Left takes you back to the beach area. Go right 0.1 mile to a four-way intersection and go left toward the park road, crossing through prairie. Straight takes you into Twin Valley Campground; the trail to the right is the horse path. At the park road, a two-tire path descends through spruces 0.1 mile to another meeting of the equestrian path. Go right here and head through prairie for the next 0.5 miles, briefly passing through a grove of locust trees and finally arriving at the horse path going left to right. Go straight across and 50 feet to another juncture. Lost Canyon Trail goes left and follows along the edge of the Cox Hollow Campground. It gradually slopes into the canyon, switches back at 0.3 miles, and takes you another 0.2 miles to a creek running through a culvert.

Now you start to see some mammoth rock outcroppings off to the left. Water flows toward you on the right, and at 0.5 miles from the culvert, you cross a wide wooden bridge over the creek. Two more bridges await before the next trail juncture at 0.15 miles.

The path to the right follows the creek 0.2 miles to Stephens Falls. This is a good cutoff option. Otherwise continue left, crossing a footbridge and following another smaller creek coming down the hill in front of you until 0.3 miles later, you arrive at the park road.

Go right here along the road's edge 200 feet as the trail cuts back into woods briefly and then out into prairie for the home stretch. Hike 0.3 miles to the asphalt trail and go left back out to the parking lot.

Note: The park is part of the state's Junior Ranger and Explorers program; activities books are available in the park office. Hiking is not allowed in winter when this trail has snow and is groomed for skiing. Consider White Oak Trail or consult the park office at (608) 935-2315 for other options.

NEARBY ACTIVITIES

The Frank Lloyd Wright Visitor Center and Taliesin Home, at WI 23 and County Road C in Spring Green, is open from May through October. This National Historic Landmark offers guided tours. Call (608) 588-7900 or go to **www .taliesinpreservation.org**.

GOVERNOR DODGE STATE PARK: White Oak Trail 43

IN BRIEF

Hike the shores and climb the rocky bluffs overlooking Cox Hollow Lake. Then visit a prehistoric rock shelter.

DESCRIPTION

From the trailhead pass to the right of the concessions stand and a trail kiosk. Go straight ahead downhill just 400 feet to where the water flows over the dam to the right. Cross a wide wooden bridge to see the water tumbling over rocks to your left. Either follow the asphalt path straight across, or better yet, climb the earthen dam to your right and follow along the top of it as it skirts Cox Hollow Lake. There are no natural lakes in the southeastern corner of the state known as the Driftless Zone; the glaciers didn't arrive here to leave damming deposits in river valleys. Off to the right, you can see rocky cliffs on the other side of the lake. That is where you are headed.

It's 0.1 mile across the dam and into the woods. To your left is the return trail for the 3.3-mile Mill Creek Trail. Several paces beyond this, the trail forks. Up to the left on asphalt is the start of Mill Creek Trail. Go right on a packed-dirt and crushed-rock footpath, which

KEY AT-A-GLANCE INFORMATION

LENGTH: 4.3 miles

CONFIGURATION: Loop

DIFFICULTY: Moderate

SCENERY: Mixed forest, cliffs, exposed rock, a lake, wetlands, rock shelter

EXPOSURE: Mostly shaded

TRAIL TRAFFIC: Light

TRAIL SURFACE: Mostly packed dirt, rocks and roots, with some grass, cedar chip, crushed rock, and asphalt

HIKING TIME: 1.5 hours

Driving distance: 45.8 miles from the West Beltline Highway (US 12/18) and Verona Road (US 18/151)

ACCESS: 6 a.m.–11 p.m. year-round

MAPS: USGS Pleasant Ridge; at the park office

WHEELCHAIR ACCESSIBILITY: None

FACILITIES: Restrooms, water, picnic tables, boat landing, concessions, campgrounds

SPECIAL COMMENTS: A 1-mile segment of this trail is a self-guided nature trail. Pets must be leashed except in designated pet swim areas, but are not allowed on the Pine Cliff Nature Trail segment. All vehicles require a park sticker ($7 daily, $25 annual for vehicles with Wisconsin plates).

Directions

From the West Beltline Highway (US 12/14) go southwest 37.4 miles on Verona Road/ US 18/151. At Exit 47 for Dodgeville, take US 18 west for 1.9 miles, and then turn right on Bequette Street/WI 23 for 3.3 miles to the park entrance on the right. Take the park road 0.25 miles past the office and go right at the first intersection 2.5 miles to the parking lot. The trailhead is to the right of the concessions building.

GPS Trailhead Coordinates

UTM Zone (WGS 84)   15T

Easting   0733112

Northing   4766893

Latitude   N 43° 00' 53.02"

Longitude   W 90° 06' 18.67"

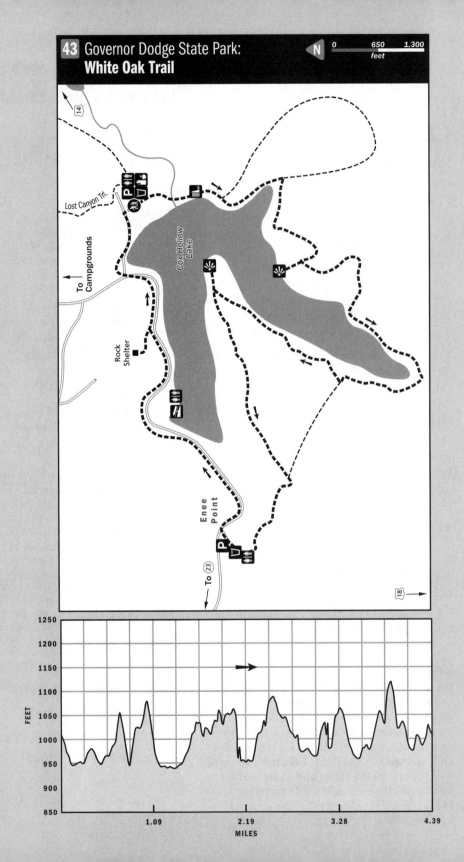

43 Governor Dodge State Park: White Oak Trail

N

0   650   1,300
feet

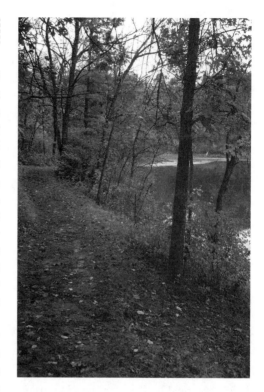

The trail skirts Cox Hollow Lake

is the White Oak Trail. Only 250 feet along is the juncture with Lakeview Trail. If you go left, this loop adds another mile to your hike and rejoins this trail just 0.15 miles farther along. White Oak continues along the lakeshore, passes the Lakeview return trail, and goes right and across a culvert before it heads back around a finger of the lake to your right. The trail becomes narrower as it heads into thicker forest and gradually turns more and more rugged with roots, rocks, and uneven surfaces.

The trail goes around a rocky outcropping to the left and starts to curl up left over tree-root steps through forest dominated by native pine. From the juncture to the top is 0.3 miles where the trail may be difficult to discern in the carpet of pine needles. Watch for it to the left where it heads back down the rocky bluff. This area at the top is Raccoon Point, and you can follow it out to the end with a drop-off to either side. Return along the opposite side to come to the trail as it continues past the point.

The path goes to the right and down with a lot of tree roots and loose sandstone. It winds around trunks and boulders 0.2 miles to the bottom, where it crosses a small wooden footbridge over a creek. The trail bends left and follows the creek, curves when it reaches the lake, and heads uphill to a smaller cliff. You are now getting looks into the marshy area at this corner of the lake, which is great for spotting waterfowl.

At 0.3 miles from the bridge, the trail comes out to an access road and a map board. To the left is the park's horse trail. Go right to continue on White Oak Trail. This area can get a little soggy in spring or during rainy periods, but the grass keeps it from getting too muddy. There is a bench here for a quiet spot to observe the marshy area. On the other side of this open stretch, the trail curves right, passing over a muddy spot with a few stepping stones or branches in wet seasons. The path widens and becomes grassy with sandy patches.

At 0.2 miles from the bench, the trail forks. You can stay left for White Oak, but better to take Pine Cliff Trail to the right. The 1-mile, self-guided nature trail offers educational signage as it climbs a bluff on a narrow footpath. It starts along the lake's edge, then climbs left moderately with some log and dirt steps. At the top go right at the map board and there is a 20-foot-high outcropping of rock. There are no easy steps, but it is climbable to the next surface, which is a flat area that offers various scenic overlooks of the lake at the end of the bluff.

Return from the point, climb back down the rocks, and follow the spine of the ridge, passing your arrival trail. The trail goes 0.5 miles back to White Oak Trail, where you go right and down into a hollow coming to a bridge over a ravine of water-smoothed stone. Across the bridge, stairs go down the other side of the ravine. From the bottom of the steps, it's 0.3 miles to a parking area. Cross a narrow footbridge and pass a lot of exposed rock as you follow a creek on your right. You go over the creek as you enter the parking lot. There is a kiosk and restrooms to the left and a water pump in season.

Go right out to the main park road. This is Enee Point rising above you ahead to the right. Straight across is Box Canyon. There are no "official" trails up to the point, but the hike is permissible for those looking for a short but challenging climb with a view at the end.

Go right on the park road and follow it back to where you started. Alternatively, you could double back the way you came on White Oak Trail. Along the park road at 0.7 miles, you come to Deer Cove Picnic Area on your left just after a boat landing area on your right. Look for a spur trail to the left when you are facing Deer Cove. A 350-foot trail leads up to a rock shelter that has evidence of being occupied by Paleo Indians between 7000 and 6000 B.C., clearly the oldest of the campsites in the park. Back on the road, it's another 0.2 miles to the road to the modern campgrounds to the left and then another 0.1 mile to the parking lot and the trailhead.

Note: The park is part of the state's Junior Ranger and Explorers program; activities books are available in the park office.

NEARBY ACTIVITIES

The House on the Rock at 5754 WI 23, Spring Green is an odd attraction containing rooms full of exotic collections and the world's largest carousel. Truly it must be seen to be believed. Call (608) 935-3639 for more information or go to **www.thehouseontherock.com**.

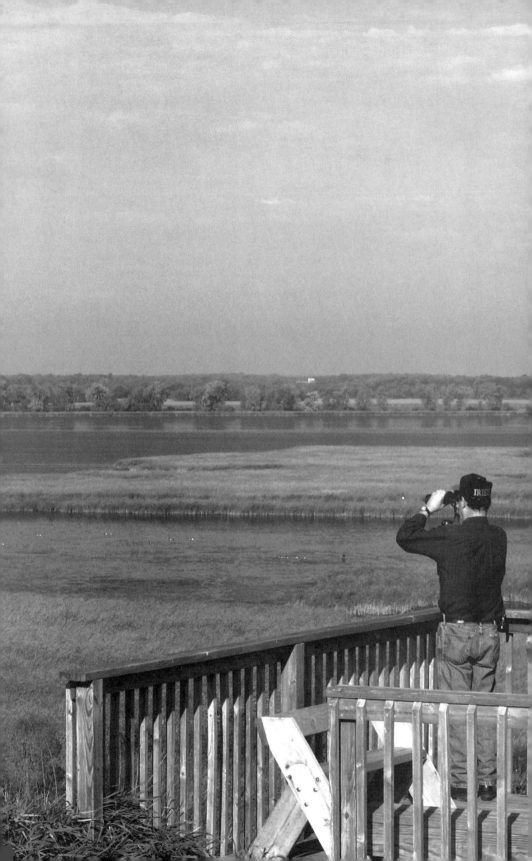

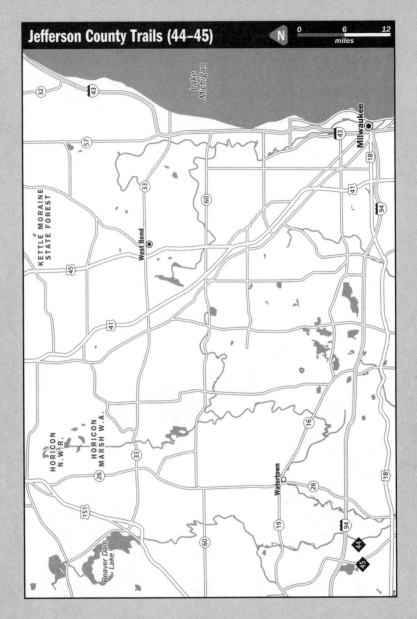

Lake Michigan

32

43

57

33

60

Milwaukee

43

18

41

94

KETTLE MORAINE STATE FOREST

West Bend

45

41

16

HORICON N.W.R.

HORICON MARSH W.A.

33

26

Watertown

26

18

151

19

94

Beaver Dam Lake

60

44

45

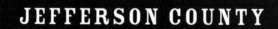

JEFFERSON COUNTY

44 AZTALAN STATE PARK

KEY AT-A-GLANCE INFORMATION

LENGTH: 1.8 miles

CONFIGURATION: Loop

DIFFICULTY: Easy with a couple of short moderate climbs

SCENERY: Flowing water, prairie with some mixed forest, Native American–built earthen pyramids and mounds

EXPOSURE: Mostly exposed

TRAIL TRAFFIC: Light to medium

TRAIL SURFACE: Mowed grass

HIKING TIME: 1 hour

DRIVING DISTANCE: 3.2 miles from the intersection of Interstate 94 and WI 89

ACCESS: 6 a.m.–11 p.m. year-round

MAPS: USGS Jefferson; archaeological maps on site

WHEELCHAIR ACCESSIBILITY: Yes, but grassy trails

FACILITIES: Water, restrooms, picnic tables, grills, and shelters

SPECIAL COMMENTS: There's a designated pet area, but pets must be leashed. Since this is a state park, visitors must pay a vehicle registration fee of $7 ($10 non-Wisconsin plates) or an hourly fee of $5. Educational signs throughout give valuable information about the history and archaeology of the site.

IN BRIEF

Climb earthen pyramids at a grassy archaeological site along the Crawfish River and learn about an advanced Native American culture that left as much mystery as artifacts.

DESCRIPTION

Thought you'd need to go to Egypt or Central America for pyramids? Think again. Two earthen step pyramids and the artifacts and evidence gathered here indicate this was a very important site for a mysterious Native American people.

There are remains of other temple-mound towns in the United States, but this is the farthest north of all of them. Probably this tribe was related to the Cahokia, whose center was near present-day St. Louis. The Crawfish River must have been attractive to the native community as a good source of fish and wild rice, and the waterway served as a transportation route flowing south to the Rock River and farther on to the Mississippi River.

The archaeological record indicates the site was occupied between 1000 and 1300 A.D. The stockade and pyramids have been reconstructed to give an idea of the size of the community. Circular mounds can be found farther up the hill and to the north. Erroneous beliefs

GPS Trailhead Coordinates

UTM Zone (WGS 84) 16T

Easting 0348399

Northing 4769540

Latitude N 43° 03' 48.33"

Longitude W 88° 51' 42.64"

Directions ———→

Exit Interstate 94 at WI 89 (Exit 259) and go south. Turn left at the traffic light on County Road V and go 2 miles to County Road B. Go left here 0.7 miles and turn right on County Road Q. The museum is on your left, and the park entrance is another 0.3 miles ahead on the left. Follow the park road to the last parking lot to find the trailhead.

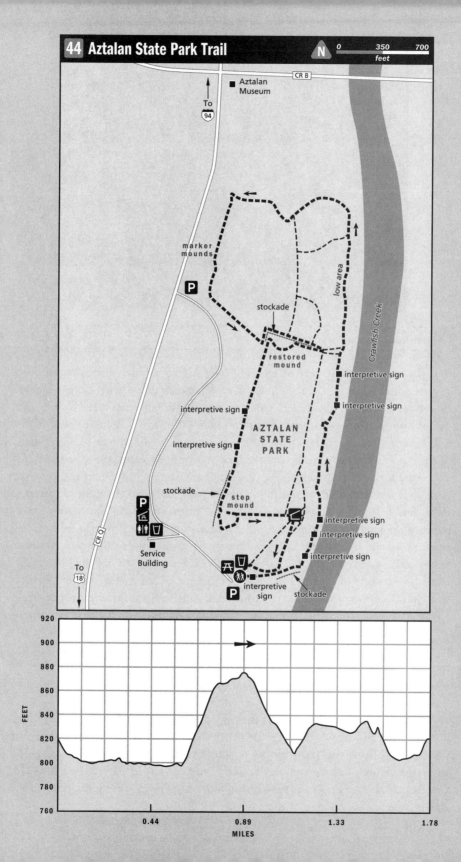

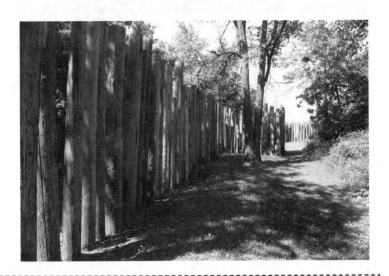

A reconstruction of the stockade

that this was somehow related to the Aztecs brought it the name Aztalan after it was rediscovered in 1835. Human bone fragments found with animal remains in refuse heaps has prompted some archaeologists to speculate if there was cannibalism occurring—ritualistic or otherwise—but there is no agreement on the significance of the findings. There were once more than 40 mounds here, but many of them fell under the plow before the land was turned over to the state in 1927.

After you pay your vehicle fee at the self-pay station in the parking lot at the park entrance, continue deeper into the park almost 0.5 miles to the last parking lot to find a picnic area with grills and some pit toilets nearby. Look for a water pump at the northeast corner of the lot; the trail starts here. From the pump, look east toward the river and find a posted map showing where other temple towns of mounds are located in the United States. Continuing toward the river, hike along the left side of a partial segment of stockades. (You might also just want to first check out the river on the right-hand side where the mowed grass goes right to the edge since your opportunities will be minimal along the trail.)

The wide trail is cut grass and passes through mixed forest as it follows the river, though not directly along the shore. There's a short spur trail that leads to the water's edge just after the main trail curves left away from the stockade. Just several steps past this is an educational sign about the importance of fishing to the natives.

Within the forested section of the trail, you are sheltered from wind by thick undergrowth and woods, but there is generally no cover from the sun above. For the next 500 feet, you pass two more interpretive signs regarding hunting and gathering before reaching an opening to the field to your left. If you face the field, you can see the largest of the mounds at about 10 o'clock. Along the river to the right of the trail, swallows swoop over the muddy waters.

Seven hundred feet from here and again 200 feet past that are two more interpretive signs. Another 200 feet brings you to some shade and another section of the stockade. A trail goes left along the inside of it, and as you pass through a "gate" in the fortifications, you also see a trail along the opposite side. These cut back to the open field if you just can't wait. Otherwise, continue straight along the path parallel to the river. Five hundred feet along is a short low area that can be soggy in wet weather and spring. A wood-chip cutoff trail cuts left back to the field 300 feet beyond that, and, finally, the main trail takes the turn away from the river—which has been hidden throughout most of the trail by foliage—about 0.2 miles from where you passed through the stockade.

The path becomes packed dirt and heads into more shaded territory, but the understory thins out, and you can see deeper into the trees. Just 500 feet later, you enter the clearing. A trail goes left along the trees back in the direction of the parking lot, but go straight and then keep following the trail as it bears right and follows the curve of the trees. The trail puts trees on your right and tall grass on your left and 300 feet later starts a moderate climb up the hillside. It's about 250 feet that brings you to the first in a row of conical mounds running south from the northwest corner of the park. Here you are at the highest point and can see the entire park and how it's laid out. Behind you are elms and locust trees, and you are a short walk from the museum. You might opt to go to the nearby county road and head north 750 feet to the museum.

Continuing from the first mound, the trail heads south alongside the uncut grass of the central field and puts the mounds to your right. You can opt to walk across the top of the mounds; it is allowed. There are ten mounds here altogether, and they are spread out along a 500-foot stretch.

You arrive at the upper parking lot. Trails head left down the gentle slope of the land through prairie, and there's an interpretive map of the site just off the edge of the lot. Go to the end of the lot and take the trail left down the hill on a direct line to the right edge of the stockade. When you reach it, follow left along the outside of the tall wooden poles until the corner and then continue along the stockade to the bottom of the hill. There are spaces between the poles, and you can cut through here and approach the mound within the walls from below rather than just come around the stockade at the very beginning. It makes more of an impression this way. If you don't cut through the stockade, you can continue into the woods to where you originally passed through the wide "gate" as you walked the forest trail, and then come back up on the other side.

Once inside the stockade, turn back up the hill. Tucked into the corner is a large squared mound with steps up the center of it. Follow the trail up the hill and climb to the top of the mound. Return to the trail either by the steps or just hiking down the steep backside. Now you can continue south off the end of the stockade, crossing the field along a series of interpretive signs until you arrive at the largest of the mounds, a sort of earthen step pyramid also shielded by reconstructed stockade. Trails crisscross the open field within the reconstructed and imagined stockades, but they will change according to park mowing patterns. Out here in the open, however, the landmarks of earth mounds and stockades and even interpretive signs are easy to spot. The distance from the first pyramid to the far side pyramid is 0.2 miles.

This second construction is the larger of the two. Originally the top was shielded from view for sacred ceremonies. Pass behind the mound to find an interpretive sign and then go around to the front to steps going up each of the two pyramid levels. The view from the top is another nice impression of the entire site and a good photo opportunity.

From the base of the front of the mound, cross the open field to a low hill where there is an interpretive shelter/kiosk. You will learn much more about the history and excavation of the site here. From here follow one of the mowed paths 600 feet back to the parking lot.

Guided tours are given on weekends April through October. Schedules for them are posted at the park, or call the park office in Lake Mills at (920) 648-8774. This National Historic Landmark shouldn't be missed.

NEARBY ACTIVITIES

The Aztalan Historical Museum is right next door and includes some area artifacts as well as a collection of antiques. It is open from mid-May through September, Thursday through Sunday, 1 to 4 p.m. You can contact the museum at (920) 648-4362.

GLACIAL DRUMLIN STATE TRAIL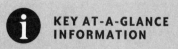

IN BRIEF

Cross the Crawfish and Rock Rivers and get a close look at a glacial drumlin on this converted rail bed that offers a mostly shaded path through rich farmland.

DESCRIPTION

A glacial drumlin is a hill of debris left by a retreating ice mass. The hill rises up sharply at the front and then tapers off at an easier slope in the direction of the glacier's retreat. You see some on this hike. Glacial drumlins contain rock and gravel all the way from Canada, and because of this, they are popular sources for the crushed rock. Quarrying has caused many drumlins to disappear.

The entire Glacial Drumlin State Trail runs 52 miles from Cottage Grove all the way east to Waukesha. In 1986 it was developed from an unused section of railway, so the grade is gentle. The section mapped out here is arguably the best part of the trail. It begins at an old railroad depot in Lake Mills where you can find a small exhibit of local history, and crosses two rivers before it ends where the trail goes on road just before the city of Jefferson.

To hike both rivers and avoid the long out-and-back, you can either use two cars,

KEY AT-A-GLANCE INFORMATION

LENGTH: 13.2 miles
CONFIGURATION: Out-and-back
DIFFICULTY: Easy
SCENERY: Farmland, wildflowers, two rivers, glacial drumlins
EXPOSURE: Mostly shaded with some exposed stretches
TRAIL TRAFFIC: Moderate
TRAIL SURFACE: Crushed limestone
HIKING TIME: Up to 5 hours
DRIVING DISTANCE: 21.1 miles east from the interchange of Interstates 39 and 94
ACCESS: Open year-round anytime
MAPS: USGS Lake Mills and Jefferson; at the trail office; www.glacialdrumlin.com
WHEELCHAIR ACCESSIBILITY: Yes
FACILITIES: None on trail. Restrooms and water at the trailhead.
SPECIAL COMMENTS: Dogs must be on a leash no longer than 8 feet. A state trail pass is required for bicyclists 16 years old and older, but hiking has no fee. Stay alert for approaching bicyclists, or when snow is present, snowmobiles.

Directions ——————————→

From the interchange of I-39/94, go east 19.1 miles to the WI 89 exit and go right (south) 2 miles to the Glacial Drumlin State Trail Office. The trailhead is across the highway on the left.

GPS Trailhead Coordinates

UTM Zone (WGS 84) 16T

Easting 0432421

Northing 4821457

Latitude N 43° 32' 34.82"

Longitude W 87° 50' 11.45"

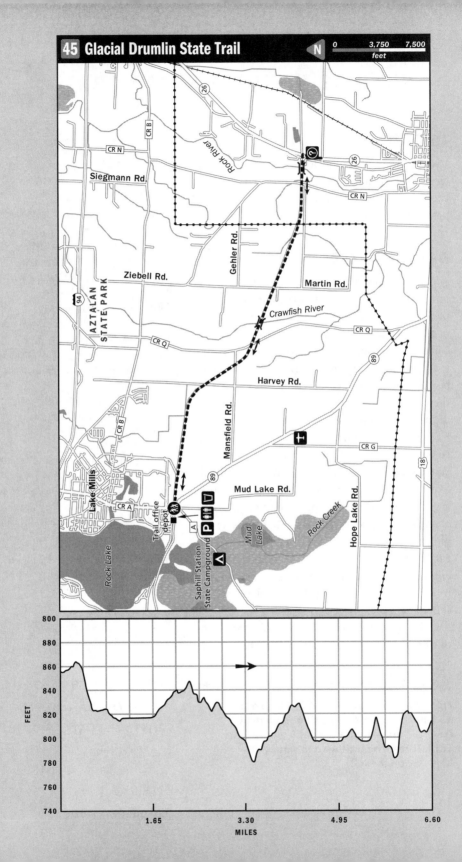

N

| 0 | 3,750 | 7,500 |

feet

26

Rock River

CR B

CR N

Siegmann Rd.

CR N

26

Gehler Rd.

Ziebell Rd.

Martin Rd.

94

AZTALAN STATE PARK

Crawfish River

CR Q

CR Q

89

Harvey Rd.

CR G

CR B

Mansfield Rd.

18

Lake Mills

89

CR A

Mud Lake Rd.

Hope Lake Rd.

Trail office / depot

A

P

Saphill Station
State Campground

Mud
Lake

Rock Creek

Rock Lake

800

880

860

840

820

800

780

760

740

FEET

1.65   3.30   4.95   6.60

MILES

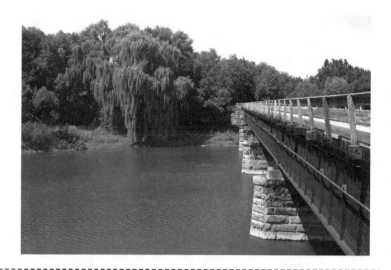

The bridge over Rock River

parking one at the other trailhead near Jefferson, or hike from the Jefferson end of the trail. The out-and-back distance to see both river crossings is 6.7 miles from that end.

The trail begins from the depot heading east across County Road A/Main Street. After 0.1 mile you enter shade as the rail bed sinks into the surrounding terrain. A short distance later, the surrounding terrain is lower and the trail then rides above it.

At 1 mile from the trailhead, you come out into the open for 0.3 miles before the trail finds shade again. At that point there is a snowmobile trail heading left. Stay straight. Though there are cornfields on either side, the trail itself enjoys a corridor of mixed forest throughout much of this hike so that exposure is less than you might expect.

You pass a stand of aspens and some big cottonwoods that border the fields to the north and then a yield sign for a farm road crossing the trail. Pass through box elders to Harvey Road. The trail continues on the other side, and 0.2 miles later, you come to an interpretive sign about glacial drumlins. You can see one to the south. The trail is exposed from here, passing through fields of goldenrod 0.2 miles to the next crossing at Mansfield Road. Beyond this road the trail goes under the canopy of black walnuts and crosses a farm road at 0.2 miles. To your right just past here, look for a drumlin covered in prairie flowers.

Cross County Road Q. To the north 1.5 miles is Aztalan State Park, an archaeological site and another nice hike. There is no official public parking on this road. On the other side, pass a small bit of wetlands on the left and soon after that, another farmer's crossing. You will go 0.3 miles from CR Q before coming to the first bridge. This is an old railroad trestle modified with wood planks to make a trail crossing 40 feet above the Crawfish River. An interpretive sign at the center of the bridge puts time and history in perspective. You can see woods on either side of the river and hear birds, crickets, frogs, the whispering wind, and even jumping fish. It's a nice place to linger a bit.

The next 0.5 miles takes you to Popp Road with open sky and a lot of wildflowers along the way. On the other side of the road, the trail heads back into forest and grows thicker, making this one of the better places to spot woodland creatures. It's another 1.7 miles to the next road crossing, mostly shaded with a few colonies of aspen along the way. Cross County Road M and enter into woods again, leading 0.2 miles to the next bridge. This is the Rock River, which eventually receives the Crawfish River downstream and continues through Illinois all the way to the Mississippi River. It was an important riverway for Native Americans, connecting communities from Wisconsin to many others far downstream in the Midwest. The trail uses another former railroad trestle to make the crossing.

Past the bridge 800 feet, you pass a gravel access road to the right, and then the trail goes under the WI 26 overpass. It turns right and follows along between the highway and agricultural fields 0.3 miles to the end of the trail. There is parking here and a map board. The overpass is a good turnaround point if you are hiking back to Lake Mills. The trail does continue from the parking lot, but this is an on-road portion heading east. This last stretch is noisy being next to the highway, but not a bad alternative starting point for the hike.

NEARBY ACTIVITIES

The Zeloski Marsh Unit of the Lake Mills Wildlife Area is a recently restored wetlands and an excellent bird-watching site. Sandhill Station State Campground has 15 walk-in tent sites in a secluded oak savannah 1 mile south of Lake Mills on Mud Lake Road. Call (920) 648-8774 for more information or to make a reservation.

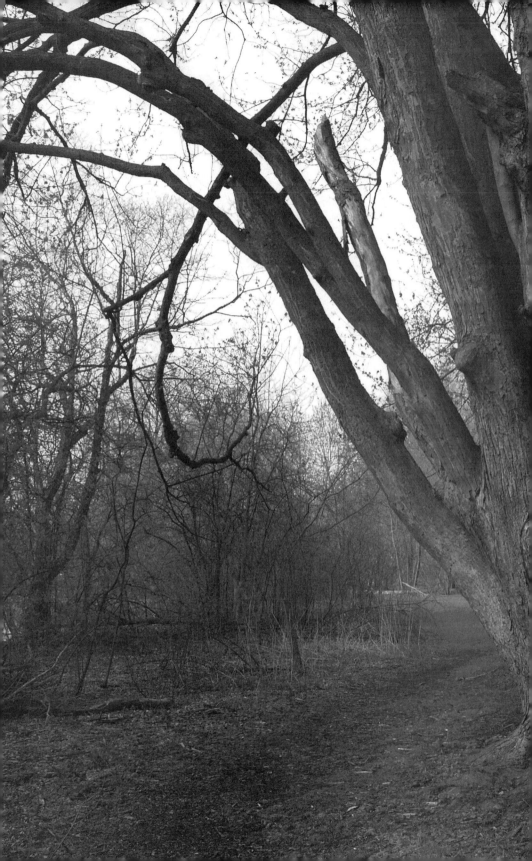

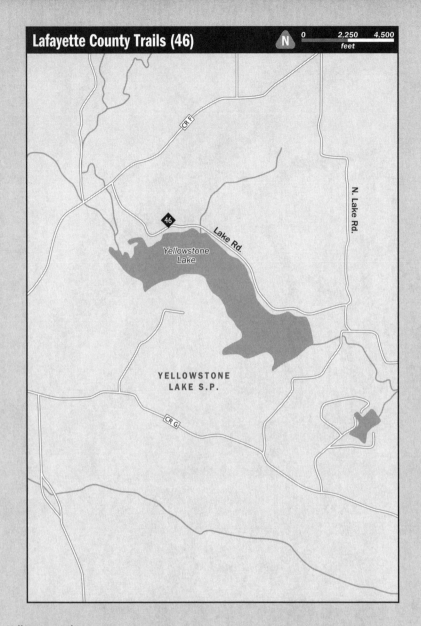

N

0   2,250   4,500
feet

CR F

N. Lake Rd.

46

Lake Rd.

Yellowstone Lake

YELLOWSTONE
LAKE S.P.

CR G

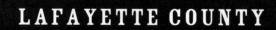

LAFAYETTE COUNTY

46 YELLOWSTONE LAKE STATE PARK

 KEY AT-A-GLANCE INFORMATION

LENGTH: 9.4 miles

CONFIGURATION: Multiple loops

DIFFICULTY: Easy to moderate

SCENERY: Wetlands, lake, mixed forest, oak savanna, prairie

EXPOSURE: Mostly shaded except prairie and along the dike

TRAIL TRAFFIC: Light

TRAIL SURFACE: Packed dirt with tree roots, mowed grass

HIKING TIME: 4 hours

DRIVING DISTANCE: 45.6 miles southwest of Verona Road/ US 18/51 and the Beltline Highway (US 12/14)

ACCESS: 6 a.m.–11 p.m. year-round

MAPS: USGS Yellowstone Lake; at the park office and on map boards at trail junctures

WHEELCHAIR ACCESSIBILITY: None, but the Wildlife Loop is passable

FACILITIES: Pit toilets, water, shelters, picnic areas, playgrounds, swimming area, boat launch, concessions, boat rentals

SPECIAL COMMENTS: All vehicles require a park sticker ($7 daily, $25 annual for vehicles with Wisconsin plates). The park participates in the Junior Ranger/Wisconsin Explorer program (see Preface, page xv).

GPS Trailhead Coordinates

UTM Zone (WGS 84)   16T

Easting   0255938

Northing   4739864

Latitude   N 42° 46' 20.86"

Longitude   W 89° 58' 59.60"

IN BRIEF

The Wildlife Loop on a dike into the lake is brimming with activity, but the prairie and oak savanna loops over rolling hills and the paths through the woods are every bit as enjoyable.

DESCRIPTION

This state park offers a lot of route options. The route mapped here ties most of the trails together for one long hike. Pass the pavilion and start up the trail into the woods. This heads 0.3 miles to a trail juncture. The 1.3-mile Oak Ridge Trail lies straight ahead; the 0.8-mile Prairie Loop is to the right. There's a map board here as well as a bench.

Go straight 200 feet for the easiest of the trails. Here you find another map board and a fork in the trail. Go straight into the prairie as the trail follows along the right edge. Just 100 feet along is a spur trail to the right out to Ronnerod Lane. The trail curves left and then ducks into the forest on a partially shaded dirt path with lots of roots and scattered acorns. Find a clearing and a bench at the turnaround point before the trail brings you back uphill through aspen. The trail comes through a bit of oak savanna before descending on crushed rock, crossing a gully, and returning to the map

----

Directions ————————————————→

From its intersection with the Beltline Highway (US 12/14), take Verona Road/US 18/151 southwest 19.3 miles to WI 78. Go 17.3 miles south on WI 78 through Blanchardville. On the south side of town, go right on County Road F and follow it 8.2 miles to Lake Road and the park entrance. Continue 0.8 miles south (left) on Lake Road until it brings you past the park office to the first parking area on the left. The trailhead is to the east beyond the pavilion.

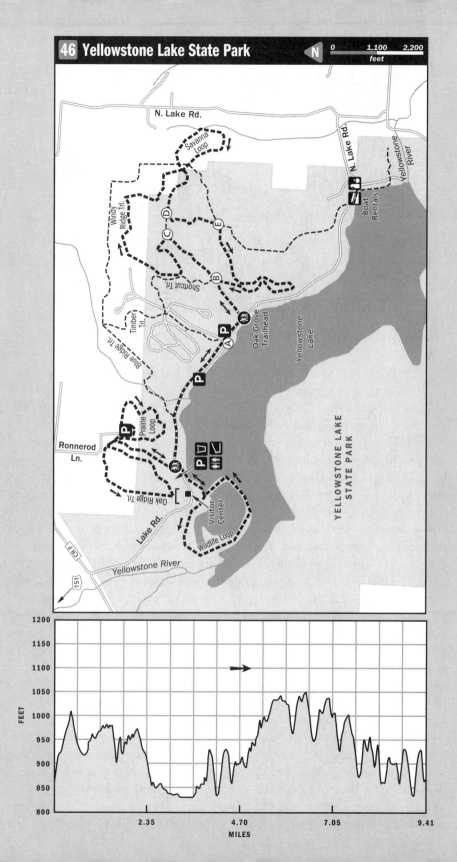

N

0   1,100   2,200
feet

N. Lake Rd.

Savanna Loop

Windy Ridge Trl.

N. Lake Rd.

Yellowstone River

Boat Rentals

D

C

E

B

Shortcut Trl.

Timber Trl.

Blue Ridge Trl.

Oak Grove Trailhead

A

P

P

P

Yellowstone Lake

Prairie Loop

P

Ronnerod Ln.

Oak Ridge Trl.

P

Lake Rd.

Visitor Center

Wildlife Loop

YELLOWSTONE LAKE STATE PARK

151

CR F

Yellowstone River

MILES

2.35   4.70   7.05   9.41

FEET

800
850
900
950
1000
1050
1100
1150
1200

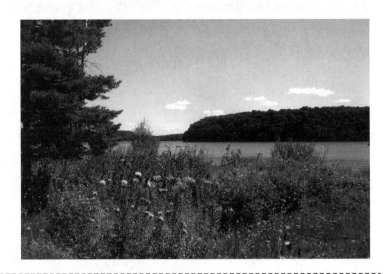

The Wildlife Loop along the lake

board. Go right back to that first map board and then go left for the Prairie Loop.

Follow the left branch of the loop out into the sunshine. Despite the name, much of the loop actually passes through the woods rather than the prairie. The path heads to the right and follows the curve of a parking loop at the end of Ronnerod Lane until it comes around again and is heading north into some pine. The path bends right to more pine and rounds the prairie, heading down on grass into mixed forest, mostly shaded. There is some moderate uphill hiking through aspen with prairie to the right and then back into thicker woods as you return to the end of the 0.8-mile loop. Go left back down the hill to the parking lot.

Cross the road from the parking lot and go right on a grassy trail alongside the road. Pass bat houses amid tall grass and wildflowers with the lake to the left. Pass the park office to a trail juncture and map board. This is the 1-mile Wildlife Loop. Follow this mowed path going right through aspens, mostly exposed, with brush on either side. You come to an old piece of asphalt and a trail that goes left; go straight across and down this corridor. Brush seems to block wildlife and initially you might think "wildlife loop" was a misnomer. You come to a juncture with a snowmobile trail that goes straight or right. Go left as the trail starts to follow a dike through marsh water, dead trees, and willows, not to mention mosquitoes. You have some shade, but then you come out to open sky to follow the curving dike into the lake and back to shore 0.5 miles later. Watch for all sorts of creatures, including herons, cranes, frogs, muskrats, and many birds.

When you complete the loop, go right, back to the parking area. You have the option of taking your vehicle to the next half of the trails or simply hiking 0.8 miles along the park road to the next trailhead. Yet another option is to take the Blue Ridge Trail up to the hills and the Timber Trail back down to create a meandering connection to the Oak Grove Trail. There is another parking area near the Oak Grove Trail on the left side of the road. From here hike on the left side of the park road and continue 0.1 mile east to the trail going left into the brush. There is a map board here, and the trail goes uphill moderately 0.2 miles to the next juncture. Your return trail comes here from the right. Stay straight, passing the Shortcut Trail on the left up to Windy Ridge Trail.

Continue another 0.3 miles to the next intersection. Straight is Oak Grove and Windy Ridge Trail. Going right reduces this section of the hike to 1.3 miles on the Oak Grove Trail. Go left up the hill through oak savanna, moderately steep, following a gully to the left. Find prairie as the path winds around the top end of the gully and crosses over. Another 0.2 miles takes you along the edge of the prairie and curves to a trail juncture just inside the woods. To the left is Timber Trail, which could take you back to that second parking lot to complete a 0.8-mile loop. Also a few steps in this direction is the other end of that Shortcut Trail. Go out into the prairie following Windy Ridge Trail. To your left are a parking area, playground, and more bat houses. The trail heads 0.8 miles over the somewhat steep and rolling hills with very nice views of the land and patches of oak savanna in the distance.

The trail follows the top of a ridge, descends to the bottom, crosses the crease, and heads back up, bearing south into oak savanna. There's a bench for a rest at the top. Round some brush and savanna, remaining in open prairie until a juncture at 0.8 miles. There is a bench and a map board here. Go left on the 0.6-mile Savanna Loop. Go straight across the intersecting trail just 150 feet past here. This is the Blue Ridge Trail, where you find another map board. With farmland and barn views, the loop descends into the crease between the hills, exposed. The path goes along the left side of a small piece of savanna before curling right around it and returning up the hill, crossing back over the Blue Ridge Trail once more to the loop's starting point.

Now go left through the prairie down to more oak savanna at the bottom. Come to Point D on the park map at 0.25 miles. Go left to pick up the Oak Grove Trail. If you go right instead, it is a shorter return back down the trail you took up into the hills in the first place. Pass a short connecting spur to the Blue Ridge Trail at Point E at 0.3 miles. This takes you to the concession stand at the southeast end of the park. The trail is mostly shaded with some open spots. As it makes its turnaround 0.6 miles later at the southernmost point of the trail, you pass a bench on the right. In the spring and fall this is a good overlook of the lake. The next 0.4 miles offers shade and a straight moderate decline just before you cross a culvert at the bottom and arrive at the trail juncture. To the left is the path you came in on. Follow this back down to the park road and go right back to the parking lot.

NEARBY ACTIVITIES

Check out River Valley Trading Co. at 204 South Main Street in Blanchardville for local art, food, antiques, and all sorts of things. Call (608) 523-1888 for current hours.

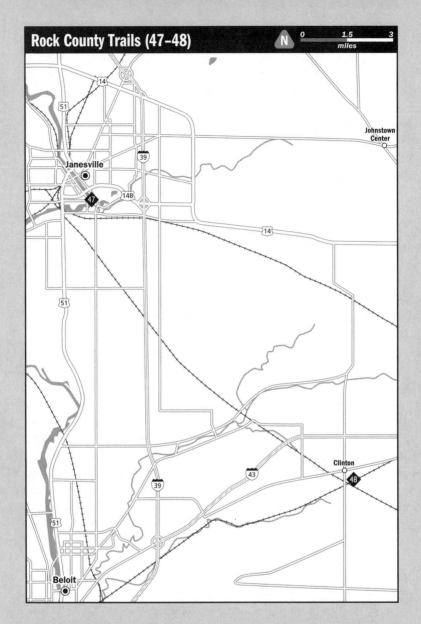

Johnstown
Center

Janesville

47

14B

14

51

Clinton

43

48

39

51

Beloit

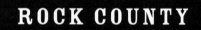

ROCK COUNTY

47 ICE AGE TRAIL: Janesville Segment

KEY AT-A-GLANCE INFORMATION

LENGTH: 10.8 miles total

CONFIGURATION: Out-and-back

DIFFICULTY: Easy

SCENERY: Urban parks, the Rock River, creeks, forest, prairie

EXPOSURE: Mostly sun, some shaded stretches

TRAIL TRAFFIC: Moderate

TRAIL SURFACE: Asphalt

HIKING TIME: Up to 4 hours

DRIVING DISTANCE: 35.7 miles south from the juncture of Interstate 39/90 and US 12/18

ACCESS: Year-round anytime

MAPS: USGS Janesville East and West; *The Ice Age Trail Companion Atlas*

WHEELCHAIR ACCESSIBILITY: Yes

FACILITIES: Restrooms, water at parks along the trail

SPECIAL COMMENTS: Dogs are allowed on leashes from September 15 to May 15 only.

IN BRIEF

Follow a scenic trail crossing the Rock River and then threading its way through the city along a creek and a wonderful green space.

DESCRIPTION

This segment of the Ice Age Trail is a much easier hike than the others as it follows asphalt its entire length with very few significant changes in elevation. Nevertheless, it is a nice bit of escape from the surrounding city.

The trail starts at Riverside Street heading south across the Rock River on a pedestrian/bicycle bridge. There is an observation deck halfway across where you can stand out of the way of traffic. Midway through the park on the other side, your trail curves left. Another trail continues straight. Follow the curve along a vine-covered fence on your right. You are now entering Jeffris Park as you cross a short bridge 400 feet before the next street crossing. To your right is where the Burr Robbins Circus made camp from 1874 until 1888. There is a historical marker here and a couple of benches.

Cross the busy Beloit Avenue. At 0.1 mile you come to a row of cedars on your right and pass under power lines another 0.1 mile later where the cedars end. There's a meandering

GPS Trailhead Coordinates

UTM Zone (WGS 84) 16T

Easting 0334747

Northing 4726317

Latitude N 42° 40' 17.68"

Longitude W 89° 01' 0.08"

Directions

From its intersection with US 12/18, take I-39/90 south 33.2 miles to Janesville. Take the 175A Exit for US Business 14 West. Go right 2.2 miles following Racine Street/US 14. Turn left on South Jackson Street and follow it for 0.3 miles to Riverside Street. Turn right to park on the street. The trailhead is at the end of Riverside Street going a short block east of Jackson Street.

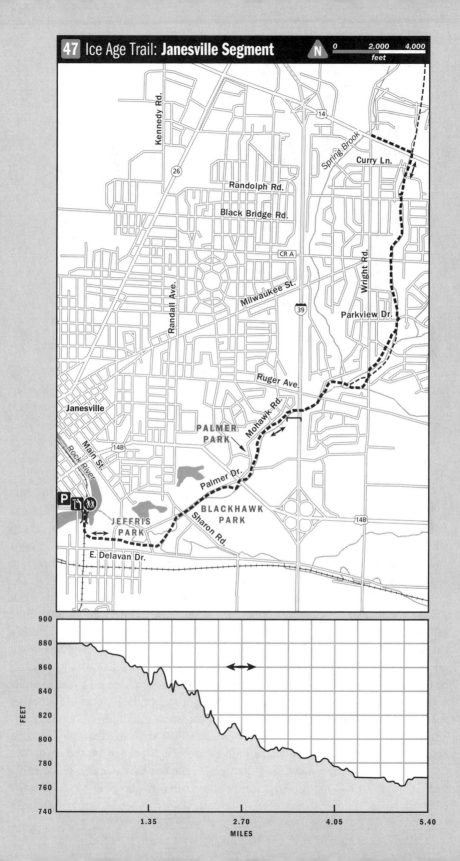

N

0   2,000   4,000
feet

Kennedy Rd.

26

Randolph Rd.

Black Bridge Rd.

CR A

Randall Ave.

Milwaukee St.

14

Spring Brook

Curry Ln.

Wright Rd.

39

Parkview Dr.

Ruger Ave.

Janesville

14B

Main St.

Rock River

Mohawk Rd.

PALMER
PARK

Palmer Dr.

P

JEFFRIS
PARK

BLACKHAWK
PARK

Sharon Rd.

14B

E. Delavan Dr.

900
880
860
840
820
800
780
760
740

FEET

1.35   2.70   4.05   5.40

MILES

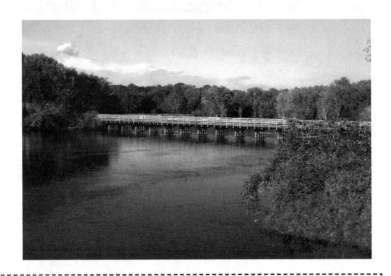

Pedestrian bridge over Rock River

creek to the left just before you cross South Main Street. The trail starts to curve left (north), and at 0.2 miles, you will pass over Spring Brook on a pedestrian bridge. A creekside trail goes off to the left and to the right. As you pass the 1-mile marker, you come out to Palmer Drive and go right. A bike path also goes left from this point. The path is unshaded through a mowed area with brush off to the right and Palmer Drive to your left. You are 0.6 miles from the next street crossing at Racine Street.

Pass in front of Blackhawk Golf Course and head into the shade of large oaks just before you arrive at a historical marker in a corner park. It recalls the 1832 Black Hawk War when 1,000 Sauk, Fox, and Kickapoo, unhappy about where the U.S. government and treaties had put them, tried to defy U.S. troops and militia. This marker accounts an attack by Native Americans on European settlements in Illinois.

The trail rounds some brush and crosses a golf course path before arriving at Racine Street. Cross Racine to Palmer Park at the lights. The trail does a 0.1-mile gentle curve through the grass toward Spring Brook to your right before crossing Palmer Drive straight ahead. After Palmer Drive, follow parallel to Mohawk Road on the left with open water to your right. At 0.2 miles you come to restrooms, benches, and a vending machine on the trail. To your right is a bridge to some tennis courts, but continue straight, passing the 2-mile marker. At another 0.2 miles, the trail bends right, where you get to some parking spots and a bench just off the street to your left. There is a trail to the right to a pet exercise area across the creek. Stay straight as the path enters woods away from the road.

The trees last 0.15 miles, and then you come out to a wooden fence and a spur trail left to the street, and another short ramp to the right to the water's edge. There is another bench here. The path passes under I-39 0.1 mile later.

Past here you are not far from residences, which are just outside the trees to either side. Another 0.2 miles takes you across Ruger Avenue. On the other side, the trail veers to the right into fragrant pines and a few other trees. At 0.15 miles, a spur trail breaks right into the woods, and 300 feet after that another goes left out to Greendale Drive.

You'll come upon the 3-mile marker just before the next intersection where a trail goes right to a local sports complex. Go left up the hill to cross Wright Road. Cross and go left (north) along the sidewalk for 300 feet. Then the trail descends the hill to the right amid prairie with pine off to the left until you cross Brunswick Lane at 0.2 miles. Cross the street and find a mowed trail out to the brook to the right that then runs parallel and rejoins the main trail farther along just before you arrive at Parkview Drive at 0.25 miles. Another 0.3 miles takes you to the 3-mile marker, and another 0.2 miles finds you at Milwaukee Road. A traffic warning light alerts drivers to slow down and allow you to cross the busy roadway in a clearly marked crossing area.

The trail continues 0.15 miles, coming out into the open with wildflowers and farmland to the left and backyards to the right. At 0.3 miles there's an exit trail to the right to Mackinac Drive and a residential area. From Milwaukee Road to the next street, Randolph Road, is 0.5 miles. Cross and find an Ice Age Trail (IAT) kiosk on the right. The trail crosses the next 0.25 miles behind Kennedy Elementary School to Curry Lane. From here it is 0.1 mile to a tunnel under US 14. On the other side, a trail goes straight out to a residential neighborhood, but the IAT continues left along the highway 0.35 miles to Wright Road, which is the end of this segment.

NEARBY ACTIVITIES

Stop in at Gray's Brewing Company at 2424 West Court Street in Janesville for a sample of local beer and very popular sodas. Call (608) 752-3552 or go to **www.graybrewing.com** for more information.

48 PELISHEK NATURE TRAIL

KEY AT-A-GLANCE INFORMATION

LENGTH: 11.1 miles

CONFIGURATION: Out-and-back

DIFFICULTY: Easy

SCENERY: Forested corridor through farmland, prairie, and wildflowers

EXPOSURE: Partly shaded, partly sun

TRAIL TRAFFIC: Light

TRAIL SURFACE: Grass and packed dirt

HIKING TIME: Up to 4 hours

DRIVING DISTANCE: 51.9 miles south from the juncture of Interstate 39/90 and US 12/18

ACCESS: Year-round anytime

MAPS: USGS Clinton; posted at the trailhead

WHEELCHAIR ACCESSIBILITY: None

FACILITIES: None

SPECIAL COMMENTS: Some might not appreciate the nearby interstate halfway down the trail. In winter, when there's snow at least, beware of snowmobilers. It is possible to park another car at the eastern trailhead in Allens Grove.

IN BRIEF

A converted rail grade offers you a country stroll through prairie and forest with wildflowers and wild apples.

DESCRIPTION

The trail follows an old rail bed, but unlike many of the other converted rail beds, this one hasn't had asphalt or crushed limestone put in. The grassy path has a nice country lane feel to it, and a variety of birds and various small animals such as groundhogs, squirrels, and chipmunks skitter around the edges.

Grain mills stand just north of the parking lot. Look for a map board at the trailhead. There is also a map box, and this may have trail maps from time to time, but don't count on it. But as this is a rather simple out-and-back trail, directions won't be much of a concern.

The trail begins heading east, and at 0.1 mile, enters light woods on either side. To the left outside the corridor of trees are residences and a school. To the right are agricultural fields, often planted with corn. Another 0.2 miles brings you to the first of several nice rest areas where you will find a couple of benches and a small overhang sheltering them. The trail is mostly open to the sky at this point, but the trees close in 0.1 mile later. Just past

GPS Trailhead Coordinates

UTM Zone (WGS 84)   16T

Easting   0347218

Northing   4712883

Latitude   N 42° 33' 11.66"

Longitude   W 88° 51' 39.52"

Directions →

From its intersection with US 12/18, take I-39/90 south 43.4 miles to Beloit. Take Interstate 43 north 6.6 miles to WI 140. Go right (south) 0.9 miles into Clinton and go left on County Road X 0.2 miles (three blocks) to Mill Street. Go right 0.4 miles to the trail parking lot on the left side of the road. The trailhead is just to the north of the lot and clearly marked.

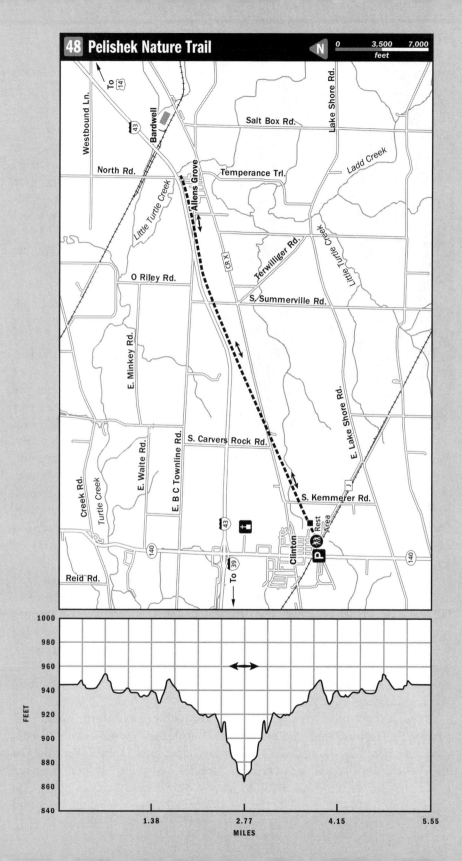

N

0   3,500   7,000
feet

To 14

Westbound Ln.

North Rd.

Bardwell

43

Salt Box Rd.

Lake Shore Rd.

Little Turtle Creek

Allens Grove

Temperance Trl.

Ladd Creek

Little Turtle Creek

CR X

Terwilliger Rd.

O Riley Rd.

S. Summerville Rd.

E. Minkey Rd.

S. Carvers Rock Rd.

E. Lake Shore Rd.

Creek Rd.

Turtle Creek

E. Waite Rd.

E. B C Townline Rd.

S. Kemmerer Rd.

J

43

Rest Area

Clinton

P

Reid Rd.

140

39

To

140

1000
980
960
940
920
900
880
860
840

FEET

1.38   2.77   4.15   5.55

MILES

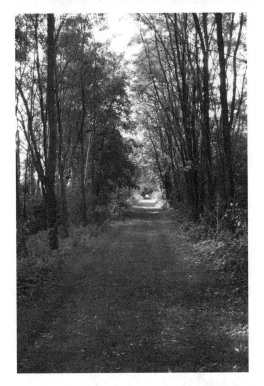

A grass-covered former railroad bed

that point is another rest area already. This also has benches. A couple of bird feeders dangle nearby to attract a bit of wildlife for those who stop here. Odds are that would mean squirrels and a few competing sparrows.

Continue 0.15 miles to the first road crossing, which is South Kemmerer Road. The path continues on the other side, entering back into mixed forest, which gives way to a corridor of locust trees after 0.1 mile. Cross an intermittent creek 0.3 miles from Kemmerer Road and then head out into the open once more. The prairie areas to either side are colorful with wildflowers in spring and summer.

Arrive at a picnic table and shelter after another 0.3 miles and then enter into the trees again. Another 0.3 miles brings you to a mowed lane coming in from the left. To the right is a deep ditch, and to your left is an aspen colony. Continue straight another 0.1 mile, passing a picnic table at Fencehoppers Snowmobile Club. This is the organization, in fact, that was behind much of the support and development of this trail. When snow is present, the trail is used primarily by snowmobile enthusiasts.

Just past the snowmobile clubhouse, cross County Road X at an angle, taking care to look back over your shoulder for traffic. The trail heads into some brush and then crosses a private drive 0.2 miles later. The next crossing is a farm path 0.6 miles from here where the brush opens to fields and farmland and you see I-43 to your left. Watch for red-tailed and Cooper's hawks in the fields. You will also find a few apple trees through this stretch, blossoming in May, and producing fruit starting in August—although it's unlikely you'll find too many that are good enough to eat.

The next 0.8 miles takes you closer to the highway, and then the trail runs parallel. At 0.8 miles you find two benches out in the sun and again 0.2 miles later. This stretch of the trail sinks below the rolling topography to keep the rail grade level. At the second set of benches, look for a loop into the prairie grasses to your left, between the trail and the highway. This mowed footpath curves into the grass for an up-close look at the wildflowers and then rejoins the main trail

200 feet farther along. A second trail does the same just after that. Another 0.2 miles takes you to the next crossing, which is Summerville Road. To your left is the interstate overpass.

Continuing along the trail, you start to see cattails at around 0.4 miles and a shelter, benches, and a picnic table at 0.6 miles from Summerville Road. Here you find another small loop trail left into the grasses and wildflowers, but also with some bluebird houses. Another 0.4 miles brings you to a spur trail right, which opens out into Clinton Street in Allens Grove. After this the trail gets more shade and the trees thicken up on either side. You start to see residences off to the right, while the interstate remains to your left. A ridge starts to rise up to your right, and at 0.3 miles, there's another trail to the right. This one explores a small patch of woods. You are now just 0.5 miles to the end of the trail at North Road. This segment features a lot of maples that show good colors come fall. There are also a lot of black walnuts here.

At the eastern trailhead, find a map board. You can go left here along the road and under the interstate overpass to get to the bridge for a view of Little Turtle Creek. There is no official parking here, though local anglers occasionally do so. From the eastern trailhead, the rail bed is undeveloped. However, a rough, packed-dirt footpath takes you 300 feet into the woods where you can see the concrete pylons of the former railroad bridge that once spanned the creek.

NEARBY ACTIVITIES

At 219 Allen Street, not far from the trailhead in Clinton, is a nice small-town diner called Sun Down Café. They serve great burgers and breakfast any time of day. Beware: It's cash only. Call (608) 676-5681 for more information.

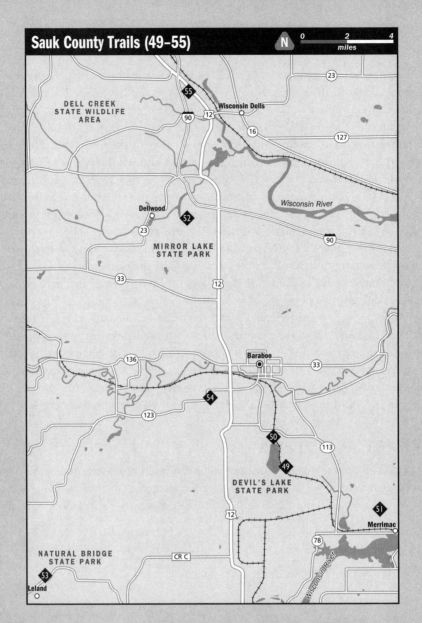

DELL CREEK
STATE WILDLIFE
AREA

23

55

Wisconsin Dells

90   12

16

127

Wisconsin River

Dellwood

52

23

90

MIRROR LAKE
STATE PARK

33

12

Baraboo

136

33

54

123

50

113

49

DEVIL'S LAKE
STATE PARK

12

51

Merrimac

78

Wisconsin River

NATURAL BRIDGE
STATE PARK

CR C

53

Leland

SAUK COUNTY

49 DEVIL'S LAKE STATE PARK:
East Bluff

KEY AT-A-GLANCE INFORMATION

LENGTH: 5.6 miles
CONFIGURATION: Loop
DIFFICULTY: Strenuous
SCENERY: Cliffs, lake overlook, mixed forest
EXPOSURE: Exposed on the steep climb, otherwise mostly shaded
TRAIL TRAFFIC: Moderate at the cliffs, light in the forest
TRAIL SURFACE: Stepping stones, asphalt, crushed rock
HIKING TIME: 2–2.5 hours
DRIVING DISTANCE: 33.2 miles from US 12 and University Avenue
ACCESS: 6 a.m.–11 p.m. year-round
MAPS: USGS Baraboo; online at www.dnr.state.wi.us; at park office
WHEELCHAIR ACCESSIBILITY: None
FACILITIES: Restrooms, campgrounds, water, changing rooms at the beach
SPECIAL COMMENTS: Devil's Lake requires some care and common sense. Over the years several people have fallen to their deaths from the cliffs. Stay on the trails and do not climb. Dogs are allowed on leashes. All vehicles require a park sticker ($7 daily, $25 annual for vehicles with Wisconsin plates). The park participates in the Junior Ranger/Wisconsin Explorer program (see Preface, page xv).

IN BRIEF

Forget the StairMaster, this is a natural workout with a view. Climb to the top of a towering bluff overlooking Devil's Lake and then explore the woods and prairie beyond.

DESCRIPTION

The hike starts with Balanced Rock Trail which zigzags up the broken rock of the bluff face. In just about 0.3 miles, you climb nearly 500 feet from the base of the bluff to the scenic overlook. The trail heads into the woods between the bluff and the parking lot, and you cross over railroad tracks and follow a packed dirt trail to where the broken rock marks the bottom of the bluff. The trail is clearly marked and steps have been fashioned using the stones and patches of asphalt along the way. You pass Balanced Rock at about 0.2 miles.

At the top of the climb is a wonderful overlook to the right from a large flat area of stone. Turkey vultures ride the thermals here. Go left to find a trail intersection with a map and an emergency box to the left. A trail to the left is your return path; the one to the right along the cliff is part of the Ice Age Trail: Devil's Lake Segment. Go straight from the cliff into the woods on the East Bluff Woods Trail. You'll be going downhill for a long way now.

GPS Trailhead Coordinates

UTM Zone (WGS 84)   16T
Easting   0279415
Northing   4810171
Latitude   N 43° 24' 43.09"
Longitude   W 89° 43' 28.21"

Directions

From University Avenue in Middleton, go north on US 12 30 miles to Ski Hi Road. Go right 1.25 miles to South Shore Road and turn right again. Follow this road 1.6 miles as it curves left and enters the park, taking you 1.6 miles to the parking lot for the south shore of the lake. Pick up the asphalt walking path at the north end of the parking lot for the trailhead.

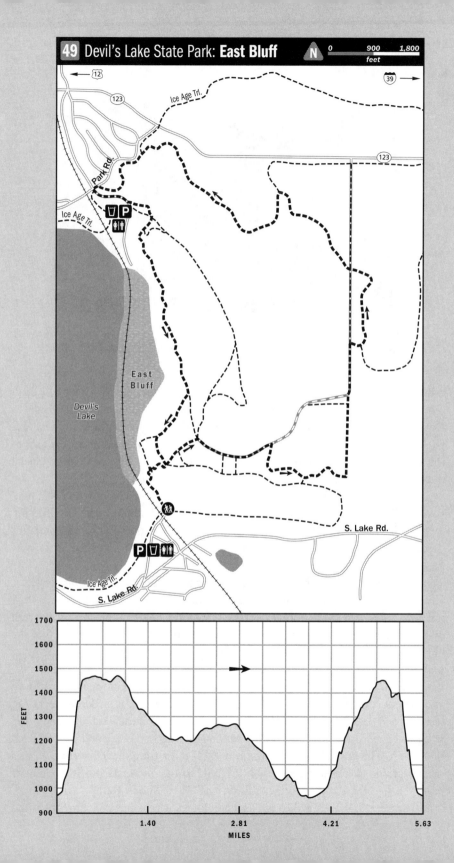

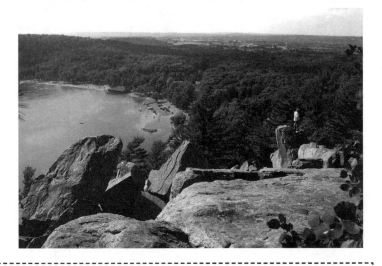

The view of the north hhore from the east bluff

Start into mixed forest with blue sky beyond the edge of the woods to your right. At 0.15 miles at the first intersection to the left is East Bluff Woods Trail. Go right on a two-tire path. Follow this 0.3 miles, passing a trail to the right to Devil's Doorway at 0.1 mile and to The Potholes at 0.15 miles. These are geological features worth exploring: a sort of gateway of stone and depressions in the stone caused by erosion from rocks swirling in the eddies of flowing glacial meltwater.

At 0.3 miles the trail leaves the access road and goes right at a large #5 sign. Pass a path to Moldy Buttress 5B, a climbing point at 0.2 miles on the right, and 5C–D'Arcy's Buttress just about 0.1 mile after that. Continue as the trail starts to descend a bit and curves left on crushed stone with occasional eroded areas until you reach a trail juncture 0.2 miles later.

There is a bench to the right. The straight trail is the Uplands Trail, but left is your course, which is East Bluff Woods Trail *and* Uplands Trail. Follow this 0.25 miles downhill and then notice a ditch joins it on the left. You then arrive at a trail marker, intersection, and bench. To the left is just the access road to the top of the bluff. East Bluff and Uplands trails become one as you continue straight 0.2 miles until you see a trail to the right. This is the East Bluff Woods Trail and the Steinke Basin Loop. Follow it and immediately come to a T. The right branch loops south and then north to the Ice Age Trail before coming back west to make the loop. Go left here and pass through a low-lying area with a bit of prairie with lilies and other wildflowers. Cross a small footbridge over an intermittent creek and pass a bench on the left. The unshaded grassy trail runs 0.25 miles from the T intersection to a second bridge in a clearing and then 0.1 mile to the intersection of the Uplands Trail. Go straight across on Steinke Basin/East Bluff Woods Trail.

The next 0.4 miles is through aspen colonies with some slender maples and hickories fighting for canopy dominance. At the next juncture, find Johnson Moraine Loop/Uplands Trail/Steinke Basin Trail to the right. Go left on East Bluff Woods Trail through scattered deadwood and rock. From here it's 0.7 miles to a bridge, and sunlight just after that at the park's amphitheater. Along the way, however, watch for spur trails to the left out over tree roots to a drop-off of 20 to 35 feet that creates a sort of canyon area behind the much larger lakeside bluff.

At the amphitheater an asphalt trail cuts behind it. Cross to a trail that goes back into the woods. Another 0.1 mile takes you to the park road. Go left and follow the serpentine road 0.25 miles all the way down to the parking lot, always staying left. Into the parking lot, follow along the left edge to find this lot's own trailhead with a kiosk and toilets.

Follow the crushed-stone path 0.1 mile into the woods to the first juncture with a map board and a place to clean off your boots. Take the East Bluff Trail to the right on rough asphalt through a cathedral of towering trees as it climbs once again to the top of the bluff and follows its edge. To the left at the juncture is the East Bluff Woods Trail, which stays far from the cliffs but nevertheless will run parallel and take you to the Balanced Rock Trail and scenic overlook where you first came up.

The East Bluff Trail climb is not as steep as Balanced Rock, but it goes on a bit longer. It is 1 mile from the juncture to the head of the Balanced Rock Trail. The first 0.7-mile climb through the rocky outcroppings offers a variety of nooks and crannies and overlooks to explore. The asphalt trail makes it easy to follow, and some places show steps of stone and asphalt. At some points it dips and rises again with the bluff and in various places it goes farther into the woods before swinging out again toward the cliffs.

At 0.7 miles there is a cutoff trail to East Bluff Woods Trail. Stay right to keep on level trail the next 0.3 miles to the lookout point and trail juncture at the head of Balanced Rock Trail. Go to the right and follow that back down to the trailhead.

NEARBY ACTIVITIES

Ski Hi Fruit Farm, at E11219A Ski-Hi Road, Baraboo, just west of the park, offers 30 different types of apples, unpasteurized cider, and various other local products. Apple season is usually late August to November, at which time the farm is open seven days a week. Call 608-356-3695 for more information.

50 DEVIL'S LAKE STATE PARK:
West Bluff

KEY AT-A-GLANCE INFORMATION

LENGTH: 2.7 miles

CONFIGURATION: Loop

DIFFICULTY: Moderate to difficult

SCENERY: High cliffs, forest, lake

EXPOSURE: Shaded along the top of the bluff, sun along the lake

TRAIL TRAFFIC: Moderate

TRAIL SURFACE: Mostly asphalt, some rocks, dirt and roots

HIKING TIME: 1 hour

DRIVING DISTANCE: 34 miles from US 12 and University Avenue

ACCESS: 6 a.m.–11 p.m. year-round

MAPS: USGS Baraboo; in the park guide available in the park office; posted at trailhead

WHEELCHAIR ACCESSIBILITY: None

FACILITIES: Restrooms, water, concessions, shelters and picnic area, campgrounds

SPECIAL COMMENTS: Devil's Lake requires some care and common sense. Over the years several people have fallen to their deaths from the cliffs. Stay on the trails and do not climb. Dogs are allowed on leashes. All vehicles require a park sticker ($7 daily, $25 annual for vehicles with Wisconsin plates). The park participates in the Junior Ranger/Wisconsin Explorer program (see Preface, page xv).

GPS Trailhead Coordinates

UTM Zone (WGS 84) 16T

Easting   0278729

Northing 4811936

Latitude   N 43° 25' 39.53"

Longitude W 89° 44' 1.25"

IN BRIEF

No less impressive than its sister bluff across the lake, this rocky outcropping offers a stroll along the lakeshore through talus and a series of overlooks 500 feet above the water.

DESCRIPTION

Devil's Lake might be a river if not for a glacier's intrusion about 15,000 years ago. The two bluffs seen today are two of the most ancient rock outcrops in North America. Estimated to be about 1.6 billion years old, they are made of quartzite, a metamorphic rock formed from grains of sand cemented in a nonporous fashion, unlike sandstone, which is porous. The rock buckled up millions of years ago to form the two ridges. Fast-forward to the most recent glacier of the Ice Age. The ice filled in the valley between the bluffs and when the glaciers retreated, moraines were left at either end, creating the bowl for the lake.

If you put the chateau between you and the north beach, look for the asphalt path before the chateau, running left to right. Take it heading west, parallel to the beach and toward the west bluff. It comes to a juncture that goes at an angle left or at an angle right. Take the right branch and follow it to the trees.

Directions

From University Avenue in Middleton, go north on US 12 31.5 miles to WI 159. Go right 1.2 miles to County Road DL and turn right again. Follow this road 0.3 miles and stay straight at the state park entrance following the park road 0.7 miles to the parking lot. For the trailhead follow the asphalt path west just north of the beach area. You will find a path that heads north toward the park entrance on crushed rock. This is the trailhead.

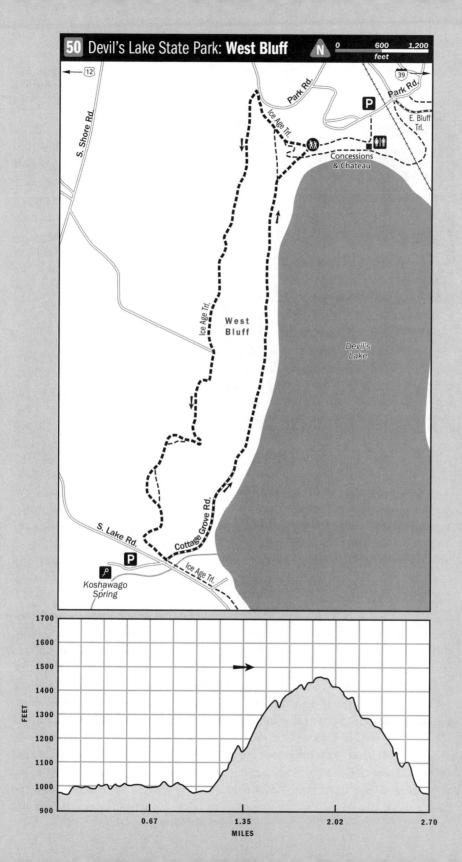

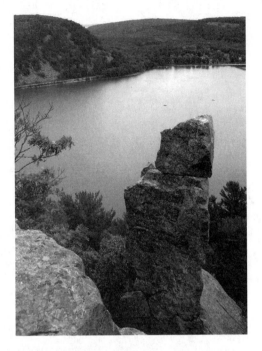

The view from the west bluff to the east bluff

The trail becomes a wide, crushed-rock path that goes in the direction of the park entrance and parallel to the incoming park road. You come to a map board and a bench on the left. Continue past to another map board at the bottom of a long series of steps up to the left 0.1 mile from the trailhead. Here's where the climbing begins, quickly giving you some altitude on the park road.

The stairs go 400 feet, and the trail becomes a roughly laid strip of asphalt from here all the way to the descent on the other side of the bluff. Another 100 feet brings you to a bench, and as you keep climbing, you find another bench 0.1 mile later at an observation point. You start to get views of the lake to the east in various places all along the top of the bluff. The path goes over a small rise after this, and you come to some steps 400 feet from the bench. Step up to a rock platform and then down again on the other side. Pass through a rock gateway on stone steps 100 feet later. Another 150 feet brings you to more steps up and over a hump and down the other side, where you continue another 0.2 miles before you find another bench. Another 150 feet past this is a clearing where you can find more benches and a call box. This is for emergencies, and there is a park access road that comes up the west side of the bluff for emergency vehicles.

Look for a good vantage point to the left here. Continuing along the trail, pass another bench 150 feet later and then arrive at another good observation point on the left 300 feet beyond that. Another 0.15 miles later is the next good place to perch and look out over the lake, and it is arguably the best overlook on this bluff. A wide, flat expanse of rock makes a natural observation deck from which you can look straight across to the equally open and prominent top-of-the-bluff lookout on the other side. You can see the south shore beach area and the moraine that bridges the southern ends of the two bluffs to close off the lake area.

The trail heads back into the woods from here and takes 0.5 miles to descend about 500 feet in elevation. The last stretch is about 0.1 mile of asphalt with long steps formed into it. At the bottom find a map board. To your right across the park road is a parking lot if you prefer to hike this from the south. You are standing where the park road passing on your right intersects with Cottage Grove Road right before you. Go right if you want to get a look at Koshawago Spring, which flows into the lake under the park road. To continue the trail, go left along Cottage Grove Road 0.35 miles to Tumbled Rocks Trail. This is an easy walk now all the way back to the north shore beach area with the lake nearby on the right, and the sloping collection of fractured rocks—known as talus—that tumbled down from the quartzite bluffs during the repeated freezings and unfreezings of the last Ice Age.

As you return to the north shore beach area, the asphalt trail angles to the right, bringing you back to where you started. This doesn't have the drama of climbing through talus like the East Bluff does, but the views are just as remarkable, and some hikers might not like the exposed feeling of Balanced Rock Trail on the East Bluff face. The Ice Age Trail shares the portion across the top of the bluff and continues around the lake at either end. The north shore beach area has concessions, boat rentals, restrooms, a nice swimming area, and even Wi-Fi in the chateau.

NEARBY ACTIVITIES

On the way north to Devil's Lake, head east 2 miles on WI 118 just before crossing the Wisconsin River to find Wollersheim Winery. Open daily from 10 a.m. to 5 p.m., the winery offers tours 15 minutes past each hour. The cost is $3.50. Check out **www.wollersheim.com** or call (608) 847-9463.

51 ICE AGE TRAIL: Devil's Lake Segment

 KEY AT-A-GLANCE INFORMATION

LENGTH: Up to 18 miles

CONFIGURATION: One way

DIFFICULTY: Moderate to difficult

SCENERY: Glacial moraines, towering cliffs, hardwood forest, Devil's Lake, creeks, prairie

EXPOSURE: Half and half, but long stretches of shade

TRAIL TRAFFIC: Light, but potentially moderate to heavy within Devil's Lake State Park bluff areas

TRAIL SURFACE: Packed dirt with roots and rocks, rough asphalt and crushed rock inside the park

HIKING TIME: Up to 8 hours

DRIVING DISTANCE: 36.3 miles from the intersection of US 12 and University Avenue/US 14 on Madison's west side

ACCESS: State park segment's hours are 6 a.m.–11 p.m. year-round

MAPS: USGS Baraboo; *The Ice Age Trail Companion Atlas*; Devil's Lake State Park office has maps of the park portions.

WHEELCHAIR ACCESSIBILITY: Only a shoreline portion at Devil's Lake State Park

FACILITIES: Within the state park are restrooms, water, concessions, boat rentals, shelters, and grills. Pit toilets and water at the Parfrey's Glen Natural Area.

IN BRIEF

Simply the grandest of the area's Ice Age Trail segments, with two dramatic bluffs overlooking Devil's Lake and an assortment of glacial formations, this hike offers a bit of everything and ends at the entrance to Parfrey's Glen, a wonder in its own right.

DESCRIPTION

Of all the Ice Age Trail segments in the area, this is, for me, the mother of them. The length alone might discourage some hikers or at least compel them to cut it in half, perhaps spending a night camping at Devil's Lake State Park, which is just past the halfway point.

From the trailhead you enter the woods on a narrow, uneven dirt path marked throughout with yellow swatches on posts and trees. You find mixed hardwoods the first 0.4 miles, and then the path heads north following the edge of a field. You get a nice view of the surrounding hills. On the other side at 0.3 miles, there is a sign indicating 1 mile to Marsh Road. Go through farmland and just before the road, go right 0.1 mile, inside the wire fence to a gate.

Cross the road to a metal gate and the trail sign near four large boulders. Follow the country lane straight, with woods to the left

---

GPS Trailhead Coordinates

UTM Zone (WGS 84)   16T

Easting   0285938

Northing   4807071

Latitude   N 43° 23' 9.51"

Longitude   W 89° 38' 34.13"

Directions

From its intersection with University Avenue/US 14, go north 23.2 miles on US 12 to Sauk City. After the bridge over the Wisconsin River, go right on WI 78 for 11.8 miles to Merrimac. Go north on Baraboo Road for 0.25 miles. Go left on Cemetery Road for 1 mile (it becomes Marsh Road as you go) and find the trailhead parking lot on your right.

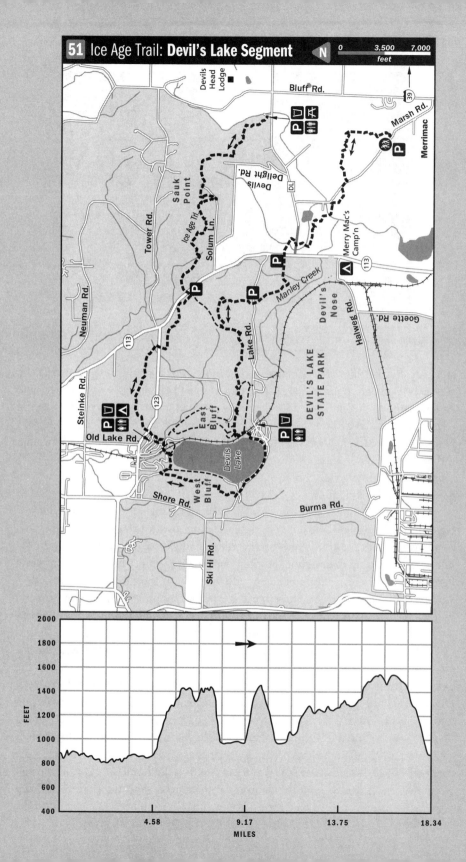

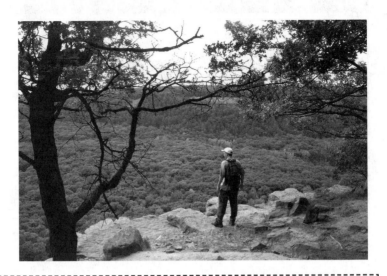

Crossing the east bluff at Devil's Lake

and crops to the right. The lane curves left in front of a small stone cabin, but the trail goes right on grass and zigzags across the field to woods on the other side. As you come to the woods 0.25 miles from the road, the trail goes right along the edge a short distance and then left into tall pines. There's a place to clean your boots and another entry point, but no parking. Go left here, continuing through the pines 0.15 miles and out onto a boardwalk through wet prairie. It rises over a creek and brings you to a footpath at the edge of some woods where you continue uphill moderately.

The next 0.8 miles takes you to CR DL. Along the way you cross a left-to-right trail in the open fields. Go straight, heading toward open water. An arrow points you left as the trail bends around the marshy area. The path heads downhill around a clump of savanna and then over the top of it. Pass over the moraine here as the trail goes right and steeply downhill with the direction of the ridge. A trail sign sends you right where there is a prairie loop to the left if you want to linger a bit. Head north and cross a small footbridge, climb the next hill to a map board and trail info, and then finish the connection to CR DL.

Cross and go right along the edge of the road until a metal gate with a No Hunting sign and a little trail arrow on a post. Squeeze around the end of the gate. The trail goes right on crushed stone and bends left 200 feet down as it crosses a field to another trail arrow. Through a gate on the other side, go left on a grassy trail down a corridor between trees 0.25 miles to WI 113. From there you can see the bluffs of Devil's Lake. Cross the highway to a parking lot. This is the state park now and would require a vehicle sticker. The trail continues past the lot through Roznos Meadow 1 mile to South Lake Road. You'll find the soil along the way is sandy from the deposits of the glaciers and the prairie has been restored to its early-1800s conditions. You will likely see bluebirds. Beyond to the west, you can see the cliffs and their characteristic talus, sloping rock fragments made by the repetitive thaws and freezes during the glacial period. Between the two bluffs is a lower moraine. This moraine, along with the one to the north of the lake, dammed what was once a river and helped form the lake when the glaciers retreated.

At South Lake Road, find another parking lot to the right—another optional starting point, but also requiring a park sticker. From the road the trail climbs up the side of a ravine at a moderate to difficult grade. The path crosses it at 0.5 miles through a lot of exposed rock under good canopy. At 1.1 miles from the road, come to a bench and a trail juncture. To the right is the Uplands Trail, and you could take it to bypass the entire lake area and bluffs if you prefer to save those for another day. Go left and continue climbing 0.4 miles from the juncture, where you'll find a bench and scenic overlook and then a spur trail left to rock-climbing areas at 0.15 miles after that. The trail then curves away from the cliff and starts downhill on crushed rock. From the spur trail to the next juncture is 0.5 miles, where you will see the East Bluff Woods Trail and Uplands Trail going to the right. Stay straight for 0.2 miles, and then the trail breaks left from the park trail at a red sign for Moldy Buttress, a rock-climbing point. Follow this path 100 feet out to the cliff on East Bluff Trail. A Civilian Conservation Corps trail goes left here, but go right on an uneven strip of asphalt. You will likely start to see a lot more trail traffic from this point on until you leave the state park.

Continue along the cliff path 0.3 miles to a stone-step trail left down to The Potholes if you want a look at unique erosion patterns formed long ago by swirling rocks in glacial runoff. Just past this trail is a map board, and another 100 feet farther along is another trail down to the left that takes you through the Devil's Doorway. On the other side of this, continue 0.2 miles to the meeting of several trails at a map board at the top of the Balanced Rock Trail. There is an emergency call box here. Look left to a rock ledge overlooking the lake and southern beach area. Look for a trail marker that leads down to the right from here, and you follow the 0.3-mile Balanced Rock Trail down the cliff face on rock steps and rough patches of asphalt. At the bottom, cross the railroad tracks, pass through the trees beyond, and come out into the south shore beach area. There is a Native American bird-shaped effigy mound to the right. You'll find water, restrooms, a beach for swimming, picnic areas, and concessions along the beach.

From the railroad tracks, the Ice Age Trail (IAT) runs 1.2 miles, following the asphalt path along the shoreline around the southern end of the lake on a board-walk and then just the park road until it arrives at Cottage Grove Road and the trailhead for the West Bluff. You can skip the climb and walk along the lakeshore by taking the Tumbled Rocks path to the right at the end of Cottage Grove Road. Otherwise, start climbing. It's 0.5 miles to the first overlook at the top of the bluff. From there you have another 0.9 miles along the top of the bluff and then down the northern end to the park road. Go right, following the trail into the park, past the park office, and east over the railroad tracks at the opposite end of the north shore beach. Follow the trail markers but essentially take the park road to the Ice Age campground, passing under the highway 1 mile from the West Bluff. Come to an intersection, and on the other side, take the trail that angles right, also the Johnson Moraine Trail. Head up the campground road into the woods, find toilets and water on the left, and take a trail into the woods on the right. Hike another mile, passing a return trail on the right and continuing to CR DL/WI 113. Cross into the woods on the other side, where you'll find a map board.

At 0.1 mile the Uplands Trail goes straight and right; go left on the IAT, crossing four bridges in 1 mile before arriving at a juncture. The Uplands Trail is to the right; your trail is to the left. Pass another spur trail to a parking lot before you arrive at CR DL/WI 113. Cross at an angle to the left to find the next trail segment. This is 4.2 miles from Parfrey's Glen. The trail is rugged once more with tree roots and rocks, passing intermittently through mixed forest and prairie and rising and falling with the hills. Two miles from the highway, come to a juncture and follow an arrow to the left, not straight. From here 0.4 miles is Solum Lane, where there are a couple of homes. Go left with the lane, being careful to follow the yellow arrows and patches where they immediately go left of the old road. Another 2.2 miles remain. This path takes you in and out of the woods and prairie uphill for a bit, but then it is mostly downhill through hardwood forest to the end. A few patches show some tricky footing, especially when the light gets low close to sundown, which may be hastened a bit by the hills behind you.

If you have time and energy, do not miss Parfrey's Glen to your left at the end of the trail. The short hike into a unique gorge holds some rare sights in terms of geology, flora, and fauna.

Note: Make sure you know when sundown is and that you start early enough to beat it. This also makes a good two-day hike with a camp-over in Devil's Lake State Park. Devil's Lake requires some care and common sense. Over the years several people have fallen to their deaths from the cliffs. Stay on the trails and do not climb. Dogs are allowed on leashes. All vehicles within the park boundaries require a park sticker ($7 daily, $25 annual for vehicles with Wisconsin plates). This is also required at the Parfrey's Glen lot at the end of the trail.

NEARBY ACTIVITIES

On your way here or home take the free car ferry across the Wisconsin River at Merrimac (considered the only nonwalking segment of the Ice Age Trail). Buy some ice cream at the stand next to the dock on the Merrimac side before the ride over. The ferry shuts down for winter; otherwise it usually runs 24 hours a day, seven days a week. Watch for flashing signs on US 12, County Road K, Interstates 90/94, and WI 60, 19, and 113, which indicate when the ferry is not running.

MIRROR LAKE STATE PARK

IN BRIEF

Take the easy way or the more difficult path through the woods along the edge of Mirror Lake. Hike to a scenic overlook when you are done.

DESCRIPTION

From the park office, go west on a gravel trail just north of the visitor center door. The trail crosses the asphalt turnaround near the park entrance. The trailhead is straight across into the woods near a trail marker. The trail on the first loop is easy through pine and mixed forest on a path of mowed grass with some sandy patches.

Just 250 feet into the woods is the first trail juncture and a trail map. Go right to begin the East Loop or continue straight to get to the less traveled loops to the west. Going right, the trail heads gently downhill through oaks with partial canopy cover and then into evergreens as it slopes up again. At 0.2 miles is the next trail juncture and another map board where a spur trail goes right into the parking lot near the visitor center. From the second map board, it is another 0.5 miles to the turnaround point of this loop. The trail turns toward Bluewater Campground and heads back in the opposite direction with no canopy coverage. A spur trail

KEY AT-A-GLANCE INFORMATION

LENGTH: 3.3 miles (plus a separate 1-mile scenic overlook trail)

CONFIGURATION: Two loops

DIFFICULTY: Easy to moderate

SCENERY: Woods, lake overlooks, some exposed sandstone

EXPOSURE: Mostly shaded

TRAIL TRAFFIC: Light to moderate

TRAIL SURFACE: Packed dirt, mowed grass, cedar chips

HIKING TIME: 1.5 hours

DRIVING DISTANCE: 45 miles north of the Interstate 39 and US 151 juncture

ACCESS: 6 a.m.–11 p.m. year-round

MAPS: USGS Wisconsin Dells South; at park office and trail junctures

WHEELCHAIR ACCESSIBILITY: A separate trail with a scenic overlook

FACILITIES: Restrooms, water, campgrounds, playgrounds, swimming beach

SPECIAL COMMENTS: At the visitor center, you can get a nice checklist for wildflowers, butterflies, and summer birds you may see in the park plus an educational guide for the Time Warp Trail. All vehicles require a park sticker ($7 daily, $25 annual for vehicles with Wisconsin plates).

Directions

From its intersection with US 151, take I-90/94 West 42.5 miles north to US 12/ Wisconsin Dells Parkway (Exit 92). Go left (south) 0.6 miles to Fern Dell Road. Turn right (west) and follow this road 1.5 miles to the park entrance. The trailhead is immediately on your left as you enter. Park to your right beyond the visitor center.

GPS Trailhead Coordinates

UTM Zone (WGS 84)   16T

Easting   0273196

Northing   4827049

Latitude   N 43° 33' 42.88"

Longitude   W 89° 48' 29.71"

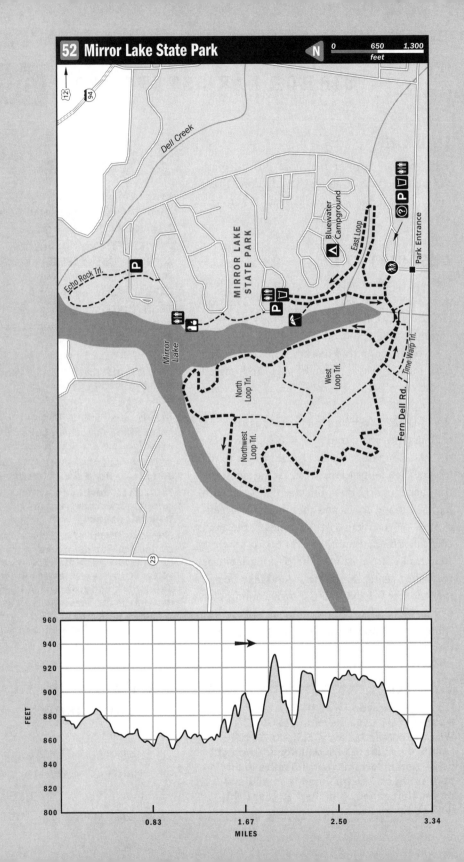

52 Mirror Lake State Park

N

0   650   1,300
feet

Dell Creek

MIRROR LAKE STATE PARK

Echo Rock Trl.

Mirror Lake

Bluewater Campground

East Loop

Park Entrance

North Loop Trl.

West Loop Trl.

Northwest Loop Trl.

Fern Dell Rd.

Time-Warp Trl.

12 94

23

960
940
920
900
880
860
840
820
800

FEET

0.83   1.67   2.50   3.34

MILES

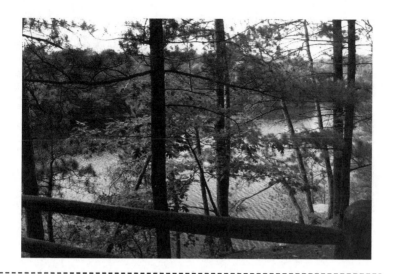

A view of the lake from Northwest Loop Trail

goes right to a picnic area. As you come up on 0.5 miles, you start to see playground equipment as you go up a short hill to the clearing. To your left you see pit toilets and a map board. There is a beach here for swimming. You can get to the Echo Rock Trail from here as well (see below). The return segment of the East Loop is also to your left, just 20 feet away right before the toilets, and it heads back into the woods in the direction you just came. On your right you pass a playground and a trail to the swimming area. There is no lifeguard. The return segment of the loop is 0.3 miles, and you can see the lake through the trees to your right.

You return to the main trail and a map board. Another 200 feet to your left is the beginning of the East Loop, and it is 0.1 mile back out to the trailhead from here. Go right (west) as the trail comes out of the woods with a nice view of one long finger of Mirror Lake to your right. Cross a small footbridge over a creek into the lake and stay right. A spur trail breaks left out to Fern Dell Road just before the bridge. Just after the bridge to your left is the Time Warp Trail, a 0.4-mile loop you can explore with a corresponding interpretive booklet from the visitor center. Go straight as the next trail juncture begins the next loop, which is a combination of the North, West, and Northwest loops. Go right at the next juncture into the woods under the thick canopy of oaks.

To your right is the lake but with better views in fall and spring when the leaves are gone. At 0.4 miles the trail bends left as you come to a map board. The trail left is a segment shared by the North and West loops and heads away from the lake into the center of the woods where you would have a choice to go north on the 1.2-mile North Loop or southwest on the West Loop for a 1.3-mile loop.

Staying on this perimeter trail, you find the trail shows some sandy spots and the tree cover becomes smaller maples. The trail bends right and goes uphill

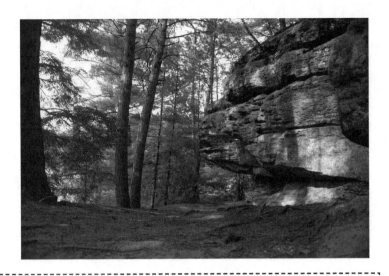

Echo Rock Trail

moderately until it arrives at a short path to a ledge on the right for a good view of the greater lake at 0.1 mile. The trail descends a bit to another good view 0.1 mile later. The path rises and falls with the terrain, and you cross a crease in the earth that slopes right to the water. The meager understory with lots of dead wood allows you to see the roll of the land and gives you a better chance of spotting deer.

Another 0.1 mile takes you into a clearing where the trail bends right and you see the foundation of an old house to your left. Just past it to the right is a railing along the curving trail with the best views of the water below. The trail rounds the point through a grassy clearing and passes a bench on the left before heading back into pine forest. From here the grade is moderately uphill on a trail of grass and pine needles. You'll notice two concrete tire paths up the hill, a previous driveway for the cottage you just saw. These continue uphill another 300 feet.

You reach another juncture 0.1 mile from the start of the concrete paths. Go right here, following the arrows. Another 0.1 mile brings you to another juncture and a trail map. The left trail is part of the North Loop. You continue right on the Northwest Loop. This portion of the trail weaves back and forth through the forest and rises up and down like a roller coaster. This is the most difficult section with short, moderate-to-steep climbs. In another 0.2 miles, you see a ridge with exposed sandstone 50 feet to your left. Ferns grow up to the bottom of it. The path climbs steeply, curves left, and then goes directly up to the top of the ridge, where you can see the exposed stone to either side of you.

From the top of the ridge, you have 0.8 miles more of a path going up and down through gullies with good shade. Follow the arrows to stay on the path as there might be park access roads or old trails visible in the brush. The trail is mostly packed dirt and grass with tree roots, though you may find cedar chips on the steep portions to cut down on erosion. At 0.8 miles the trail emerges into a clearing. Go straight across to the trees and at 0.1 mile come to another map board. A trail goes left here right through the middle of the loops. Another trail 300 feet after this goes right out to Fern Dell Road and is the return path of the Time Warp Trail. From the map board if you stay straight, it will take you 0.3 miles out to the trailhead, retracing your steps starting just before you reach the footbridge.

Be sure to go check out Echo Rock Hiking Trail, a 1-mile loop with an optional 0.4 miles out-and-back asphalt segment that is accessible. It is the best scenic overlook of the lake, and the trail from the viewing area down into the woods takes you up close to the eroded sandstone. You can drive to the north end of the park and pass the Cliffwood Campground for parking at the trailhead. Another option is to hike there from the northern turnaround point on the East Loop Trail. If you continue straight through the playground/picnic area there and north through the parking lot, a trail will connect you to the concessions area. Follow along the north side of the concessions parking lot to the right and a paved trail will take you to the trailhead of the Echo Rock Trail. Other park loops include a 0.7-mile interpretive trail to the east and more than 9 miles of bike trails to the south of Fern Dell Road that are also hikeable.

Note: The park participates in the Junior Ranger/Wisconsin Explorer program (see Preface, page xv).

NEARBY ACTIVITIES

The Aldo Leopold Legacy Center features exhibits and guided tours for those interested in the life and work of the conservationist and author of *A Sand County Almanac*. It's open 10 a.m. to 4 p.m., Thursdays and Fridays, and noon to 4 p.m. on Saturdays. Call (608) 355-0279.

You can see all 15 species of cranes at The International Crane Foundation at E11376 Shady Lane Road, Baraboo, Wisconsin. Call (608) 356-9462 or go to **www.savingcranes.org** for more information.

53 NATURAL BRIDGE STATE PARK

KEY AT-A-GLANCE INFORMATION

LENGTH: 2.4 miles

CONFIGURATION: Loop

DIFFICULTY: Moderate to strenuous

SCENERY: Sandstone bluffs, a stone arch, mixed forest, some prairie

EXPOSURE: Mostly shaded

TRAIL TRAFFIC: Light to moderate near the arch; more deer than people in the southern section

TRAIL SURFACE: Packed dirt, some mowed grass and steps

HIKING TIME: 1–1.5 hours; 30 minutes for just the arch

DRIVING DISTANCE: 10.9 miles west of US 12 on County Road C

ACCESS: 6 a.m.–11 p.m. year-round

MAPS: USGS Blackhawk; posted on the trail at trail junctures but not at the trailhead; nearby Devil's Lake State Park also has the map in their own park brochure.

WHEELCHAIR ACCESSIBILITY: None

FACILITIES: Restrooms, water pump, picnic tables

SPECIAL COMMENTS: The hike can be shortened to take in just the bridge. Signs along the path identify medicinal plants used by Native Americans. You must pay a state park daily-use fee at the self-service box in the parking lot if you haven't got an annual sticker.

GPS Trailhead Coordinates

UTM Zone (WGS 84) 16T

Easting 0262502

Northing 4803351

Latitude N 43° 20' 43.72"

Longitude W 89° 55' 48.64"

IN BRIEF

A magnificent sandstone arch, the largest in the state, is the star of the show typically overshadowing a nice challenging hike across a neighboring bluff. Educational signage makes this a minicourse in medicinal plants.

DESCRIPTION

This quiet, out-of-the-way state park draws visitors to see its 35-foot-high sandstone arch, but most people don't realize that between 9000 and 8000 B.C., this place was already occupied, making this one of the oldest confirmed settlements in northeastern North America. Archaeologists found artifacts and animal remains—15 different types of mollusks and 50 vertebrates, ranging from passenger pigeon to mountain lion—in and around a rock-shelter at the base of the arch. Tribes such as the Fox and the Sauk also occupied the area prior to the arrival of white settlers, but even they are relatively late arrivals.

From the end of the parking lot, head north across the open mowed area, where you see pit toilets to the right and a water pump to the left. At the other end of the clearing, there are two trails into the woods. Take the one to the left with a trail sign about invasive species. You can clean your footwear here before and after the hike.

Directions ➛

Just about 8 miles north of the bridge in Sauk City on US 12, find CR C heading west. Take this 10.9 miles west and find the park entrance on the right side of the road. Follow the short road to the parking lot; the trailhead is at the north end of the lot.

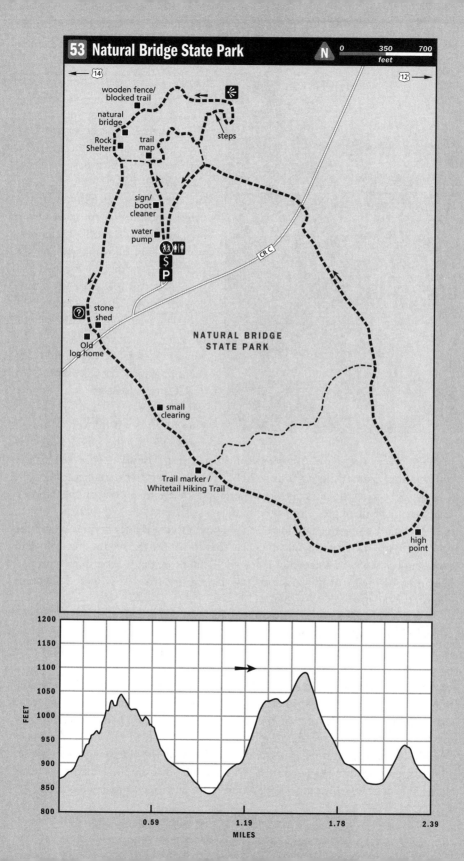

N

0   350   700
feet

14

12

wooden fence/
blocked trail

natural
bridge

Rock
Shelter

trail
map

steps

sign/
boot
cleaner

water
pump

CR C

$
P

stone
shed

Old
log home

NATURAL BRIDGE
STATE PARK

small
clearing

Trail marker /
Whitetail Hiking Trail

high
point

FEET

1200
1150
1100
1050
1000
950
900
850
800

0.59   1.19   1.78   2.39

MILES

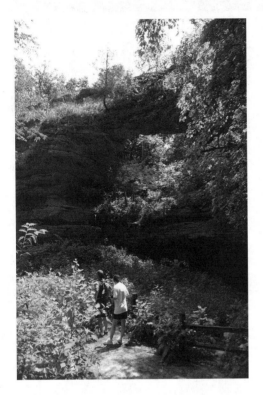

Indian Moccasin Nature Trail takes you up around the top of a bluff and then down past the arch. Oak, maple, hickory, and the occasional clump of aspen dominate the forest, and throughout most of the arch portion of the trail, the understory is thin, allowing you to see the rolling earth that escaped the glaciers in this region of Wisconsin known as the Driftless Zone.

The trail rises into the woods to a trail juncture. Those looking for the path of least resistance to see the natural bridge should go and return along the trail to the left. Otherwise, stay right on packed dirt with frequent exposed roots. The climb is moderate, and in many places there are railroad-tie and earth steps. Another 600 feet up the trail, another path breaks right downhill. This is a cutoff to the return trail. Continue straight to a wooden staircase with railings that goes directly up the exposed sandstone near the high point of the bluff.

The stairs come to a landing and then go up to the right, curving around the rocky outcropping but bringing you close to it to admire the separating layers laid down millions of years ago. Look for shelf fungi on the trees around you and lichens across many of the rock surfaces and tree trunks. A sign here enlightens you on the culinary uses of lichen.

At the top the canopy opens up to sky and a few cedars occupy the level crown of the bluff, surrounded by small remnants of prairie with Indian grass, little blue-stem, and grama grasses. Go to the wooden railing along the right side of the trail and find a bit of a scenic overlook. At the peak of summer, some of the greenery here may be cropping the picture, but you should be able to see the hills beyond and a narrow strip of farmland between them and you. You are at the highest point of this section of the trail (but the southern half will climb even farther and faster without the benefit of steps).

As the trail continues, it curves around top of the ridge and then crosses the axis, passing into thicker brush. To your left see how the land slopes away while the crest of this ridge is to your right and only about another 6 feet higher.

You come to a sign about blackberries and the uses of their leaves. If you come in late summer, you can sample them here for yourself. More railroad-tie steps bring you a bit lower, and you come to an area of slender-trunked maples packed together and struggling to compete with the taller oaks that have taken away most of the sunlight. On your left pass a wooden fence blocking an old spur trail. This was once a path to the top of the bridge, but entry here is now prohibited to preserve the formation.

Look for witch hazel, which flowers in late fall after all the other trees have dropped leaves. A sign marks its location on the right side of the trail past the wooden fence.

The path descends left with a lot of exposed sandstone. Just a few steps more and you are confronted by the naturally formed bridge of sandstone. The space within the arch is 25 feet across and 15 feet high. A wooden fence keeps visitors from getting too close; in the past many people carved their names into the soft stone.

The bridge was formed when the mineral deposits holding the sand together dissolved unevenly, and wind and weather erosion left what you see. Look down and to the right to find a large sheltered space in the rock. Excavations of this site in 1967 found charred wood believed to be as old as 12,000 years.

The trail continues on the other side and is shorter and gentler than your first climb. More railroad ties and railings lead to the bottom, where you find another trail map and a sign about poison ivy, hopefully not too late. The trail to the left goes back to where you found the original trail map and then out to the parking lot. In July look for black caps (also known as black raspberries) on this cutoff trail.

Stay straight on a wide mowed path through wildflowers in the tall grass to the sides. The trail quickly enters into shade, and the brush closes in around you. Come to a bench on the left. The right side of the trail is another area good for black caps in early July and some raspberries a few weeks later. This path goes only 900 feet before entering back into sunlight via a corridor of sumac. Look for the map board to your right. This mowed area is right on the side of the road, and you see an old log cabin on your right and a smokehouse on your left. Just past the smokehouse is a short wooded trail back to the parking lot.

Cross the road to the hay field on the other side and pick up the trail that crosses straight to the trees 400 feet from the asphalt. The cut-grass path begins a moderate climb into mixed forest. Soon the trail gets a bit more rugged with tree roots, and by the time you reach the trail marker for the Whitetail Hiking Trail, it has become a narrow footpath. The trail to the left goes to the edge of the ridge you are climbing and drops down. That segment is difficult and even less developed than the one you are faced with, but it doesn't climb as high.

Keep straight. Underbrush will grab at your ankles, and the shelter of the canopy means dew and previous rains linger longer. Your feet may get wet. The understory rarely rises above the knee, so you can see deep into the woods.

You're likely to find far more deer here than fellow hikers. Be sure to check for deer ticks once you complete the hike.

The trail climbs steeply and starts to head left as it comes upon the highest point of the hike just less than 0.4 miles from the trail marker. The terrain descends gently at first, and then you come to a patch of ferns and a switchback where the trail goes down even more steeply. The ferns often hide where you are stepping.

There's 0.3 miles of this between the apex and the exit to the hay field. From there the trail cuts a gentle serpentine path through the field to the road. Cross the road and go right to pick up the trail again. Duck back into some thick woods and go uphill again, crossing a small prairie to arrive at the cutoff trail that you passed at the beginning of the hike just before the staircase on the Indian Moccasin Trail. Continue on the mowed path until you soon find yourself at the clearing next to the parking area.

Some may prefer to do this trail in reverse, preserving the sandstone bridge as a big finale.

NEARBY ACTIVITIES

Dr. Evermore (aka Tom Every) is a local artist who has created a menagerie of exotic animals and devices out of scrap metal and odds and ends. His Historical Artistic Memorial Metal Sculpture Park is located on the west side of US 12 just north of CR C and shouldn't be missed.

PEWIT'S NEST

IN BRIEF

Hike to the mouth of a water-filled gorge, then climb to the top for views of a creek and a few cascades.

DESCRIPTION

The humble Skillet Creek was once a rush of runoff from the melting glaciers that cut a gorge 30 to 40 feet across and almost as deep through fine sandstone that dates back to the Cambrian period, 490 million years ago. Hikers can walk right up to the edge and look down on the gently flowing water that tumbles over three small cataracts. The hike is short but moderately strenuous in a couple of stretches, but most will come here for the view.

Pewit's Nest was given its name by the pioneers who observed a local man who had fashioned a dwelling out of small cave in the cliffside just above the water. It resembled the nest of a bird called a pewit, also known as a phoebe. The man allegedly used the flowing water of the creek to power lathes. If you stop and ask for directions, be aware that the locals often refer to the area as "Peewee's Nest." It was once just a secret spot known by people from the area, but now the 36 acres form a State Natural Area.

The trail cuts into tall grass and passes through a small meadow where crabapples blossom in spring.

Directions

On the south side of Baraboo on US 12 heading north into town, turn left onto CR W and drive 1.5 miles to a small gravel parking area on the left side of the first big curve in the road. The trail starts at the parking lot.

KEY AT-A-GLANCE INFORMATION

LENGTH: 0.9 miles

CONFIGURATION: Out-and-back

DIFFICULTY: Moderate with a few difficult parts

SCENERY: Towering oaks, wildflowers, flowing water, a gorge

EXPOSURE: Mostly shade

TRAIL TRAFFIC: Light

TRAIL SURFACE: Packed dirt, exposed roots and rocks

HIKING TIME: 0.5 hours for the trail, longer for a swim or exploring the ledges

DRIVING DISTANCE: 1.5 miles west from US 12 and County Road W

ACCESS: 6 a.m.–8 p.m. year-round

MAPS: USGS North Freedom

WHEELCHAIR ACCESSIBILITY: None

FACILITIES: None

SPECIAL COMMENTS: Dogs allowed on a leash. The water is highest in the spring.

GPS Trailhead Coordinates

UTM Zone (WGS 84)   16T

Easting   0274300

Northing   4814853

Latitude   N 43° 27' 9.21"

Longitude   W 89° 47' 22.36"

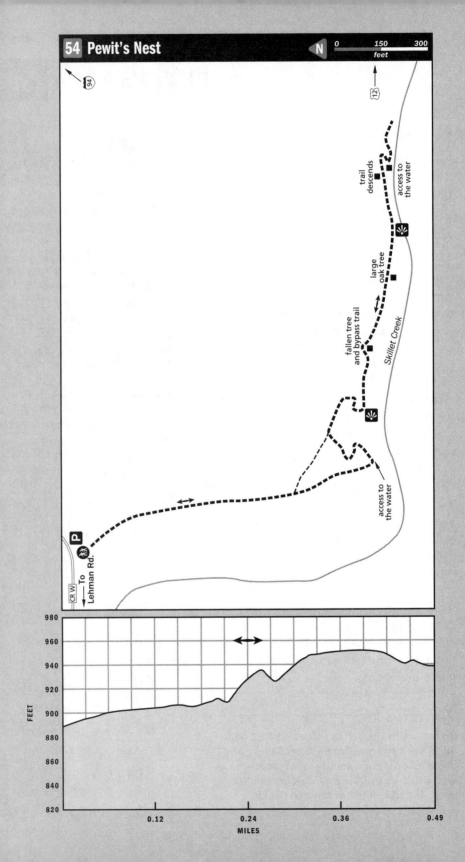

N

0   150   300
feet

94

12

trail
descends

access to
the water

large
oak tree

fallen tree
and bypass trail

Skillet Creek

access to
the water

P

To
Lehman Rd.

CR W

980
960
940
920
900
880
860
840
820

FEET

0.12   0.24   0.36   0.49

MILES

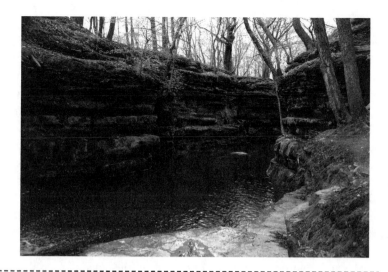

Skillet Creek passes through a gorge

The packed-dirt footpath can get quite muddy in the spring or rainy moments. To the left some of the underlying sandstone layers emerge from the ridge that runs parallel to the trail. Foliage blocks most of this view in the summer, but the trail itself is open to the sky at this point. Another 700 feet from the trailhead, the trees start to close in on the path, and another trail breaks off to the left and rises up into the ridge where the older growth is. This is a short cutoff path and your return trail, so continue straight.

Cross a small clearing and come to a stand of maple saplings with larger trees beyond. Here you find Skillet Creek. There is often a lot of fallen timber here to step over. To your left is the outlet of the gorge. In nice weather people sometimes swim down here, but low water levels and questionable farm runoff might make that inadvisable.

Go right up to the rising rock at the creek edge and go left along the bottom. The rock will be at your right, and the path gets a little tricky as it climbs with natural steps formed by rocks and tree roots and strewn with fallen pine needles. If this sort of climb is not your thing, don't worry, you can backtrack the 300 feet to the cutoff point and take the moderate sloping path up.

Climbing here, however, takes you beneath tall pines and through a short rocky pass until you arrive halfway up the cutoff path. Take this up to the right. Be careful of tree roots here under decaying leaves and needles.

The trail is moderately steep but not treacherous. As you get to the top, the area opens into a wide space beneath the tall oaks and maples and then reaches a fork. Go to the left and head to the ledges overlooking the gorge. The trail continues to the left, but you are going to want to stop here and wander around the ledge to take in the view. The water gurgles softly and foams white below but can get quite a rush on when water is high in the spring or a few hours after a heavy rain.

Straight across you can see more woods that run another 50 feet past the edge before suddenly becoming rolling farmland extending away from this sudden cut in the earth.

Go right along the upper ledge, which is not quite over the water, until you come to a good place to step down a few feet to the lower ledge, where you can look directly down into the gorge. Take some pictures and take a breather.

Follow the ledge west and see the sandstone supporting the upper levels of the ledge up close at your left hand. The trail rises up again to the upper ledge just 30 feet later. Watch your step here, especially as you make the few steps up the narrow trail to the packed-dirt trail. Back on the main trail, the edge is not so near and you continue on through the forest.

Another 200 feet later, the trail breaks into a short loop to the left that merely bypasses a massive fallen trunk that you have to duck under if you remain on the main trail. Another 200 feet beyond that, it goes both ways around a massive oak trunk that occupies a lookout point on the ledge.

Besides the usual suspects of crows, robins, and blackbirds, kingbirds and the occasional kingfisher will make an appearance here. Squirrels and chipmunks are quite common, and around dusk deer may lurk in the nearby cornfields. On some days the wind will moan through the gorge.

Another 150 feet past the large oak is another good overlook that offers views of the still waters where the creek widens and the silt that lies just below the surface.

The trail heads down a steep and tricky path 100 feet beyond the overlook. This footpath can get slippery in wet seasons. Remember that you'll be climbing back up it to return. At the bottom find a narrow path over a rock ledge to your right when you are facing the creek. This skirts along the water for about 40 feet to where rock forms a natural dam across the creek. You can step down to the level of the water at the end of this and look down the gorge toward the other end. This isn't a bad place to get your feet wet a little.

Back at where you left the trail, continue only another 100 feet to find a farmer's cornfield to your left and the bend in the creek. This is the turnaround point. On your return stay right; the cutoff trail back at the ledges takes you directly to the main path in the clearing and the parking lot beyond.

In May the crabapples blossom along the first portion of the trail, and in fall this area is a good place to see the colors.

NEARBY ACTIVITIES

Circus World celebrates the history of the American circus with restored train cars and a variety of exhibits, as well as some circus acts during the summer season. It is located in nearby Baraboo at 550 Water Street (Highway 113). Call (866) 693-1500 for more information.

ROCKY ARBOR STATE PARK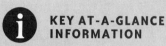

IN BRIEF

Walk along the former bed of the Wisconsin River and see where the glacial runoff and resulting river once dug deep into ancient sandstone, and then climb to the top of the ridge looking over it.

DESCRIPTION

The Wisconsin River once ran through this gorge now rich with a fine mix of forest and wetlands and an assortment of wildflowers. The waterway, which now flows about 1 mile to the east, originally formed at the end of the last Ice Age. As the massive sheets of ice retreated north, a glacial lake formed in the area that is now central Wisconsin, and the outer edges of the ice contained it. When these waters broke through the ice barrier, they rapidly carved paths through the land, exposing and reshaping sandstone laid down during the Cambrian period more than 400 million years ago. Many of the resulting formations that are characteristic of the Wisconsin Dells area are perhaps reminiscent of the Grand Canyon, but geologically speaking, these were formed "suddenly."

The trailhead is at the far end of the parking lot just past the park office. The trail follows along the edge of the old river bed and then climbs to the top of the ridge for the return trip. The rock formations along the way make a lovely setting for a short hike, and the

KEY AT-A-GLANCE INFORMATION

LENGTH: 1.1 miles
CONFIGURATION: Loop
DIFFICULTY: Moderate to difficult
SCENERY: A gorge, sandstone cliffs and rock formations, mixed forest and wetlands
EXPOSURE: Mostly shaded
TRAIL TRAFFIC: Light
TRAIL SURFACE: Packed dirt with rocks and tree roots
HIKING TIME: 0.75–1 hour
DRIVING DISTANCE: 0.8 miles southeast on US 12 from Exit 85 off Interstate 90/94 north of Wisconsin Dells
ACCESS: Memorial Day weekend to Labor Day, 6 a.m.–11 p.m.
MAPS: USGS Wisconsin Dells North; map available at park office
WHEELCHAIR ACCESSIBILITY: No
FACILITIES: Campgrounds, restrooms, water, park office, playground
SPECIAL COMMENTS: Dogs allowed on leashes. Be sure to check for ticks after this one.

Directions

From Exit 85 on I-90/94, take US 12 heading east (actually southeast) 0.8 miles to the park entrance on the right. Pass the office and go straight into the parking lot near the restrooms. The trailhead is at the end of the lot.

GPS Trailhead Coordinates

UTM Zone (WGS 84)   16T
Easting   0273822
Northing   4835734
Latitude   N 43° 38' 24.76"
Longitude   W 89° 48' 14.92"

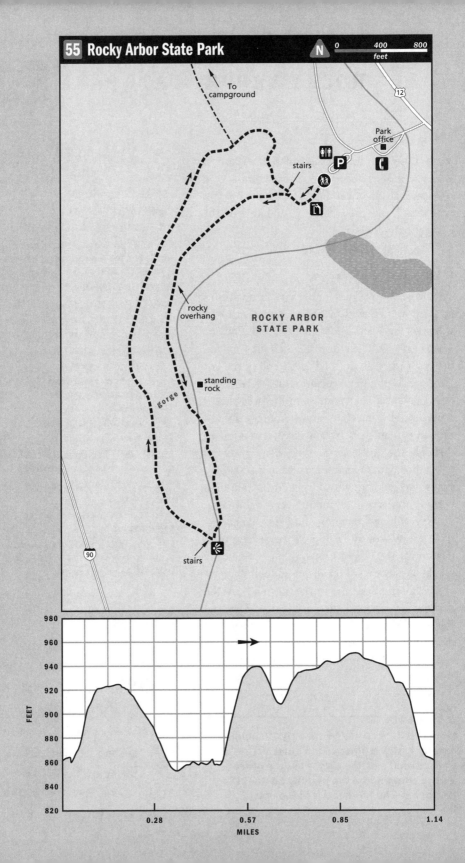

55 Rocky Arbor State Park

N

0   400   800
feet

To campground

12

Park office

stairs

rocky
overhang

ROCKY ARBOR
STATE PARK

gorge

standing
rock

90

stairs

FEET

980
960
940
920
900
880
860
840
820

0.28   0.57   0.85   1.14

MILES

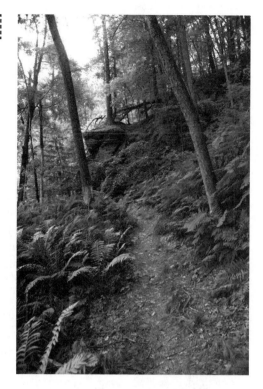

A trail through an old river bed

wildflowers and wildlife are cause to linger. The mosquitoes, however, enjoy the benefit of shelter from the wind and moist conditions, so be sure to prepare for them.

Just 150 from the trailhead, take the short trail to the left and have a look straight down the gorge from an observation deck there. Return to the main trail and go left, following the bend of the gorge slightly to the left. Another 150 feet from here, wooden steps go up the cliff face. This is your return route from the upper portion of the trail, but it is also a direct route to the campgrounds up over the ridge and about 0.3 miles away.

Continue past and expect lots of fern in the understory to the left while to the right you are looking deep into the past when, during the Cambrian period, this was all sediment at the bottom of a warm sea. The narrow trail is coated with rusty pine needles that seem out of place among the green deciduous trees you see around you. Only by looking straight up do you see the pines that tower above the rest of the treetops and grow farther up the ridge as well.

As you progress, the area to your left becomes marshy, and you see cattails. The trail is narrower still and rather tricky with rocks and tree roots and a lot of rise and fall. Cross a big flat piece of sandstone as you pass under a rocky overhang.

In the height of summer when the ferns are at their largest, there is almost a prehistoric feel to this area.

To your right look for vertical cracks where tree roots have dug deep into natural fissures in the stone and widened them as they took hold. Some of the trees seem impossibly large to be grasping the rock.

Watch to your right for a sloping gulley that cuts down from the upper level of the ridge to the trail below. Not far past this is a 25-foot-high standing rock to your left, which must have been an island in the middle of the river a long time ago. About 200 feet past this island, look to your right and observe a vertical fissure in the stone.

From here the trail is wide open to your left. Watch for columbine in the late spring. Flower aficionados will find a few species here that are not found elsewhere in the area.

At just about 0.5 miles into the hike, the trip down the river ends, and you must take the steps up to the right, passing close to moss-covered shelves in the sandstone. Stop halfway up the staircase to admire the view, because at the top, foliage often prevents a good look. The last portion of the ascent is logs laid in the earth for steps.

When you reach the trail at the top, the highway is just on the other side of the ridge and traffic noise can be a distraction. The return trail immediately starts to put distance between you and the road hum.

The trail is level through the forest and well shaded by a thick canopy. The trail surface is leaf-covered, and this can hide tree roots, so watch your step. The path begins narrow and widens as you go. About 900 feet down the trail from the top of the steps, look for the channel sloping down to the right, which is the same one you saw from below on the outbound trail. But you won't see that lower trail because it is directly beneath the ridge.

Fine grass growing beneath the trees makes the trail clearer in summer. You come to a juncture where a trail heads left 0.5 miles from the stairs. This takes you to the campgrounds. Go right instead as the trail slopes down gently to a trail marker with an arrow. Here the trail dips again. To the left you can see the lot below in the distance. The path, littered with rust-colored pine needles and show-ing some shelflike rocks, turns a corner going left down a railroad-tie staircase with a wooden handrail. When it comes around the bend, there's another hand-rail. Take the steps descending with handrails on both sides to the original trail.

Look up to your left at the bottom and marvel at how little soil lies beneath the trees there. Seeds somehow managed to find a tiny amount of soil to sprout atop these rocks, and the root system grew into whatever cracks were present, widening and allowing other soil and nutrients to gather there. The persistence and unlikely strength of these expanding roots eventually widens fissures in the rock, and the most ambitious trees finally destroy their own perches by breaking off the rock. Every once in a while park managers must take down a tree that is literally teetering on the edge.

Mammals run the gamut here from woodchucks and squirrels to deer and foxes, and even black bear have been sighted this far south, albeit rarely. It's a short hike so far from Madison, but not to be missed.

NEARBY ACTIVITIES

Mirror Lake State Park is just south of here off the same interstate, and, of course, Wisconsin Dells, where the present-day river runs, is a tourist mecca for the state. Take a tour down the river and see the wonderful sandstone formations from aboard an amphibious "duck" at Dells Glacial Park Tours at 1550 Wisconsin Dells Parkway, Wisconsin Dells, 53965. Go to **www.dellsducks.com** or call (608) 254-6080 for more information.

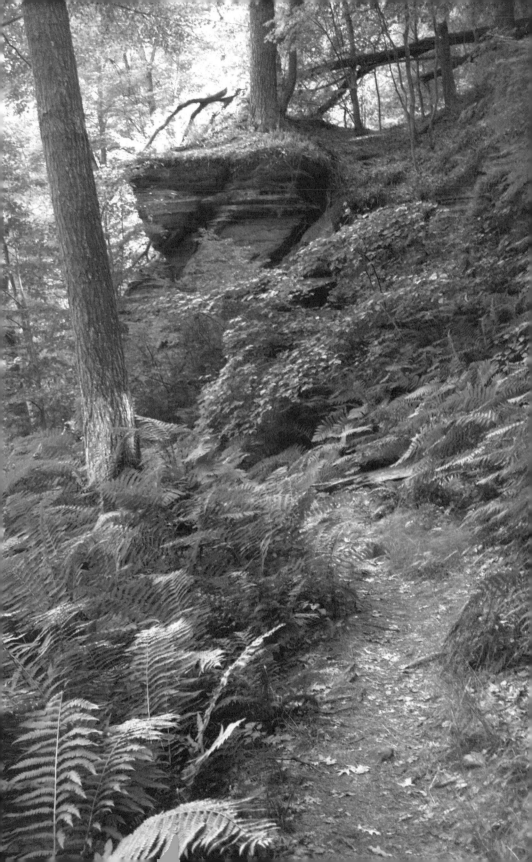

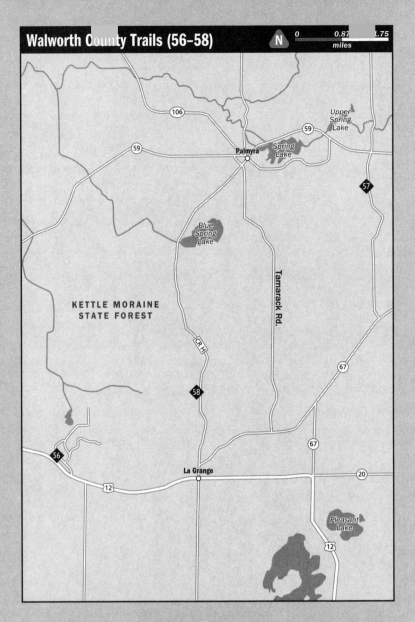

Walworth County Trails (56–58)

N

0   0.87   1.75
miles

106

59

Upper Spring Lake

Palmyra   *Spring Lake*

57

Blue Spring Lake

KETTLE MORAINE
STATE FOREST

Tamarack Rd.

CR H

67

58

67

56

La Grange

12

20

Pleasant Lake

12

WALWORTH COUNTY

56 ICE AGE TRAIL: Whitewater Lake Segment

KEY AT-A-GLANCE INFORMATION

LENGTH: 8.9 miles

CONFIGURATION: Out-and-back

DIFFICULTY: Moderate to difficult

SCENERY: Moraines, mixed forest, Whitewater Creek and Lake

EXPOSURE: Mostly shaded

TRAIL TRAFFIC: Light

TRAIL SURFACE: Packed dirt with abundant rock and tree roots

HIKING TIME: 4 hours

DRIVING DISTANCE: 45.2 miles from the juncture of Interstate 39/90 and US 12/18

ACCESS: 6 a.m.–11 p.m. unless you are a registered camper

MAPS: USGS Whitewater; *The Ice Age Trail Companion Atlas*

WHEELCHAIR ACCESSIBILITY: None

FACILITIES: Portable toilet at trailhead; toilets, water, telephone, campsites at Whitewater Lake Campground

SPECIAL COMMENTS: Dogs are allowed on leashes. All vehicles require a park sticker ($7 daily, $25 annual for vehicles with Wisconsin plates) to park in either Whitewater Lake Campground or the Ice Age Trail lot on US 12.

GPS Trailhead Coordinates

UTM Zone (WGS 84)   16T

Easting   0364870

Northing   4740370

Latitude   N 42° 48' 14.26"

Longitude   W 88° 39' 9.38"

IN BRIEF

Another excellent segment of the national scenic trail, this path climbs moraines through Kettle Moraine State Forest's Southern Unit before ending at Whitewater Lake.

DESCRIPTION

This segment of the Ice Age Trail (IAT) heads south from US 12, but another portion heads north from the parking lot as well. Cross the highway with care as traffic comes quickly through here. From the end of Sherwood Forest Road, go directly across to the trail marker and a metal gate across the entrance. Just after it, the trail forks. To the left is the Moraine Ridge Trail, a state horse and snowmobile trail. The narrow footpath to the right is the Ice Age Trail. It climbs a ridge through brush and on broken rock and packed dirt, moving parallel to the highway and offering good elevation in only about 400 feet.

The path then turns south, quickly leaving traffic behind. Find wood-beam and earth steps to an aspen colony, and then enter a clearing with a bench overlooking the surrounding area from the top of the ridge. Head back into the woods 100 feet later via steps down through more aspen. Brush thins out and 0.25 miles

Directions

From its intersection with US 12/18, go south 20.8 miles on I-39/90 to Exit 163 for Milton/Edgerton. Take WI 59 east (right at the end of the ramp) 2.8 miles to County Road N for 10.8 miles where it becomes Walworth Avenue outside Whitewater. Turn right on US 12 and follow it 6.5 miles to the intersection of Sherwood Forest Road. The Ice Age Trail parking lot is on the left. The trailhead is on the south side of the highway, opposite the lot.

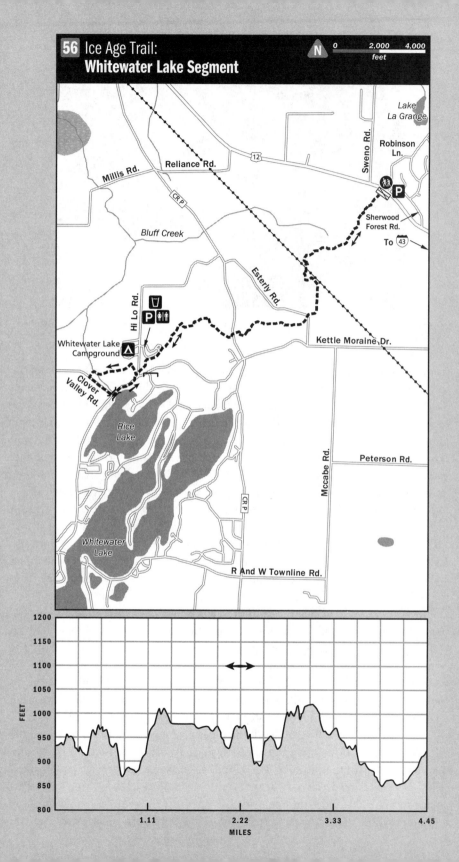

N

0   2,000   4,000
feet

Lake
La Grange

Robinson
Ln.

Sweno Rd.

Reliance Rd.

12

Millis Rd.

CR P

Sherwood
Forest Rd.

Bluff Creek

To 43

Esterly Rd.

Hi Lo Rd.

P

Whitewater Lake
Campground

Kettle Moraine Dr.

Clover
Valley Rd.

Rice
Lake

Mccabe Rd.

Peterson Rd.

Whitewater
Lake

CR P

R And W Townline Rd.

1200
1150
1100
1050
1000
950
900
850
800

FEET

1.11   2.22   3.33   4.45

MILES

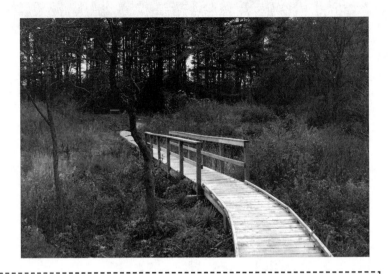

A boardwalk over Whitewater Creek

from the bench and overlook, oaks start to dominate. The path follows along the top of moraines with good shade and nice views into the creases between them. Wildflowers appear along the trail from spring to fall. The path has a lot of stray rocks, which can make footing tricky when the leaves fall and cover them. The first moraine is about 0.2 miles long. When you arrive at the end of it, follow the trail down and then up again along the back of another lower and shorter moraine. Another 100 feet brings you to the next one. As the moraines shrink, continue downhill until you come to the edge of a clearing 1.1 miles from the trailhead.

The trail then starts left up the hill along the clearing where high-tension lines come over the hills. The trail passes partly through the brush and hardwood forest along the edge of the clearing before cutting right across under the lines and back into forest on the other side. Cross to the other side of the hill there and then walk along the edge of a ridge heading east until the path heads right, away from the hill and into pine forest. The path is carpeted with needles, easy, and level. Come to an access road that heads to the right (south) along the edge of these tall pines. Follow it 0.1 mile to another intersection where the taller pines end on your right. Continue straight and pass through shorter pines as you follow the road to where it bends right and takes you out to Esterly Road, 0.2 miles from the last juncture. The IAT joins the horse and snowmobile trail through here. Cross the road and continue to follow the yellow trail patches. Pass through a clearing amid a lot of brush and then take steps down through a corridor of pine.

At 0.4 miles from Esterly Road, the pines give way to oaks and aspen on the left. You can look down the ridge on both sides. Another 0.3 miles brings you to another crossing of the Moraine Ridge Trail. Take a soft right down a path marked with a sign that reads HORSES AND SNOWMOBILES PROHIBITED IN THIS AREA. Pass sumac to your left under an open sky and continue downhill 0.1 mile on rocks and more wood-beam and earth steps before the path switches back to lead you to County Road P. Go straight across to pick up the trail which heads into another clearing full of sumac followed closely by pine forest. Just 0.15 miles from CR P, the trail starts uphill on wood-beam steps through mixed hardwoods to pine at the top of the bluff. This segment of the trail again climbs moraines, and the path shows a lot of roots and rocks and some occasional wood-beam steps, but also offers good shade.

It's a total of 0.9 miles from the road to where you come off the back of the ridge to a scenic overlook. There is a bench here with a view of Whitewater Lake where you'll end up. Steps to the right lead down the slope 300 feet to a spur trail that enters the campgrounds. Continue past, passing the edges of the campsites just up to the right. From the spur trail, you have 0.3 miles to hike until you come to Hi Lo Road. Pass a trail to the park office, a map box, likely unstocked, and a couple of small kettles to the right and left before you come to the road crossing. To the left 200 feet is Kettle Moraine Drive. Go straight across Hi Lo Road and up into pine forest to a trail juncture 150 feet into the trees. The straight path is your return; go right into oak and pine. The trail is easier through here and mostly shaded. At 0.3 miles cross the horse path once more, and then 0.1 mile takes you out of the forest at Whitewater Creek, which meanders through wet prairie. There is a bench here. Go right along the edge of the forest to reach a boardwalk and bridge over the small stream. On the other side is another bench. The trail goes left and bends right into the trees, crossing 200 feet to Clover Valley Road. There is an area map on the back of the road sign. Your choice now is to either turn around and head back the way you came or continue to the lake to make a small end-loop before hiking back on the IAT.

Go left 0.25 miles on the shoulder of the road to the edge of the lake on Kettle Moraine Drive. Go left again toward Whitewater Lake Recreation Area. Be careful: there's not much of a shoulder on the road here. Be sure to walk facing traffic. The lake drains under the road into Whitewater Creek, a stream with waters favorable for trout. Just past the creek, the horse trail heads left into the woods. Then 0.2 miles from Clover Valley Road, find a blue-marked trail left into the pine forest. Two hundred feet into the trees, find the IAT once again. Go right and retrace your steps to the trailhead. Alternatively, you could park a second vehicle here at the campgrounds or even stay the night if you packed equipment. The campground has pit toilets but no showers.

NEARBY ACTIVITIES

Old World Wisconsin at S103 W37890 Highway 67 in Eagle is a 600-acre outdoor museum dedicated to Wisconsin rural history. Various farmsteads represent several of the cultures that settled near here, and trams connect them. It is open from May 1 to October 31. Go to **www.wisconsinhistory.org/oww** or call (262) 594-6300.

57 KETTLE MORAINE STATE FOREST:
Emma Carlin Trail

KEY AT-A-GLANCE INFORMATION

LENGTH: 4 miles

CONFIGURATION: Loop

DIFFICULTY: Moderate to difficult

SCENERY: Hardwood and pine forest, glacial formations, scenic overlook

EXPOSURE: Mostly shaded

TRAIL TRAFFIC: Light to moderate

TRAIL SURFACE: Uneven packed dirt and sand, abundant rocks and tree roots

HIKING TIME: 2 hours

DRIVING DISTANCE: 49.7 miles from the juncture of Interstate 39/90 and US 12/18

ACCESS: 6 a.m.–11 p.m. year-round

MAPS: USGS Little Prairie; at Kettle Moraine State Forest offices; posted at trail junctures

WHEELCHAIR ACCESSIBILITY: None

FACILITIES: Pit toilets, water

SPECIAL COMMENTS: This trail is popular with mountain bikers. Bikers must ride in one direction; be sure to go the opposite way. All vehicles require a park sticker ($7 daily, $25 annual for vehicles with Wisconsin plates). Hiking is free, but bikers must purchase a state trail pass ($4 daily, $15 annual).

GPS Trailhead Coordinates

UTM Zone (WGS 84) 16T

Easting 0373876

Northing 4747607

Latitude N 42° 52' 14.32"

Longitude W 88° 32' 38.86"

IN BRIEF

Trek along the upper ridges of kettle moraines in this remarkable state forest full of oaks and red pine and some of the most graphic examples of glacial deposits you're likely to see.

DESCRIPTION

The state forest takes its name from kettle moraines, glacial deposits left by receding ice. As the glaciers melted, the debris of the earth-moving sheets of ice accumulated in the form of ridges and hills. But pockets of ice became trapped beneath some of them. When that ice melted, the land took on a bowl shape. This trail system is riddled with the feature.

From the trailhead you must hike 0.2 miles before arriving at the actual loop. It starts into woods, primarily pine, on a packed-dirt trail. You can expect a lot of mountain bikers here, especially on weekends. Be sure to go against traffic and give way to bikers.

There is a trail map on the right and a bench on the left 200 feet along the entry trail. Cross an open grassy area that is part of a glacial sand plain and then reenter trees to find the juncture where the loop runs left to right for bikers. Go left against the one-way signs.

Directions

From its intersection with US 12/18, go south 17.6 miles on I-39/90 to Exit 160 for Edgerton. Take WI 73 east (left) 0.9 miles to WI 103. Turn right and follow it carefully (there are a couple turns) for 28.2 miles to Palmyra. Turn left on Main Street/WI 59 and follow it 2.4 miles to County Road Z. Go right 0.6 miles to the Emma Carlin Trail parking lot on the right. The trailhead is opposite the entrance to the parking lot next to a kiosk.

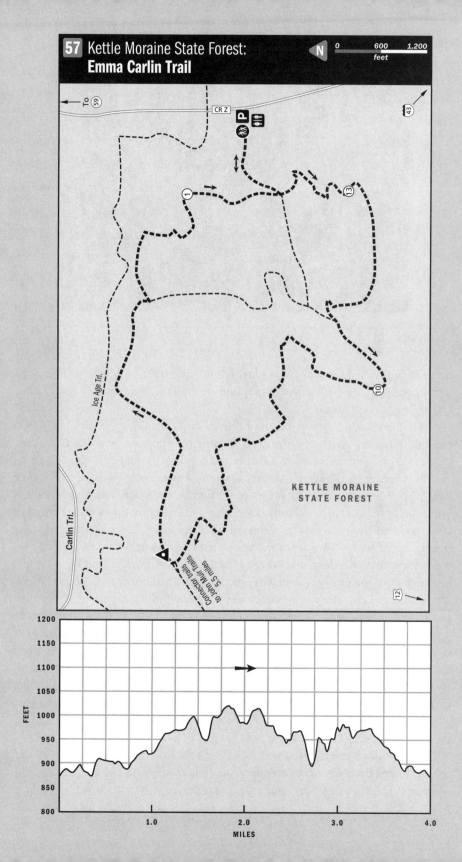

57 Kettle Moraine State Forest:
Emma Carlin Trail

N

0	600	1,200

feet

To 59

CR Z

P

43

1

13

10

Ice Age Trl.

Carlin Trl.

**KETTLE MORAINE
STATE FOREST**

Connector trails
to join Muir Trails
5.5 miles

12

FEET

1200
1150
1100
1050
1000
950
900
850
800

1.0   2.0   3.0   4.0

MILES

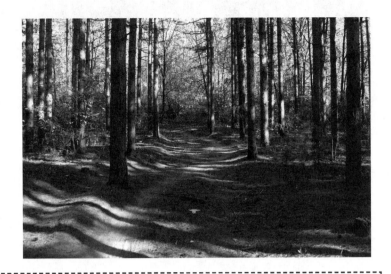

A pine plantation

Another trail straight across and slightly left is marked DO NOT ENTER. This is the Red Loop, which runs 2 miles. Going left you follow the "return" path of the Orange and Green Loops.

The first 0.3 miles is mostly uphill into moraines taking you to a signpost marking Point 13 on the trail map. Just past this you pass between two kettle depressions on what is in effect a natural land bridge to the next ridge. The trail dips here before you climb. From here the trail is quite rocky and not to be taken lightly by those without good ankles or supportive footwear. The next 0.4 miles bring you to the bottom of a basin. Thereafter the trail climbs on a wide S through the woods and up the next moraine another 0.1 mile. You see a trail coming steeply and directly down from the upper path of a switchback. Best to stay on the main trail and follow that where it will pass this shortcut and come to the intersection of the Orange Loop. Go right to reduce your hike to 2.4 miles. If you do this, the next juncture is 0.1 mile, and you should remain straight rather than going right at that point to follow the Orange Loop.

Continuing on the Green Loop, climb over the highest points within the center of the park. Another 250 feet up a steep slope, you come to the first and continue for 0.2 miles until Point 10, all the while enjoying views into the depressions around you and toward other high ridges across them. Continue 0.15 miles to Point 9 and just 100 feet later, Point 8. Cross some erosion-prevention bars along the way. Point 9 offers great views down either side, and you can see why the ridge is called a "razorback."

From Point 8 the trail follows the edge of the ridge and then crosses over to the right edge 0.1 mile later. At Point 7 the trail switches back, and you continue another 0.15 miles to where you pass along the edge of a rock wall. The trail bends left and ascends easy to moderate. Just beyond that the land dips once more to either side. The next 0.35 miles continue to follow the razorback of the ridge overlooking a kettle to your right until you arrive at a low rock wall across the path. These are beachball-size stones. You are surrounded by oak and aspen in this area. Another 50 feet takes you across another wall sunk into the land and crossing your path.

Past the rock wall, you have another 0.1 mile of cedar and sumac with little shade before you come to an aspen colony. From the aspens it's another 0.1 mile through the more open cedar and sumac terrain until you arrive at a trail intersection and a scenic overlook. To your left you see two trails, one of which is marked DO NOT ENTER. These are two outlets of the same connecting trail, which join the Emma Carlin Trail with the John Muir Trail 5.5 miles away. The terrain is arguably more challenging than either of the two. Traffic for bikes is two-way, so if you decide to hike it, be aware riders may come quickly from behind you. This clearing and intersection also offer a map board and a scenic overlook. Look out northwest over Lower Spring Lake where on a clear day you can also see Holy Hill in the distance. This area offers some great colors in fall, and updrafts off the overlook draw hawks and turkey vultures.

Go right from the clearing and into brush to continue on the Green Loop. The narrow bike path cuts a groove into the sandy terrain, and there is grass on either side of it if you prefer. The trail continues another 0.7 miles through cedar and sumac with no shade before arriving at a trail juncture. To the right is the path shared by the Red and Orange Loops coming at you for hikers (going away for bikes). Stay left on the Green Loop and the trail bends left through a clearing with thick brush and some oaks as it heads uphill. You find yourself once again along the edge of a ridge with the deep depression of a kettle to your right.

From the trail juncture to the next is 0.4 miles, where you find a trail bearing left out of the system. Go right and pass Point 1 100 feet later. The trail passes through aspen before it arrives at a marshy area on your left, a good place to spot a heron. The path takes you to the right, following the edge of the wetlands and then heading into partial cover of mixed forest. When you come to the entry trail and intersection 0.2 miles later, go left and follow the path back through the grassy field to the parking lot.

Note: Hunting is allowed September to May. Be aware that during gun deer-hunting season at the end of November, you should wear bright-colored clothing, especially blaze orange. Call (262) 594-6200 if you are unsure about when the hunters are present.

NEARBY ACTIVITIES

The Turner Museum, operated by the Palmyra Historical Society, features historic artifacts and exhibits about Palmyra's past. A gift shop is also located at the museum. Stop in at 112 North Third Street, Palmyra, or call (262) 495-2412.

58 KETTLE MORAINE STATE FOREST:
John Muir Trail

KEY AT-A-GLANCE INFORMATION

LENGTH: 9.5 miles

CONFIGURATION: Loop

DIFFICULTY: Moderate to difficult

SCENERY: Mixed forest, some prairie, glacial landscape

EXPOSURE: Mostly shaded with some stretches of sun

TRAIL TRAFFIC: Light to moderate

TRAIL SURFACE: Packed dirt, abundant rocks and tree roots, some sand

HIKING TIME: 4 hours

DRIVING DISTANCE: 45.2 miles from the juncture of Interstate 39/90 and US 12/18

ACCESS: 6 a.m.–11 p.m. year-round

MAPS: USGS Little Prairie; at park office; posted at trail junctures

WHEELCHAIR ACCESSIBILITY: None

FACILITIES: Pit toilets, water, picnic shelters and grills, vending machine, pay phone

SPECIAL COMMENTS: This trail is popular with mountain bikers. Bikers must ride in one direction; be sure to go the opposite way. All vehicles require a park sticker ($7 daily, $25 annual for vehicles with Wisconsin plates). Hiking is free, but bikers must purchase a state trail pass ($4 daily, $15 annual).

GPS Trailhead Coordinates

UTM Zone (WGS 84) 16T

Easting 0368924

Northing 4742082

Latitude N 42° 49' 12.30"

Longitude W 88° 36' 12.41"

IN BRIEF

A challenging trail climbs up and down through oak and pine forests along the rubble deposits of the last glaciers.

DESCRIPTION

Don't let the mountain bikers discourage you: This is a hiking trail as well. The abundance of ridges and kettles offer challenges to boots and wheels alike, and the extensive trail system leaves plenty of room for everyone. Watch for deer and turkey as well as many songbirds.

Walking into the trail system from the trailhead, take the first right. You must go against bike traffic for safety. This trail cuts 0.1 mile to the actual loop in the same way that the left-bound trail does in the opposite direction. Between the two trails is 0.1 mile of the trail. At the juncture, go right to stay in the proper trail direction, heading north.

At 0.15 mile the Red Trail comes from the left. You could cut 1.5 miles off the hike by going west here, taking a right 0.4 miles later on the Orange Trail and following that up and across to connect back to the Blue Trail. This is one route (but not the only one) that can get

Directions

From its intersection with US 12/18, go south 20.8 miles on I-39/90 to Exit 163 for Milton/ Edgerton. Take WI 59 east (right at the end of the ramp) 2.8 miles to County Road N for 10.8 miles where it becomes Walworth Avenue outside Whitewater. Turn right on US 12 and follow it 9.2 miles to La Grange. Go left (north) on County Road H 1.6 miles to the John Muir Trail park entrance on the left. The trailhead is at the southwest corner of the parking lot near a map board kiosk.

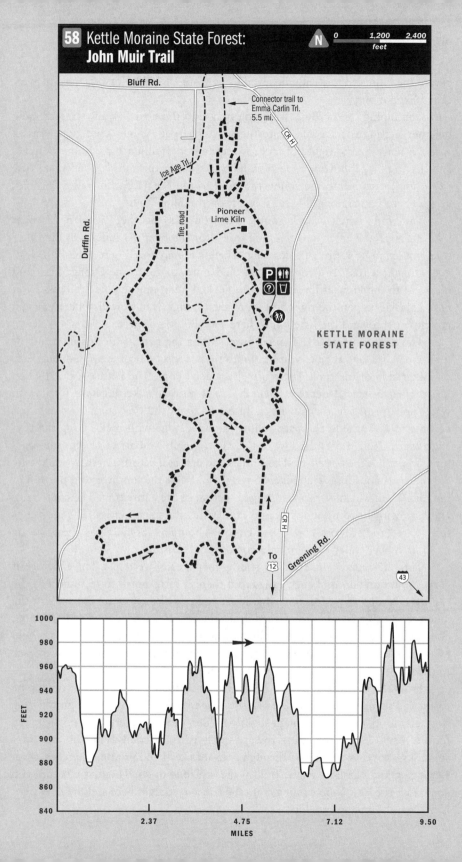

58 Kettle Moraine State Forest:
John Muir Trail

N   0   1,200   2,400
        feet

Bluff Rd.

Connector trail to
Emma Carlin Trl.
5.5 mi.

CR H

Ice Age Trl.

Duffin Rd.

fire road

Pioneer
Lime Kiln

P ♦♦ ♂♀
? 🗑

🚶

KETTLE MORAINE
STATE FOREST

CR H

To
12

Greening Rd.

43

FEET

1000
980
960
940
920
900
880
860
840

2.37   4.75   7.12   9.50

MILES

you to the Pioneer Lime Kiln, believed to be from an 1843 Norwegian settlement called Skoponong.

Continuing on the Blue Trail, you may find the next 0.4 miles rather tame but then getting rockier and more rugged as the path climbs up a ridge. Pass a wooden fence on the right 0.5 miles from the Red Trail juncture. From there it's another 1 mile, following a few switchbacks along the mostly shaded narrow ridge, until it comes to the connecting trail to the Emma Carlin trail 5.75 miles away. There's a map board here; stay left on the Blue Trail.

The trail switches back south, and you pass another wooden fence at 0.15 miles as you enter into red pine forest for the next 0.3 miles. On the other side, you come to a fire lane crossing. There's a map board here. The Blue Trail goes straight across. You could go left 0.25 miles to get to the Orange Trail and then east to the Pioneer Lime Kiln. Another 0.4 miles on the Blue Trail takes you past a glacial bog on the right and on to the Orange Trail as well, where you can go left (east) toward the lime kiln. There's a map board there.

The next juncture is 1.1 miles away. Along the path you cross intermittent prairie patches, and then as you head into the woods, you come upon open water on either side of the trail. These are also glacial bogs. The kettles formed when ice trapped in glacial deposits melted. These particular kettles have filled with water and formed leatherleaf bogs. Just past them the trail starts to climb and become more rugged. The path follows along a ridge with rocks along the trail edge overlooking a deep hollow to the right. Finally you arrive at the trail juncture. To the left the Green Trail continues and acts as a cutoff trail that would take 2.8 miles off your Blue Trail hike. Stay right and hike the southwestern portion of the Blue Trail, which is the most rugged section of the entire trail. The course zigs and zags with hairpins and rises and falls with ridges and kettles. The surface is full of tree roots, loose rocks, and exposed boulders. Some areas show plastic mesh or rubber water dams to help combat trail erosion.

This 2.9-mile segment starts south, then heads west in a bulge before it curves south and around back east. From there it turns north to reconnect to the rest of the trail system, forming what looks roughly like a boot on the map. At the juncture, go right. Left is the Green Trail, the cutoff segment for this boot loop. You could go a few paces in this direction to find a trail to the north that would take you back to the Red Trail, where you could go right and find your way back to the trailhead for a total distance of 0.8 miles.

From the juncture you have 2.6 miles left to go. Start downhill through pine forest and then head straight across a small open field. The trail takes another big southerly loop, this time through slightly milder, though nevertheless challenging, terrain. As you make the return toward the north, the woods thin a bit and offer some sky above, and you pass through areas of brush and prairie. There's a bit of zigzagging and climbing to the trail in the last mile or so. The first juncture you come to is the Red Loop coming from the left. Go straight here and the next right is the exit 0.1 mile to the lot.

NEARBY ACTIVITIES

Stop in at the LaGrange General Store, Café, and Deli on US 12. Besides good sandwiches and something to drink, the place offers bicycle rentals and repairs. Call (262) 495-8600 or go to **www.backyardbikes.com.**

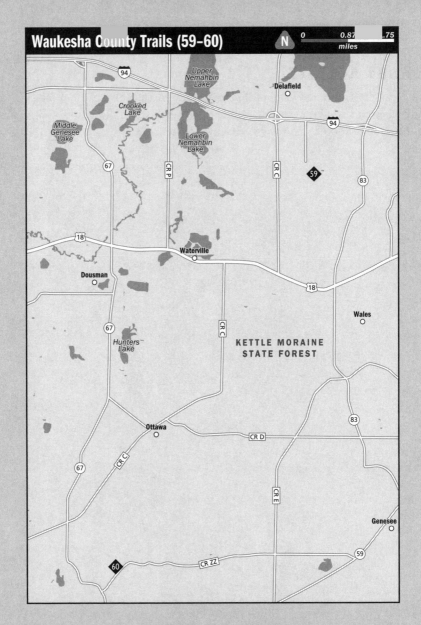

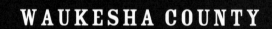

WAUKESHA COUNTY

59 KETTLE MORAINE STATE FOREST:
Lapham Peak Unit

KEY AT-A-GLANCE INFORMATION

LENGTH: 6.9 miles

CONFIGURATION: Loop

DIFFICULTY: Moderate to difficult

SCENERY: Mixed forest, prairie, kettle moraine, high-point overlook

EXPOSURE: Mostly shaded

TRAIL TRAFFIC: Light

TRAIL SURFACE: Packed dirt, grass, some crushed rock

HIKING TIME: 3 hours

DRIVING DISTANCE: 46 miles east from interstates 39/94 interchange

ACCESS: 7 a.m.–9 p.m. (until 10 p.m. in winter)

MAPS: USGS Oconomowoc East; at park office; map boards at trail junctures; www.dnr.state.wi.us

WHEELCHAIR ACCESSIBILITY: A separate 1.5-mile paved nature trail and a viewing platform near the observation tower

FACILITIES: Restrooms, water, park office

SPECIAL COMMENTS: Dogs allowed. There is a state park vehicle registration fee ($7 daily, $25 annual for vehicles with Wisconsin plates; $10 daily, $35 annual for out-of-state plates).

IN BRIEF

Climb a tower at the highest peak in Waukesha County and be prepared to work as you hike the glacial roller coaster around this park that features a kettle moraine.

DESCRIPTION

Lapham Peak is named for Increase A. Lapham, a scientist and naturalist who came to Wisconsin in 1836 and wrote much about the state's wildlife and geology. All combined there are 17 miles of loop trails here. The easiest trails are the Purple and Green loops. The course mapped out here is a loop of the entire park primarily following the Black Loop, which has some rather strenuous up-and-down climbs. The asphalt Plantation Trail is accessible for wheelchairs.

Begin from Parking Lot 9. The trailhead is not clearly marked, but look beyond the trail kiosk for a wide stretch of mowed trail—just to the left of the paved trail—with an arrow going away from you. Go straight to the woods. The trail goes up steeply on packed dirt into pine forest. At 0.2 miles you pass a bench to the right. You find benches at nearly all trail junctures in fact. Downhill to the right is a cutoff to the Plantation Trail, but follow the trail signs with a black circle on them.

GPS Trailhead Coordinates

UTM Zone (WGS 84) 16T

Easting 0386564

Northing 4766160

Latitude N 43° 02' 22.78"

Longitude W 88° 23' 33.34"

Directions

From the interchange of I-39/94, drive east 45.2 miles to Exit 285 to County Road C. Turn right (south) on CR C and drive 0.8 miles to the park entrance on the left. Follow the park road 0.7 miles to the Homestead Hollow parking area on the left. The trailhead is to the right of the restrooms behind the trail map kiosk.

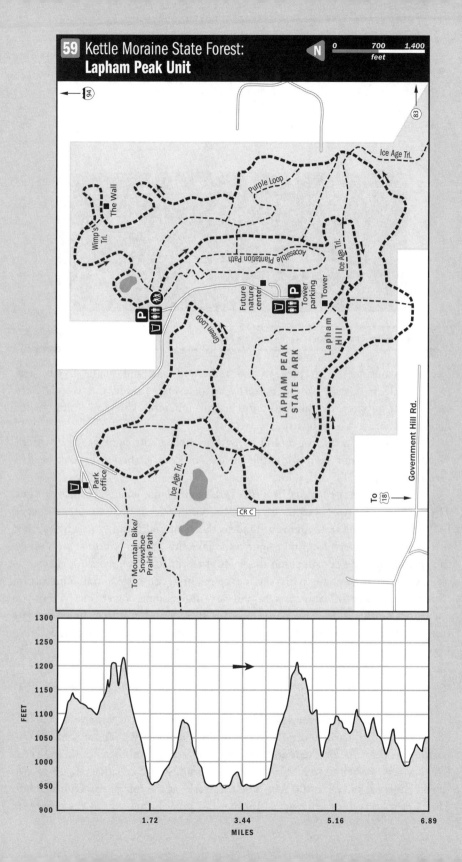

N

0   700   1,400
feet

94

83

Ice Age Trl.

Purple Loop

The Wall

Wimp's Trl.

Ice Age Trl.

Accessible Plantation Path

Future nature center

P

Tower parking

Tower

Lapham Hill

P

Green Loop

LAPHAM PEAK STATE PARK

Park office

Ice Age Trl.

Government Hill Rd.

To 18

CR C

To Mountain Bike/ Snowshoe Prairie Path

1300
1250
1200
1150
1100
1050
1000
950
900

FEET

1.72   3.44   5.16   6.89
MILES

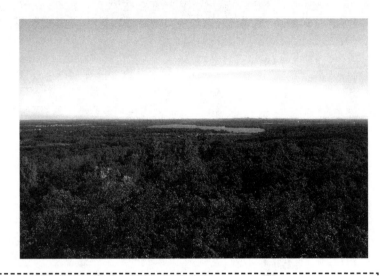

The view from the observation tower on Lapham Peak

The trail continues with pine to the right and oak and maple to the left. At 0.1 mile is a trail to the butterfly garden just outside the woods here. Go straight another 0.2 miles to another trail juncture. The easy trail goes left here, and there is a map board.

A hard right takes you uphill to parking and a soft right heads downhill. Watch for your trail symbol on the posts. The trail is shaded by oak-hickory forest, and the terrain rolls a lot.

You will cross the Ice Age Trail (IAT) 0.2 miles later, which goes left to right. The observation tower is to the right here if you prefer to take the more rugged IAT. Regardless, the trail curves around to the right and brings you within a few feet of the IAT, where you find a spur trail. Take this and go left up some steps to the clearing where you can climb the 45-foot tower for some amazing views.

Return to the main path via the steps. You come to a trail juncture at "Stairway to Heaven." Stay straight and pass under some power lines where you come to The Big Slide. This path descends steeply and curves right where you find a cutoff heading up and back to the left if you want to skip the Green Loop/Meadow Trail. Stay right and hike another 0.1 mile before crossing the Ice Age Trail once again. To the right is the campsite for that trail and beyond that the tower again. Enter a clearing at 0.2 miles and go right. The trail left here cuts off the meadow.

Another 0.1 mile brings you into the woods, and on your left you find Native American marker trees, which look like bent elbows. There is an accompanying storyboard for them and another map board. Another cutoff trail goes left, but stay straight here. This is Two Tier trail, and the path goes up in two steep climbs for the next 800 feet. The trail forks at the top as you continue left. The park road is out to the right. Another 0.2 miles brings you to the other end

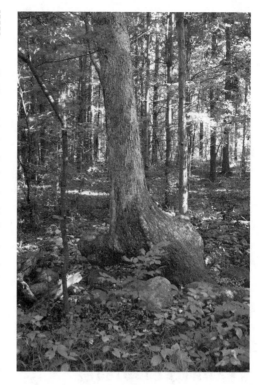

A Native American marker tree

of the last cutoff trail, and you continue out into an open field 0.2 miles after that.

This segment follows around prairie on mowed-grass paths. Stay on the main trail and don't take spur trails off to the right as they lead out of the trail system or to parking. The first spur to the left just 100 feet into the meadow cuts off the loop. Otherwise it is 0.5 miles around to the other end and back into the woods where the cutoff trail rejoins the main trail. You will pass the Evergreen Grove picnic area and parking, where there are toilets and water.

When the trail comes back around to the woods, go right into the shade along some pines with oak savanna to your right. Pass the other end of a previous cutoff trail on your left at 400 feet. Go right as the trail takes a little elbow deep to the right along the edge of prairie with oak savanna still to the right. Cross the Ice Age Trail, which leads right to a pond overlook 1.25 miles to Menahbim Spring.

Crossing the IAT brings you to South Field. Follow along a rock wall to your right. Then the trail goes left along a long row of cedars. The path enters the woods once again, and you come to a trail map and juncture. To the left is part of the Green Loop. Go straight to a steep climb at South Hill, bringing you to another juncture. Stay right here. It's another 0.5 miles with a bit of climbing, and then you come to a bench. Another 300 feet brings you across a ski trail where there's another map board. Go straight. The trail dips down another 0.1 mile to another map board. The trail from the left is the end of the Stairway to Heaven trail which came directly from the tower area. Keep going past this, and you pass Target Tree after another 0.2 miles.

At 0.2 miles you come to another juncture. The black trail goes left here and enters a short loop of some of the more challenging short climbs of the trail. But to the right is Pete's Pass, which offers a view of a kettle moraine. I recommend going right here, which is the only time you part from the Black Loop. (This is a part of the Blue Trail). Alternatively you could have a peek and come back for the challenge.

Pete's Pass ends 0.2 miles later, passing the kettle moraine on the right. The Black Loop joins again from the left, and the Ice Age Trail crosses just a few steps later. Just 250 feet later is still another juncture with a trail map. Left is the easy Purple Trail coming from where you began your hike near the butterfly garden. Go right and at 0.1 mile, find a map board and the Purple Trail heading left into prairie. Continue right and down into woods. At 0.2 miles you pass the remains of a settler's cabin to your left. The trail continues along the top of a ridge with oak forest, and 300 feet later gives you another option. Left is a cutoff that would take you 0.4 miles back to the trailhead bearing right at the first intersection along its length. Stay right on the Black Loop and face the steepest climb of the hike. Pass along Rock Ridge and cross a ravine to the left. The first juncture is at 0.6 miles. Go left on The Wimp's Trail to cut off the steepest climb. Go right to face The Wall. It's steep, but only about 200 feet long. The trail loops back around and comes to the end of the 400-foot Wimp's Trail cutoff 0.3 miles later.

The trail continues 0.3 miles to a juncture. Go straight to go out to the parking lot. Go right to wrap around a small scenic pond before coming back around and out alongside a shelter house. Follow the park road up to the parking lot where you began.

NEARBY ACTIVITIES

Nearby Delafield offers a historic downtown area and a variety of shops and boutiques. Find out more at **www.delafield-wi.org.**

KETTLE MORAINE STATE FOREST: Scuppernong Trail

60

IN BRIEF

Rolling hills through pine forest and a view for miles from a scenic overlook are the highlights of this hike through some of southeastern Wisconsin's finest post-glacier terrain.

DESCRIPTION

The short climbs over rolling terrain and a generally good trail surface makes this trail popular with cross-country runners. The trail outlined here follows the Green Loop, the outermost and longest loop in this section of the forest. On the black-and-white maps from the park office, all trails appear the same, but the overlap can be clarified against the color-coded map boards at trail junctures.

From the trailhead the path turns left just inside the trees. A park access road continues straight from here. The first trail juncture is 200 feet farther along, and this is where the loop will return. Go right and follow a sandy lane strewn with pine needles. The lane goes straight through an orderly pine plantation for 0.1 mile, where it bends left a little and leaves orderly pines for scattered spruces for a moment before heading back into pine plantation.

Another 0.15 miles later, hardwoods enter the mix, though pine is still the dominant

KEY AT-A-GLANCE INFORMATION

LENGTH: 5.4 miles
CONFIGURATION: Loop
DIFFICULTY: Easy to moderate
SCENERY: Pine forest, hardwood forest, overlooks
EXPOSURE: Mostly shaded
TRAIL TRAFFIC: Light to moderate
TRAIL SURFACE: Packed dirt, sand, crushed rock, some tree roots and stones, some grass
HIKING TIME: 1.5–2 hours
DRIVING DISTANCE: 52 miles east of Interstates 39/94 interchange
ACCESS: 6 a.m.–11 p.m. year-round
MAPS: USGS Eagle; in map box at park office; posted at trail junctures
FACILITIES: Restrooms, water, picnic tables, grills
SPECIAL COMMENTS: Dogs allowed on leashes. No hiking or dogs when snow is present. All vehicles require a park sticker ($7 daily, $25 annual for vehicles with Wisconsin plates). Trail activities other than hiking incur a $4 daily fee. There is a small park office that is often closed, but you can self-register there. Parts of the park are open to gun hunting; during deer season at the end of November, be sure to wear bright clothing, especially blaze orange. Call (262) 594-6200 to know for sure if the hunt is on.

Directions

From where I-94 departs from I-39 and heads east toward Milwaukee, take I-94 41.2 miles to WI 67. Go south 9.9 miles to County Road ZZ and go left 0.4 miles to the park entrance. The trailhead is at the north corner of the lot.

GPS Trailhead Coordinates

UTM Zone (WGS 84) 16T
Easting 0380750
Northing 4755275
Latitude N 42° 56' 26.82"
Longitude W 88° 27' 41.87"

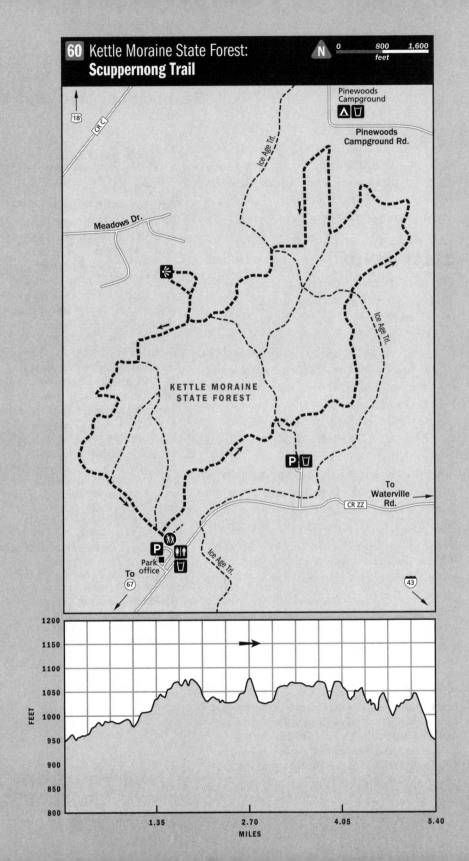

60 Kettle Moraine State Forest:
Scuppernong Trail

N

0   800   1,600
feet

18
CR C

Pinewoods
Campground

Pinewoods
Campground Rd.

Ice Age Trl

Meadows Dr.

Ice Age Trl

KETTLE MORAINE
STATE FOREST

P

To
Waterville
Rd.

CR ZZ

P

Park
office

Ice Age Trl

To
67

43

FEET

1200
1150
1100
1050
1000
950
900
850
800

1.35   2.70   4.05   5.40

MILES

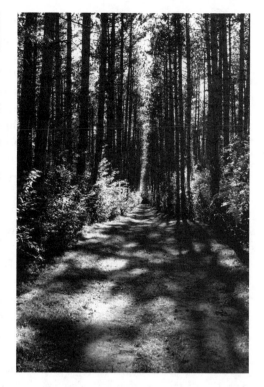

A trail through a pine plantation

species and the trail doesn't offer much shade. After 0.15 miles you pass a bench, and then the rolling terrain really starts offering more of a workout than the flat stretch at the beginning.

From the bench to the next juncture is 0.25 miles. If you choose to go straight, it is the easy Red Loop that offers an inner loop back to the parking lot for a total of 2.3 miles. A hard right turn takes you down the short trail to D. J. Mackie group picnic area, where there is also water and parking. Take the soft right on the Green/Orange loops. The forest offers an abundance of chipmunks and squirrels, and you are likely to see a deer or two the farther you are from the parking areas and the open pine plantation. Sand gives way to a lot more scattered rock, and the up and down climbs are slightly steeper and more frequent from this point.

From this juncture at 0.75 miles, cross the Ice Age National Scenic Trail (IAT) on your right. Before you is a map board with #6 on it. To the left is the Ice Age Trail and a bench. The IAT is marked with yellow patches on trees and trail posts and it is a narrow footpath of packed dirt. You have the option to go left here on the IAT, which would present a bit more rugged hiking and take 1.3 miles off the Green Loop. Otherwise continue right on the Green Loop.

Another 0.6 miles takes you to the edge of a small clearing. The trail bends around left here, passing a bench on the left, and then continues down old fire lanes. The trail goes south 0.2 miles, passing a picnic table and fire pit amid pine and brush on your right. Occasionally turkey vultures roost here, so step softly and scan the branches. The trail bends right, and on your left you find the return path for the Orange Loop. Take this to cut your hike down to 4.2 miles.

There is a map board labeled #9 and a bench. Go right down a 0.3-mile-long corridor heading back north under pine and on the other side of those fire pits you just passed. Climb a short incline at the end to reach Point #10. Across this small field is a road into Pinewoods Campground, where you can find water and toilets.

Go left with the prairie on your right and woods on your left. The trail reenters the pines. You find some fern, wildflowers, and the occasional oak tree.

Raspberries can be found here in midsummer during a good year. From Point #10 it's 0.5 miles through the pine until you cross the IAT once again. Continue straight as the canopy opens up. The trail curves right and downhill through short pines on a grassy trail 0.4 miles until the next juncture and map board at Point #14.

The left path is the return on the Orange Loop and backward on the Red Loop. Go right on crushed rock into shade. About 300 feet along, you come to the Observation Loop, a short 0.4-mile lollipop to the right. It's 0.1 mile to the fork where you go right and follow the loop as it becomes a bit narrower and more rugged with roots and rocks. Another 0.2 miles from the fork is an overlook with a couple of benches and the valley beyond. What you see is a glacial sand plain and a couple of small lakes, as well as a long view to the horizon.

Return to the head of the Observation Loop and continue right on the main trail. At 0.25 miles you come to a wide intersection with a map board. Straight ahead are the Red and Orange loops. Go right on the Green Loop where a sign indicates this is the hardest trail for skiers. This jagged portion of the loop heads west, passing a scenic overlook under oak trees. These will be the steepest climbs, and the descents can be slippery in wet weather. The Red Loop, which parts left from the Orange Loop 0.15 miles down the trail, would bypass the steepest parts.

On the Green Loop you find a scenic overlook at 0.2 miles. From there the trail takes a sharp left and heads downhill. Another 0.25 miles takes you up another hill and then down a 200-foot moderately steep decline. You start to see pine once again on your left. Pass another bench at 0.15 miles and yet another 0.1 mile after that, where there is also a map board where the Orange Loop comes in from the left. After a bend in the trail, you come to a 50-foot, steep and uneven descent. Be cautious of loose rock. Another 75 feet later is a similar ramp with tree roots and potentially slippery mud. You reach pine plantation for the final 0.2 miles to the end of the trail. Just before you arrive there, you see the Red Loop joining from the left, then the beginning of the loop going left just after that. Head straight out and follow the bend to the right to return to the trailhead.

NEARBY ACTIVITIES

The State Forest Visitor Center is on WI 59, 3 miles west of Eagle. Call (262) 594-6200 for more information. Scuppernong Springs is a 1.5-mile, self-guided nature trail nearby. Pick up a booklet at the trailhead.

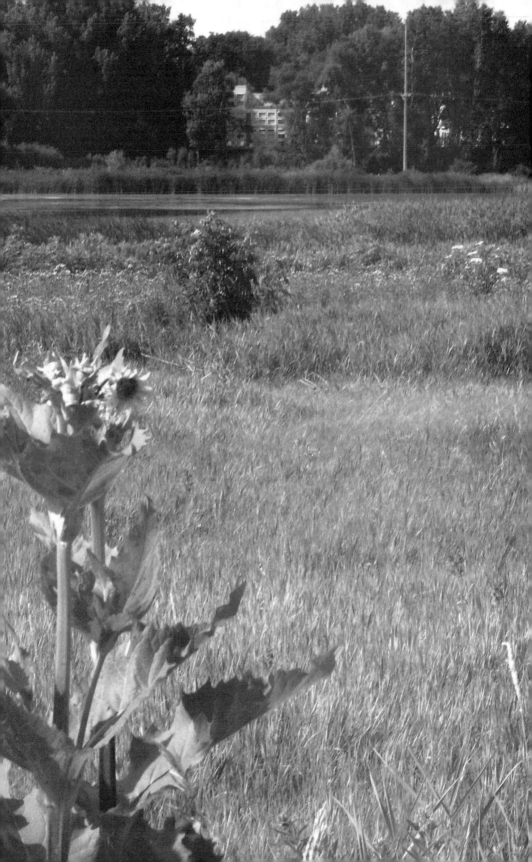

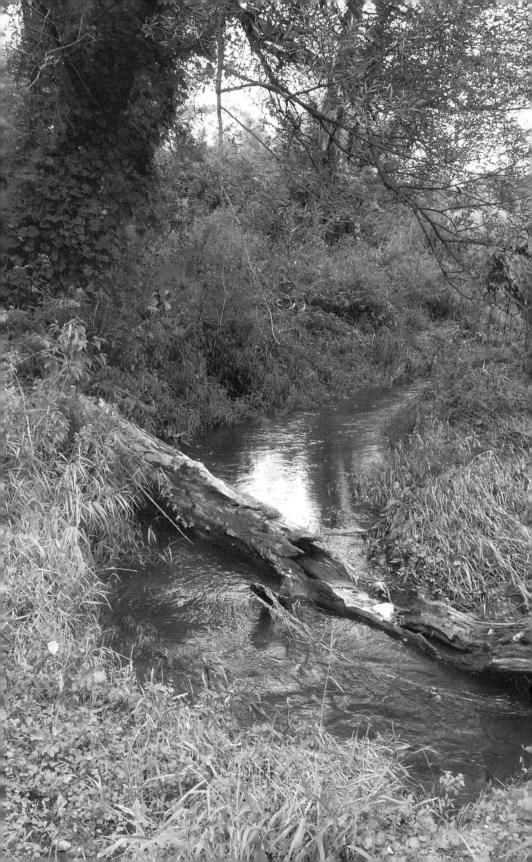

APPENDIXES
AND INDEX

APPENDIX A:
HIKING STORES

Fontana Sports: Downtown
216 Henry Street
Madison, WI 53703
(608) 257-5043
www.fontanasports.com

Fontana Sports: West Madison
231 Junction Road
Madison, WI 53717
(608) 833-9191
www.fontanasports.com

Gander Mountain
6199 Metra Drive
DeForest, WI 53532
(608) 242-9532
www.gandermountain.com

Gander Mountain Outlet
7349 West Towne Way
Madison, WI 53719
(608) 827-6608
www.gandermountain.com

REI
7483 West Towne Way
Madison, WI 53719
(608) 833-6680
www.rei.com

The Shoe Box
US 14 (at the stoplight in Black Earth)
Black Earth, WI 53515
(608) 767-3447
www.theshoebox.com

The Shoe Box: Baraboo Outlet Store
141 Third Avenue
Baraboo, WI 53913
(608) 356-1224
www.theshoebox.com

APPENDIX B:
MAP STORES

Eagle Eye Maps
50 Merlham Drive
Madison, WI 53705
(608) 233-9037
www.eagleeyemaps.com

Ice Age Park and Trail Foundation
306 East Wilson Street, Lower Level
Madison, WI 53703
(800) 227-0046 or (608) 663-8278
www.iceagetrail.org (Click: STORE)

Mad City Maps
100 South Baldwin Street
Madison, WI 53703
(608) 260-9626

Mapping Specialists, Ltd.
1319 Applegate Road
Madison, WI 53713
(608) 274-4004
www.mappingspecialists.com

Wisconsin Geological and Natural
    History Survey
3817 Mineral Point Road
Madison, WI 53705
(608) 263-7389
www.uwex.edu/wgnhs

APPENDIX C:
HIKING CLUBS

Glacial Drifters Hiking Log and
   Award Program
116 Merton Avenue
Lodi, WI 53555
(608) 592-5666

Ice Age Park & Trail Foundation
306 East Wilson Street, Lower Level
Madison, WI 53703
(800) 227-0046 or (608) 663-8278
www.iceagetrail.org/join.htm

Various chapters of the organization have
occasional hiking and volunteer work
events.

John Muir Chapter Sierra Club
222 South Hamilton Street #1
Madison, WI 53703-3201
(608) 256-0565
www.wisconsin.sierraclub.org

Wisconsin Hoofers Outing Club
800 Langdon Street
Madison, WI 53706
(608) 262-1630
www.hooferouting.org

INDEX

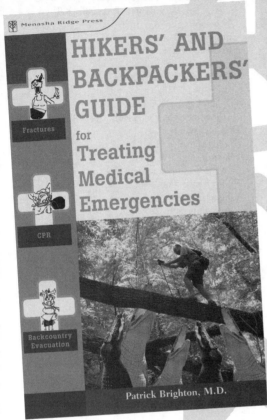

HIKERS' AND BACKPACKERS' GUIDE FOR TREATING MEDICAL EMERGENCIES

by Patrick Brighton, M.D.
ISBN 10: 0-89732-640-7
ISBN 13: 978-0-89732-640-7
$9.95
116 pages

By keeping descriptions and remedies for injury and illness simple, this book enables participants in a particular sport to be informed, stay calm, and appropriately treat themselves or fellow participants. Reading this book before initiating the activity also enhances awareness of potential problems and fosters prevention of accidents and disease. With a refreshing splash of humor, this guide is as informative as it is entertaining.

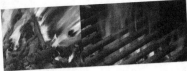
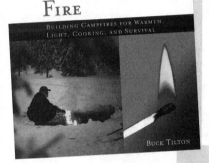
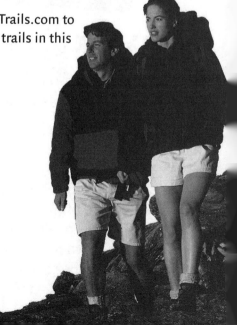
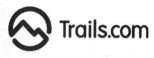

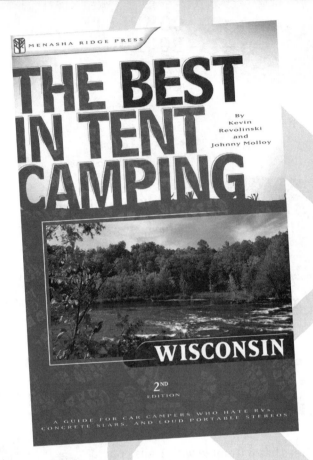

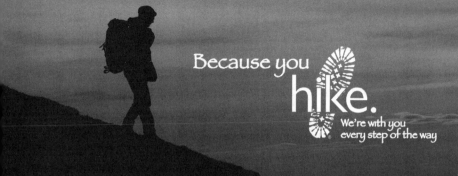
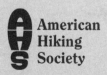

DEAR CUSTOMERS AND FRIENDS,

SUPPORTING YOUR INTEREST IN OUTDOOR ADVENTURE, travel, and an active lifestyle is central to our operations, from the authors we choose to the locations we detail to the way we design our books. Menasha Ridge Press was incorporated in 1982 by a group of veteran outdoorsmen and professional outfitters. For 25 years now, we've specialized in creating books that benefit the outdoors enthusiast.

Almost immediately, Menasha Ridge Press earned a reputation for revolutionizing outdoors- and travel-guidebook publishing. For such activities as canoeing, kayaking, hiking, backpacking, and mountain biking, we established new standards of quality that transformed the whole genre, resulting in outdoor-recreation guides of great sophistication and solid content. Menasha Ridge continues to be outdoor publishing's greatest innovator.

The folks at Menasha Ridge Press are as at home on a white-water river or mountain trail as they are editing a manuscript. The books we build for you are the best they can be, because we're responding to your needs. Plus, we use and depend on them ourselves.

We look forward to seeing you on the river or the trail. If you'd like to contact us directly, join in at www.trekalong.com or visit us at www.menasharidge.com. We thank you for your interest in our books and the natural world around us all.

SAFE TRAVELS,

Bob Sehlinger

BOB SEHLINGER
PUBLISHER